Preoperative Evaluation

Editors

DEBRA DOMINO PULLEY
DEBORAH C. RICHMAN

ANESTHESIOLOGY CLINICS

www.anesthesiology.theclinics.com

Consulting Editor
LEE A. FLEISHER

March 2016 • Volume 34 • Number 1

ELSEVIER

1600 John F. Kennedy Boulevard • Suite 1800 • Philadelphia, Pennsylvania, 19103-2899
http://www.theclinics.com

ANESTHESIOLOGY CLINICS Volume 34, Number 1
March 2016 ISSN 1932-2275, ISBN-13: 978-0-323-44229-9

Editor: Patrick Manley
Developmental Editor: Kristen Helm

Anesthesiology Clinics (ISSN 1932-2275) is published quarterly by Elsevier Inc., 360 Park Avenue South, New York, NY 10010-1710. Months of issue are March, June, September, and December. Periodicals postage paid at New York, NY and at additional mailing offices. Subscription prices are $100.00 per year (US student/resident), $330.00 per year (US individuals), $400.00 per year (Canadian individuals), $596.00 per year (US institutions), $753.00 per year (Canadian institutions), $225.00 per year (Canadian and foreign student/resident), $455.00 per year (foreign individuals), and $753.00 per year (foreign institutions). To receive student and resident rate, orders must be accompanied by name of affiliated institution, date of term, and the *signature* of program/residency coordinator on institutions letterhead. Orders will be billed at individual rate until proof of status is received. Foreign air speed delivery is included in all *Clinics'* subscription prices. All prices are subject to change without notice. POSTMASTER: Send address changes to *Anesthesiology Clinics,* Elsevier Health Sciences Division, Subscription Customer Service, 3251 Riverport Lane, Maryland Heights, MO 63043. Customer Service (orders, claims, online, change of address): Elsevier Health Sciences Division, Subscription Customer Service, 3251 Riverport Lane, Maryland Heights, MO 63043. **Tel:1-800-654-2452 (U.S. and Canada); 314-447-8871 (outside U.S. and Canada). Fax: 314-447-8029. E-mail: journalscustomerservice-usa@elsevier.com (for print support); journalsonlinesupport-usa@elsevier.com (for online support).**

Reprints. For copies of 100 or more of articles in this publication, please contact the Commercial Reprints Department, Elsevier Inc., 360 Park Avenue South, New York, NY 10010-1710. Tel.: 212-633-3874; Fax: 212-633-3820; E-mail: reprints@elsevier.com.

Anesthesiology Clinics, is also published in Spanish by McGraw-Hill Inter-americana Editores S. A., P.O. Box 5-237, 06500 Mexico D. F., Mexico.

Anesthesiology Clinics, is covered in *MEDLINE/PubMed (Index Medicus), Current Contents/Clinical Medicine, Excerpta Medica, ISI/BIOMED*, and *Chemical Abstracts*.

Contributors

CONSULTING EDITOR

LEE A. FLEISHER, MD, FACC, FAHA
Robert D. Dripps Professor and Chair of Anesthesiology and Critical Care, Professor of
Medicine, Perelman School of Medicine at the University of Pennsylvania, Philadelphia,
Pennsylvania

EDITORS

DEBRA DOMINO PULLEY, MD
Associate Professor, Department of Anesthesiology, Washington University School of
Medicine in St Louis, St Louis, Missouri

DEBORAH C. RICHMAN, MBChB, FFA(SA)
Section Chief and Director, Pre-operative Services, Clinical Associate Professor,
Department of Anesthesiology, Stony Brook University Medical Center, Stony Brook
Medicine, Stony Brook, New York

AUTHORS

MATTHIAS BOCK, MD, Priv-Doz
Department of Anesthesia and Intensive Care Medicine, Central Hospital, Bolzano, Italy;
Department of Anesthesiology, Perioperative Medicine and Intensive Care, Paracelsus
Medical University, Salzburg, Austria

ARVIND CHANDRAKANTAN, MD, MBA, FAAP
Clinical Assistant Professor of Anesthesiology, Stony Brook University Medical Center,
Stony Brook, New York

BEVERLY CHANG, MD
Department of Anesthesiology, Perioperative and Pain Medicine, Stanford Hospital and
Clinics, Stanford, California

ANA COSTA, MD
Clinical Assistant Professor, Department of Anesthesiology, Stony Brook Medicine, Stony
Brook, New York

ANGELA F. EDWARDS, MD
Associate Professor of Anesthesiology, Section Head of Perioperative Medicine, Wake
Forest Baptist Health, Wake Forest University School of Medicine, Winston Salem, North
Carolina

LEE A. FLEISHER, MD, FACC, FAHA
Robert D. Dripps Professor and Chair of Anesthesiology and Critical Care, Professor of
Medicine, Perelman School of Medicine at the University of Pennsylvania, Philadelphia,
Pennsylvania

GERHARD FRITSCH, MD, Priv-Doz
Department of Anesthesiology, Perioperative Medicine and Intensive Care, Paracelsus Medical University, Salzburg, Austria; Department of Anesthesiology and Intensive Care, UKH Lorenz Boehler, Vienna, Austria

TONG J. GAN, MD, MHS, FRCA
Professor and Chair, Department of Anesthesiology, Health Science Center, Stony Brook University School of Medicine, Stony Brook, New York

RUCHIR GUPTA, MD
Assistant Professor, Department of Anesthesiology, Health Science Center, Stony Brook University School of Medicine, Stony Brook, New York

DAVID L. HEPNER, MD, MPH
Department of Anesthesiology, Perioperative and Pain Medicine; Associate Director, Weiner Center for Preoperative Evaluation, Brigham and Women's Hospital; Associate Professor of Anaesthesia, Harvard Medical School, Boston, Massachusetts

RICHARD HUH, MD
Department of Internal Medicine, Rush University Medical Center, Chicago, Illinois

SELMA ISHAG, MBBS, MD
Assistant Professor, Division of General Anesthesiology, Barnes-Jewish Hospital, Washington University, St Louis, Missouri

AMIR K. JAFFER, MD, MBA
Department of Internal Medicine, Rush University Medical Center, Chicago, Illinois

ANKIT J. KANSAGRA, MD
Chief Fellow, Department of Hematology/Oncology, Baystate Medical Center, Tufts University, Springfield, Massachusetts

JISU KIM, MD, MSc
Department of Internal Medicine, Rush University Medical Center, Chicago, Illinois

JUSTIN G. KNITTEL, MD
Instructor, Department of Anesthesiology, Washington University School of Medicine in St Louis, St Louis, Missouri

ANAND LAKSHMINARASIMHACHAR, MBBS, FRCA
Assistant Professor of Anesthesiology, Division of Cardiothoracic Anesthesiology, Barnes-Jewish Hospital, Washington University School of Medicine in St Louis, St Louis, Missouri

HEATHER McKENZIE, MD
Instructor in Anesthesiology, Washington University School of Medicine in St Louis, St Louis, Missouri

JOSHUA D. MILLER, MD, MPH
Assistant Professor of Medicine, Endocrinology and Metabolism, Department of Medicine, Stony Brook Medicine, Stony Brook, New York

DEBRA DOMINO PULLEY, MD
Associate Professor, Department of Anesthesiology, Washington University School of Medicine in St Louis, St Louis, Missouri

DEBORAH C. RICHMAN, MBChB, FFA(SA)
Section Chief and Director, Pre-operative Services, Clinical Associate Professor, Department of Anesthesiology, Stony Brook University Medical Center, Stony Brook Medicine, Stony Brook, New York

TRACIE SAUNDERS, MD, MDiv
Professor of Anesthesiology, Stony Brook University Medical Center, Stony Brook, New York

BARBARA SLAWSKI, MD, MS, FACP, SFHM
Associate Professor of Medicine and Orthopaedic Surgery, Chief, Section of Perioperative and Consultative Medicine, Department of Medicine, Froedtert Hospital Clinical Cancer Center, Froedtert and Medical College of Wisconsin, Milwaukee, Wisconsin

GERALD W. SMETANA, MD
Professor of Medicine, Division of General Medicine and Primary Care, Beth Israel Deaconess Medical Center, Harvard Medical School, Boston, Massachusetts

MIHAELA S. STEFAN, MD
Academic Hospitalist; Clinician Researcher; Director, Perioperative Clinic and Medical Consultation, Division of Hospital Medicine, Department of General Medicine, Tufts University, Springfield, Massachusetts

CHARUHAS V. THAKAR, MD, FASN
Professor of Medicine, Director, Division of Nephrology, Kidney CARE Program, University of Cincinnati; Chief, Renal Section, Cincinnati VA Medical Center, Cincinnati, Ohio

STEPHAN R. THILEN, MD, MS
Assistant Professor, Department of Anesthesiology and Pain Medicine, University of Washington, Seattle, Washington

MIRIAM M. TREGGIARI, MD, PhD, MPH
Professor, Director of Clinical Research, Departments of Anesthesiology and Perioperative Medicine, and Public Health and Preventive Medicine, Oregon Health and Science University, Portland, Oregon

RICHARD D. URMAN, MD, MBA
Associate Professor of Anesthesia, Department of Anesthesiology, Perioperative and Pain Medicine, Brigham and Women's Hospital, Boston, Massachusetts

DUMINDA N. WIJEYSUNDERA, MD, PhD, FRCPC
Li Ka Shing Knowledge Institute of St Michael's Hospital; Associate Professor, Department of Anesthesia, Toronto General Hospital, University of Toronto, Toronto, Ontario, Canada

TROY S. WILDES, MD
Assistant Professor, Department of Anesthesiology, Washington University School of Medicine in St Louis, St Louis, Missouri

Contents

Section I: Introductory Articles

Preoperative evaluation clinics have been shown to enhance operating room efficiency, decrease day-of-surgery cancellations, reduce hospital costs, and improve the quality of patient care. Although programs differ in staffing, structure, financial support, and daily operations, they share the common goal of preoperative risk reduction in order for patients to proceed safely through the perioperative period. Effective preoperative evaluation occurs if processes are standardized to ensure clinical, regulatory, and accreditation guidelines are met while keeping medical optimization and patient satisfaction at the forefront. Although no universally accepted standard model exists, there are key components to a successful preoperative process.

Preoperative consultation is an important intervention that likely has most benefits for intermediate-risk to high-risk patients undergoing major surgery. Consultation rates are likely increasing and there is significant practice variation in the use of consultation. Consultations should be available within a well-organized and coordinated process of preoperative assessment. Preoperative consults should be accessible to anesthesia and surgical teams involved in the procedure and to the providers involved in postoperative care. The role of preoperative consultation should evolve as a rational approach and emerge as a value-based service. New payment methodologies are likely to facilitate appropriate use of this important resource.

Shared decision-making is a paradigm of patient engagement that is assuming greater importance in the era of value-based health care. The basic tenets include patient engagement on clinical decisions, taking into account multiple factors that influence physician and patient decision-making. Understanding and reconciling diametrically opposed views of care are important tenets of shared decision-making. Because many decisions are made preoperatively, the applicability of these principles may be useful especially in the situation of a higher risk surgical candidate. Many patients with Do-Not-Resuscitate (DNR) orders are undergoing procedures to improve quality of life. This article explores shared decision-making and DNR.

Routine preoperative testing is not cost-effective, because it is unlikely to identify significant abnormalities. Abnormal findings from routine testing are more likely to be false positive, are costly to pursue, introduce a new risk, increase the patient's anxiety, and are inconvenient to the patient. Abnormal findings rarely alter the surgical or anesthetic plan, and there is usually no association between perioperative complications and abnormal laboratory results. Incidental findings and false positive results may lead to increased hospital visits and admissions. Preoperative testing needs to be done based on a targeted history and physical examination and the type of surgery.

Section II: Evaluation of Major Organ Systems

The American College of Cardiology/American Heart Association has published Guidelines on Perioperative Evaluation. Preoperative evaluation should focus on identifying patients with symptomatic and asymptomatic coronary artery disease. The guidelines advocate using the American College of Surgeons National Surgical Quality Improvement Project Risk Index to determine perioperative risk. Diagnostic testing should be reserved for those at increased risk with poor exercise capacity. Indications for coronary interventions are the same in the perioperative period as in the nonoperative setting. In patients with a prior coronary stent, optimal antiplatelet therapy and timing of elective noncardiac surgery is evolving.

Postoperative pulmonary complications (PPCs) are common after major non-thoracic surgery and associated with significant morbidity and high cost of care. A number of risk factors are strong predictors of PPCs. The overall goal of the preoperative pulmonary evaluation is to identify these potential, patient and procedure-related risks and optimize the health of the patients before surgery. A thorough clinical examination supported by appropriate laboratory tests will help guide the clinician to provide optimal perioperative care.

stratify and measure improvement after a training program allow a personalized preoperative program to be developed for each patient.

Section IV: Special Considerations

screening, the evaluation should include an assessment of the effects of the substance abuse, associated diseases, end-organ damage, and an awareness of the potential perioperative risks so appropriate plans are developed to minimize the risks. Intraoperatively, anesthetic management needs to be appropriately modified. Signs and symptoms of withdrawal should be monitored for postoperatively. Pain management is particularly challenging. After discharge, this patient population is vulnerable and requires close follow-up and early referral to appropriate specialists when needed.

Pathologic changes can occur during pregnancy requiring diagnostic tests and procedures. A preoperative assessment and perioperative planning are essential. Normal physiologic changes include increased cardiac output and decreased functional residual capacity. Perioperative care should follow American Congress of Obstetricians and Gynecologists guidelines. Anesthetic concerns include desaturation during periods of apnea, aspiration, difficult intubation, friable nasal tissue, decreased MAC, and hypotension and/or decreased uterine perfusion from the uterus. Anesthesia and medications must be individualized and given only as needed. Limit exposure to multiple drugs and monitor for fetal wellbeing and premature labor per consultation and guidelines.

A significant number of anesthetics are performed outside of the operating room (OR). Despite the increased requirement for anesthesia services, the framework to perform the necessary preprocedural anesthesia assessments to optimize patients has not been uniformly developed. Performing anesthesia in non-OR locations poses significant and distinct challenges compared with the procedures in the OR. Anesthesiologists are faced with patients with increasingly complicated comorbidities undergoing novel, complex interventional procedures. With unique training in preoperative triaging, and an expertise in intraoperative and postoperative management of complex patients, anesthesiologists can contribute to greater efficiency and patient safety in the non-OR setting.

ANESTHESIOLOGY CLINICS

Foreword

Preoperative Evaluation—Can We Really Make a Difference in Outcomes?

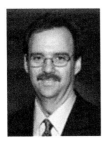

Lee A. Fleisher, MD, FACC, FAHA
Consulting Editor

One of the most important roles of the anesthesiologist is to perform a preoperative evaluation of the patient and "clear" them for anesthesia. Initially, the focus was to assess risk for morbidity and mortality based on the presence of clinical factors and to ensure that medical conditions were stable prior to elective surgery. More recently, there has been a concerted effort to identify interventions that result in improved outcomes in patients with specific comorbidities. While testing was initially performed routinely prior to surgery, it is now clear that testing should only be performed in those patients in whom the test will likely change management. In addition, there is increasing evidence for the value of "prehabilitation" prior to surgery as a means of reducing risk. The current issue of *Anesthesiology Clinics* focuses on all of these issues.

Perioperative management truly requires a multidisciplinary team. The Society for Perioperative Assessment and Quality Improvement (SPAQI) was founded with the goal of bringing together a variety of professionals in various disciplines to work together on all facets influencing optimal surgical outcomes. Therefore, the leadership of SPAQI was asked to assemble a group of experts from the Society to write on the topics. Debra Pulley, MD, is President of SPAQI and Associate Professor of Anesthesiology at Washington University School of Medicine. She was previously the Medical Director of the Center for Preoperative Assessment and Planning at Barnes-Jewish Hospital. Deborah Richman, MBChB, is Vice-President of SPAQI and Associate Professor of Clinical Anesthesia at Stony Brook University. She is also Medical Director

Anesthesiology Clin 34 (2016) xiii–xiv
http://dx.doi.org/10.1016/j.anclin.2015.12.002
1932-2275/16/$ – see front matter © 2016 Published by Elsevier Inc.

anesthesiology.theclinics.com

of the Pre-Operative Clinic at Stony Brook. The issue should provide a guide to the current state of the art concerning preoperative evaluation.

Lee A. Fleisher, MD, FACC, FAHA
Perelman School of Medicine
at University of Pennsylvania
3400 Spruce Street, Dulles 680
Philadelphia, PA 19104, USA

E-mail address:
Lee.Fleisher@uphs.upenn.edu

Preface

Preoperative Evaluation

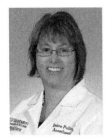 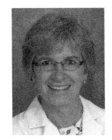

Debra Domino Pulley, MD   Deborah C. Richman, MBChB, FFA(SA)
Editors

Full Knowledge Which Alone Disperses the Mist of Ignorance
—Sir William Osler (1849-1919)

Although the above quotation from Sir William Osler referred to chauvinism in medicine, it was used by Dr Charles Barbour in a 1958 Editorial in the journal *Anesthesiology* to describe the importance of a preoperative evaluation in providing a safe anesthetic.[1] Dr Barbour argued that "untoward reactions may develop during management of anesthesia that are conceived and bred in *failure to prepare the patient adequately.*" Over fifty years later, this is still a true statement. The key to improving perioperative patient outcomes is to have a comprehensive process with preoperative risk stratification and interventions performed preoperatively, intraoperatively, and postoperatively. Dr Barbour cautioned against complacency. He stated the importance of "seeing what lies ahead" and doing something about it "with zeal."

In this issue of *Anesthesiology Clinics*, we have invited physicians in internal medicine and anesthesiology to review the latest literature and discuss various aspects of preoperative evaluation. The last time this subject was published in the *Anesthesiology Clinics* was in 2005. In the interim, there have been updates of guidelines by the ACC/AHA on cardiovascular evaluation and the ACP on pulmonary evaluation.[2,3] In addition, there has been a real focus on improving perioperative care by using the best available evidence, applying protocols, and engaging all members of the perioperative team to minimize morbidity and mortality. Many medical institutions are applying these Enhanced Recovery after Surgery principles.[4] This issue includes articles on preoperative clinics, the role of preoperative consultations, and ethical issues such as shared decision-making and Do-Not-Resuscitate orders. There is an article on preoperative testing that discusses the typical laboratory tests used in the past, but also highlights a few novel tests, such as high-sensitivity troponin and genetic testing. There are articles discussing preoperative assessment of the major organ systems: cardiovascular, pulmonary, renal, and hematologic.

Anesthesiology Clin 34 (2016) xv–xvi
http://dx.doi.org/10.1016/j.anclin.2015.12.001
1932-2275/16/$ – see front matter © 2016 Published by Elsevier Inc.

There are two articles devoted to potentially useful programs to optimize patients preoperatively: one on the assessment and management of anemia and the other covering nutritional optimization and prehabilitation. There are also several articles devoted to patient groups that require special consideration, such as the diabetic patient, the geriatric patient, the patient with implanted devices, the substance use disorder patient, and the pregnant patient. Last, there is an article related to the increasing number of non-operating room anesthetics and how best to evaluate this patient population.

We hope you will enjoy this issue and find it a useful reference in your clinical practice: to provide you with knowledge in your quest for "seeing what lies ahead" and improving patient outcomes.

Debra Domino Pulley, MD
Department of Anesthesiology
Washington University School of Medicine
660 South Euclid Avenue
Campus Box 8054
St Louis, MO 63110, USA

Deborah C. Richman, MBChB, FFA(SA)
Department of Anesthesiology
Stony Brook University Medical Center
Stony Brook, NY 11794-8480, USA

E-mail addresses:
pulleyd@wustl.edu (D.D. Pulley)
deborah.richman@stonybrookmedicine.edu (D.C. Richman)

REFERENCES

1. Barbour CM. Editorial: preoperative evaluation. Anesthesiology 1958;19:275–8.
2. Fleisher LA, Fleischmann KE, Auerbach AD, et al. 2014 ACC/AHA guideline on perioperative cardiovascular evaluation and management of patients undergoing noncardiac surgery: a report of the American College of Cardiology/American Heart Association Task Force on Practice Guidelines. J Am Coll Cardiol 2014; 64(22):e77–137.
3. Qaseem A, Snow V, Fitterman N, et al. Risk assessment for and strategies to reduce perioperative pulmonary complications for patients undergoing noncardiothoracic surgery: a guideline from the American College of Physicians. Ann Intern Med 2006;144:575–80.
4. Mython MG. Spread and adoption of enhanced recovery from elective surgery in the English National Health Service. Can J Anesth 2015;62(2):105–9.

Introductory Articles

Preoperative Clinics

Angela F. Edwards, MD[a],*, Barbara Slawski, MD, MS, SFHM[b]

KEYWORDS

- Preoperative assessment • Preoperative evaluation • Preoperative clinic
- Perioperative • Anesthesia • Surgery

KEY POINTS

- The primary goal of a preoperative program is to provide safe, reliable preoperative medical optimization in a comprehensive manner to preprocedural patients.
- Preoperative care is best delivered in a centralized but highly matrixed multidisciplinary environment.
- Communication and collaboration across service lines are essential to programmatic success.
- Although there is no single universally accepted model, a preoperative program with evidence-based protocols supported by institutional consensus ensures that goals and objectives will be met.

INTRODUCTION

Each year, more than 200 million people undergo surgery worldwide, and this population is becoming increasingly medically complex.[1] In the United States, 26% of all inpatient adverse events within the Medicare population are attributable to surgery and procedures.[2] The number of procedures performed in ambulatory surgery centers now exceeds those done on an inpatient basis.[3,4] In this progressively challenging environment, with an estimate that 44% of adverse perioperative events are preventable, it is essential that the risk of perioperative complications be mitigated. Also, the financial solvency of operating rooms in a fragmented health care system may be jeopardized by incomplete patient information that leads to delayed and cancelled surgeries.[5] The preoperative clinic is an ideal setting to optimize patients' medical

Disclosures: none.
[a] Department of Anesthesiology, Wake Forest Baptist Health, Wake Forest University School of Medicine, Medical Center Boulevard, 9 CSB, Winston Salem, NC 27157, USA; [b] Section of Perioperative and Consultative Medicine, Department of Medicine, Froedtert Hospital Clinical Cancer Center, Froedtert and Medical College of Wisconsin, Suite 5400, 9200 West Wisconsin Avenue, Milwaukee, WI 53226, USA
* Corresponding author.
E-mail address: afedward@wakehealth.edu

Anesthesiology Clin 34 (2016) 1–15
http://dx.doi.org/10.1016/j.anclin.2015.10.002
1932-2275/16/$ – see front matter © 2016 Elsevier Inc. All rights reserved.

anesthesiology.theclinics.com

conditions, ensure patient safety, and maximize economic efficiency within the pre-procedural arena.

HISTORY/BACKGROUND

Through the years, the process of preoperative evaluation has evolved significantly. What began as a presurgical hospital admission with initial evaluation the day before surgery has transformed into a multidisciplinary, team-based approach of medical optimization and care coordination occurring weeks before the procedure. Standardizing the process has helped ensure that regulatory, accreditation, and reimbursement requirements were met. Careful triage through prescreening helped identify which patients should be referred for telephone screens, clinic visits, or to specific providers for further evaluation.[6,7] Such tools have also been used to discern whether additional testing or patient education might be necessary. Historically, the organizational structure of preoperative clinics has varied by institution. Several examples of unique clinic designs, optimal physical locations, and ideal staffing models have been well described.[8] Details regarding appointment scheduling and the proportion of patients triaged to alternate visits often depended on the systems put into place and the institutional practice.[9]

In his seminal article in 1949, Dr Alfred Lee[10] recognized that "the anesthetist is frequently confronted with patients who are not in the best possible state for the operation." Lee[10] recognized the need for medical optimization and acknowledged it was "inadequate for the anesthetist to see the patient the evening before the operation, or even two to three days beforehand." Lee[10] also noted that preoperative clinics were not best suited for "perfectly fit patients…nor those undergoing trivial surgical procedures." Since his initial observation and the inception of rudimentary preoperative clinics, additional approaches have been developed using clinical data to risk stratify patients and triage accordingly.[11] The first example, provided by Chase in 1977,[11] used a software-based, computer-assisted screening program to triage patients according to risk of postoperative respiratory complications. This single-organ-system approach proved inadequate, neglecting global medical optimization, patient education, and appropriate testing.

A subsequent study of patients undergoing 4 distinct surgical procedures at 3 separate institutions analyzed preoperative testing patterns[12] and found an increase in unnecessary laboratory testing when patients were not first examined in a preoperative clinic. According to Macario and colleagues,[13] 26% of the laboratory tests were unwarranted based on physical examination findings noted by the clinician at the time of the appointment. Further studies supported more cost-effective diagnostic testing within a formal preoperative clinic setting in which all testing decisions were made following physical assessment of the patient.[14–18] These initial observations set the stage for the progressive development of preoperative clinics with standardized systems identifying high-risk patients to reduce inappropriate testing.[13–15]

In the 1990s, Fischer[19] expanded on these ideas by creating a comprehensive preoperative evaluation process. He used concepts previously proposed with goals of increasing operating room efficiency, streamlining testing, coordinating subspecialty consultations, and retrieving medical records. Fischer's[19] preoperative clinic was highly successful in reducing unnecessary testing by 55%, reducing subspecialty consultations, and decreasing day-of-surgery cancellations by 88%, which resulted in estimated cost savings of $112/patient.[19] By focusing on elements directly related to optimizing patient health, Fischer[19] created one of the first highly effective preoperative clinics.[19]

Further improvements continued, using prescreening questionnaires to designate patients for different types of appointments, telephone screens, or same-day surgery evaluations.[6,7,20–22] Badner and colleagues[20] proposed that most healthy surgical candidates did not require a comprehensive clinic visit. In order to alleviate strain on resources, they described a hybrid process in which prescreening questionnaires established patients' health status before scheduling the visit. This process permitted triage to specific clinicians and/or subspecialty consultations. Patients who met criteria were referred to preoperative clinic faculty, anesthesiologists, and internists, who then coordinated further tests or consultations. This process resulted in a more efficient, cost-effective use of medical personnel during the preoperative process. Vaghadia and Fowler[6] continued development by using their previously described nurse-based screening questionnaire as the initial diagnostic filter for patients who might require further evaluation. Their nurse-based screening model had an accuracy of 81%, specificity of 86%, and a negative predictive value of 93% compared with anesthesiologists' recommendations. Subsequent investigators[7] further quantified the effectiveness of using such tools by recognizing that nurses required 80% more time than physicians to complete the process, but their conclusions were often similar to those of the physicians. This finding validated the use of additional medical personnel to prescreen patients and proved highly useful in eliminating unnecessary visits and improving patient satisfaction.[23]

Digner[21] described a phone screen to assess "patient fitness" before scheduling the preoperative clinic appointment. This process permitted the preoperative clinic to "assess greater numbers of patients with more complex medical and social issues." Likewise, a subsequent study provided telephone screens instead of clinic visits for all American Society of Anesthesiologists (ASA) 1 and 2 patients scheduled for ambulatory surgery.[22] This method had the "advantage of identifying potential medical, anesthetic, and social issues that might delay or cancel the procedure on the morning of surgery."[21] In both instances, the use of prescreening questionnaires and telephone screens to determine assessment needs improved efficiency and patient satisfaction, and expanded preoperative service options.[24]

The aforementioned tools enhanced the effectiveness of earlier preoperative clinics to the same degree that information technology and clinical decision support systems have subsequently improved documentation, regulatory compliance, and perioperative communication.[25] Integrating institutional electronic health records into the preoperative process has improved standardization, eliminated redundancy, and provided a database for research.[20,25,26] One of the first examples of this was provided by the National Health Service (NHS) Greater Glasgow Health Board while "implementing an electronic preoperative care pathway (e-Form) that allowed all hospitals to access comprehensive patient medical history through a clinical portal on the health-board intranet."[27] Their previously fragmented, nonstandardized presurgical process was streamlined as part of a global planned care improvement program. With the development and implementation of their Web-based e-Form, they improved clinical documentation and "informational task sharing across multidisciplinary teams."[27] This e-Form subsequently enhanced the cost-effectiveness of their preoperative process. By the end of 2013, all NHS Greater Glasgow hospitals could access the preoperative e-Form through the hospital's clinical portal. This e-Form successfully transformed preoperative practices and facilitated communication to limit day-of-surgery delays, cancellations, and hospital costs. Flamm and colleagues[27] realized additional benefits by implementing electronic decision support tools into their preoperative evaluation process. Use of clinical decision support logic to suggest appropriate testing successfully led to a "reduction in unnecessary tests, improved guideline adherence, and reduced patient burden and costs,"[26] thus demonstrating the ability of Web-based electronic health records with clinical decision support tools to enhance preoperative clinical decision making and accurately identify patients requiring comprehensive evaluations.

The availability of newer technologies continues to improve the presurgical optimization process. Patient-driven Web-based applications that permit patients to upload clinical data and answer a series of questions have been viewed as the next step to improve clinical efficiency and minimize costs. Newly designed Web applications permit patients to upload personal data into clinical assessment tools using decision support logic to suggest appropriate next steps for preoperative evaluation. Such systems enable institution-wide algorithms to combine the patient's medical information and ASA classification with the planned procedure to recommend a further course of action. In all likelihood, such technology will continue to develop and reshape patients' preoperative experiences by permitting remote access to preoperative clinicians.[28]

BENEFITS AND OUTCOMES

Preoperative identification of high-risk patients with complex medical and social issues before their surgical admission has been shown to increase patient safety and satisfaction[23,24] as well as improve efficient use of operating room resources.[29] Preoperative clinic visits have been shown to reduce unnecessary testing, subspecialty consultations, and hospital stay.[19,24,30] Further, preoperative interventions that reduce the risk of postoperative complications have led to significant cost savings.[31] It has been well documented that centralizing and standardizing even part of the preoperative process through obtaining outside records; completing history and physical examinations; and finalizing surgical, anesthesia, and nursing assessments increases operating room efficiency and decreases costs. Optimizing a patients' medical conditions before surgery decreases operating room delays and cancellations, which have significant negative financial implications for the operating suite.[30–32] One estimate suggested revenue loss of approximately $1500 per hour with any unanticipated delay or cancellation on the day of surgery.[31] With such expense, last-minute changes have significant financial impacts on operating margins.[30,33,34] The direct and indirect savings achieved by minimizing redundancy, avoiding delays and cancellations, and ensuring appropriate documentation and coding offset the expense of establishing and maintaining a preoperative assessment clinic.[8,35]

Overall, the benefits to developing an effective preoperative clinic include the following:

- Decreased surgical delays and cancellations caused by nonmedical issues
- Decreased perioperative morbidity and mortality
- Reduction in excessive and unnecessary testing
- Reduction in subspecialty consults
- Increased patient and surgeon satisfaction
- Increased regulatory compliance and operating room efficiency
- Improving information transfers; clean charts (eg, consents, history and physical examinations)
- Improved patient satisfaction
- Improved compliance with preoperative instructions
- Implementing care coordination in a multidisciplinary context

Well-established preoperative clinics can coordinate services such that most, if not all, components of perioperative optimization are brought to the patient and discharge planning initiated before the patient leaves the clinic. These components include but are not limited to medical optimization, chart completion, shared decision making, and postoperative care coordination with discharge planning. These benefits provide added value, patient-centered care, and a clinical launch site for perioperative care pathways serving as a segue to the development of a perioperative surgical home.

DEVELOPING PREOPERATIVE PROGRAMS

Developing a preoperative program or clinic can seem like an insurmountable task. However, the key to successful implementation is a well-defined and institutionally supported plan. The continuum of preprocedural care is expansive, so it is important to differentiate between preprocedural processes and the preoperative clinic. Preoperative processes include not only direct patient evaluation in a clinic setting but also standardization of preprocedural care and associated administrative, educational, and leadership tasks. To be truly successful in providing superior patient care, perioperative services require significant effort beyond traditional prescreening. In addition to providing clinical care, it is increasingly recognized that efficient perioperative management requires standardized, streamlined processes to address chart completion (eg, consent forms, surgical orders, power of attorney), financial authorization, medication reconciliation, case management, quality control, and coordinated surgical services leadership. Ideally, the preoperative clinic sets the standards for care and is the model of delivery for all preoperative processes in a given health care system.

Vision and Goals

One of the first steps in developing a new preoperative program or expanding an existing program is to define the vision of the program and goals of care. The primary goal of a preoperative program is to provide safe, consistent, and reliable preoperative care to procedural patients in a universal, streamlined, comprehensive manner. Because preoperative clinics are specifically intended to improve the quality of care, service, satisfaction, and fiscal responsibility, preoperative programs must be aligned with the strategic goals of their clinical institutions. A broad vision of how this will be accomplished and the benefits to the enterprise should be shared with administrative leaders to gain organized programmatic support.[34,36] An important aspect to the initial success of the program is identification of the key stakeholders who will provide budgetary support and clinical leadership. When making the business case for the program and requesting resources, the support of these administrators is invaluable.

Alignment regarding the specific model for the program may be challenging during initial stages of development. However, successful examples with specified leadership are provided throughout the literature.[8,19,37–39] Although certain models have led to reduced health care costs,[37] reduced levels of patient anxiety,[40] and improved patient acceptance of regional anesthesia, the specific design chosen by a health care system remains open to debate and depends on the surgical population needs.[32,41–43] What remains clear is that an experienced perioperative clinical leader is required to establish and maintain the process. That leader should emphasize collaboration, commitment, and teamwork as necessary components to successful implementation. The preoperative clinic must develop as a partnership between the departments of surgery, anesthesia, medicine, nursing, and administration.

After establishing a common vision, detailed goals of a preoperative program need to be defined. The goals may result from a list of specific problems that require resolution. Beyond any immediate problems, it is useful to consider the general goals applicable to most perioperative programs and to determine whether those are within scope. The Perioperative Surgical Home model includes goals that may be useful when planning preoperative programs.[44] A modified list of these objectives is presented in **Box 1**.

As well as the goals related to an in-person preoperative assessment, many preoperative programs have associated objectives that are not related to direct patient care. These objectives are summarized in **Box 2**.

The visionary goals of preoperative programs as outlined in **Boxes 1** and **2** may not be specifically task oriented or related to precisely defined outcomes. To create the operational plan for a functional preoperative program, it is necessary to determine how program goals will be defined, accomplished, and measured. For example, the safety goal of minimizing patient-specific risks of surgery and anesthesia may be more precisely defined as reducing postoperative mortality and myocardial infarction. Deciding how a preoperative program will meet and measure such metrics is challenging. Standards of practice and disease-specific care algorithms may make these goals achievable.

SCOPE

Once the goals of a perioperative program are identified, scope can be determined. As noted previously, the scope of the preoperative process is expansive, obliging the design process to be thoughtfully planned and inclusive of all components. Preoperative care begins when the decision is made to proceed with surgical intervention and extends to admission for surgery.

Potential stakeholders in the preoperative process include:

- Patients
- Physicians: surgeons, anesthesiologists, and internists

Box 1
Goals of the preoperative program: direct patient care

Provide comprehensive preoperative evaluation

- Identify, communicate, and minimize the patient-specific risks of surgery and anesthesia
- Consistently apply evidence-based, standardized, consistent, condition-specific protocols for preoperative diagnostic testing
- Use goal-directed patient medical optimization to reduce case delays and cancellations
  ○ Develop and implement individualized perioperative care plans
- Perform detailed review of patient medications and give patient-friendly preoperative medication instructions
  ○ Include any new preoperative medications and maintenance of the patient's chronic medications, including analgesics

Initiate transitional care planning

- Plan the appropriate postoperative level of care
- Provide case management services to plan for postdischarge needs

Provide patient education and counseling

- To reduce anxiety, increase participation, and enhance recovery after surgery

Consent

- Confirm surgical consent before surgery

Box 2

Goals of the preoperative program: indirect patient care and nonclinical goals

Model process improvement

- Create standardized protocols to improve patient outcomes and decrease unnecessary testing
- Distribute protocols as the standard of care for all periprocedural patients

Centralize medical information and coordinate perioperative care

- Provide leadership in the perioperative services across service lines and departments
- Manage tasks associated with perioperative patient care
  ○ Coordinate chart readiness, control information systems, other pertinent tasks
- Comply with regulatory standards

Improve perioperative efficiency and finance

- Improve periprocedural resource use and contribute to surgical growth

Perform research

- Study outcomes related to periprocedural care and disseminate findings

Provide education

- Train relevant learners in the practice of perioperative medicine

---

- Operating rooms, ambulatory surgery centers, and procedural areas
- Inpatient units
- Ambulatory clinics

The broad scope of potential services presents a significant challenge when considering the expertise, workforce, and other resources currently available to perform the potential tasks at hand, along with the needs of the patients and institution. In addition, the demand for the number and types of preoperative services tend to increase with time and surgical growth, so planning should consider so-called scope creep, as well as an awareness of which services may be in and out of scope, both present and future.

TACTICAL AND OPERATIONAL PLANS

The operational plan is the specific action plan developed to meet the goals and objectives of the preoperative program. The goals noted in **Boxes 1** and **2** can be used as a springboard for determining which services will be delivered by the preoperative program, keeping current and future scope in mind. Furthermore, the design and development of the preoperative clinic must serve the goals and objectives of the program well. Important considerations in the development and structure of the clinic are as follows:

A preoperative clinic may provide the following services[45]:

- Preoperative medical optimization and preanesthesia evaluation via review of medical records, history, physical examination, and relevant ancillary testing, followed by risk optimization through appropriate interventions and consultations
- Discussion of the risks and benefits of anesthetic options and pain management strategies
- A private location for collaborative comanagement review and postoperative care planning

- Care coordination and social work review
- Alleviation of anxiety through counseling and education
- Obtaining informed consent
- Patient and family education on day of surgery–related topics: nil-by-mouth status, medications for the day of surgery, special nursing requirements, anticipated duration of stay, transportation issues, and contingency planning
- Validation of consent and documentation of advanced medical directives (if any)
- Reduction of day-of-surgery delay, no-show risk, or risk of cancellations through phone call confirmations the day before surgery

The physical design and location of the clinic should focus on services to be delivered:

- Location is ideally accessible from the main entrance of hospital, near referring surgical clinics or the operating rooms
- Location should be near electrocardiogram, laboratory, and radiology services
- Registration, reception, medication reconciliation, and financial clearance ideally occur within clinic
- Private areas for patient interview, examination, and education
- Rooms should be designed for patients with mobility limitations or using assistive devices
- Private areas should be available for medical record organization and chart review

SPECIFIC SERVICES DELIVERED
Triage

It is important to determine which patients are recommended to have in-person visits to the preoperative clinic. Preoperative clinic leaders develop triage systems that assist referring surgeons and proceduralists to choose appropriate patients for clinic visits. These triage systems may be either paper or electronic tools, depending on the resources of the health care system. Historically, triage has been proposed using medical comorbidities and/or ASA classification to assess physical status and risk.[46] Using such tools, ASA class 1 and 2 patients might be triaged to phone screens, whereas ASA class 3 and 4 patients require a clinic visit and consultation.

- In some patients, in-person visits can be avoided based on triage, surgical case severity, and patient physical status
- Further triage may occur to appropriate staff or physician specialist based on degree of comorbidity management required
- Skilled trained nursing staff may be used for this purpose

Triage systems developed by the preoperative program need to be accurately used by patients or providers to be effective, so design of the tool needs to take the intended user into account. If the intended user of a triage tool is a patient, it must be worded accordingly in patient-friendly language. Triage tools used in surgeons' offices may be used by physicians or by ancillary staff who have limited medical knowledge. Understanding end-users can determine the success of the triage system. In order for the triage system to be used effectively and to have patient referrals to the preoperative clinic, surgeons not only need to agree with the content of the triage system but they must also think that there is added value in referring patients for evaluation and optimization.

When developing triage systems, it is important to communicate with surgeons regarding:

- Appropriate use of triage systems
- Protocol development for referral and transfer of information based on medical comorbidities, engaging all teams in the process of innovation
- Identify which aspects of preoperative evaluation surgeons will retain
- Develop protocols to ensure consistent transfer of clinical information
- Develop external feedback systems to measure implementation
- Streamline span of care and look for cross-departmental opportunities
- Engage all teams in the process of innovation

Phone Calls

Patients who do not meet criteria for in-person preoperative clinic visits may benefit from telephone-mediated evaluation. This approach is cost-efficient and time-efficient, allowing the preoperative clinic to evaluate a larger volume of patients. Logistically, it may be difficult to reach some patients by phone. Gathering detailed information in complex patients may be more difficult, and these patients still need to meet regulatory requirements of a history and undergo physical examination performed within 30 days of surgery.[47]

In-person Clinic Visits

Services delivered during an in-person visit may include the preoperative nursing assessment, provider (Doctor of Medicine or Advanced Practice Provider) history and physical evaluation, pharmacist interview, diagnostic testing, education and consent.

Algorithms

In developing a preoperative program, it is essential to initiate and disseminate standard protocols for the delivery of patient care not only in the preoperative clinic but throughout the health care system. In some situations, national guidelines are available for preoperative evaluation[48]; however, in many clinical scenarios, perioperative expertise is needed to interpret current literature and develop local care algorithms. Agreement about the content of said algorithms, as well as their widespread adoption and adherence to them, may produce some challenges. In addition, there can be disagreement on medical judgment between the staff performing preoperative evaluations and the staff in the operating room.[46] This disagreement has the potential to lead to surgical delays or cancellations, so inclusion of multiple stakeholders when developing such protocols can help prevent these discrepancies.

Communication

Collaborative interaction between preoperative consultants, the operating room staff, referring surgeons, primary care physicians, and subspecialists is imperative to providing patient-centric preoperative care.

IDENTIFYING RESOURCES
Workforce

As preoperative programs have developed across the nation, the providers that deliver services under the preoperative umbrella have expanded. The use of anesthesiologists, internists, advanced practice providers, and nurses to deliver preoperative care depends on the available resources and the degree of patient complexity within a health care system. Each provider brings unique skills, strengths, and subject matter expertise. Recruiting and retaining a dynamic workforce with expertise and interest in perioperative medicine may prove challenging. This difficulty is especially notable among specialties with higher paid physicians, because the return on investment for physician services may be higher when care is delivered outside the preoperative clinic, which may be particularly common in community practice.[49]

Another concern is that primary care physicians will lose financial or continuity opportunities with their patients when they are referred to a centralized preoperative clinic. Although primary care physicians and external referring physicians have the ability to provide preoperative history and physical examinations or evaluations, their office resources are often insufficient to provide the comprehensive experience that a preoperative program provides. After determining a generalized staffing model, a workforce plan can be developed based on projected patient volumes and the planned staffing model for the clinic.

Preoperative staff typically consist of the following:

The medical director serves a primary role to establish clinical protocols
- Serves as clinical liaison with all engaged services
- Provides clinical accountability
- Acts as collaborating physician to clinical staff
- Maintains and updates preoperative evidence-based protocols

Clinical personnel (determine the subset most appropriate for the clinical setting)
- Anesthesiologist
- Internal medicine; hospitalist
- Nurse practitioners, physician assistants
- Registered nurse (phone screen, triage, patient education)
- Pharmacy technician (medication reconciliation)
- Residents and house officers (preanesthesia assessment, medical optimization)

Administrative leadership
- Administrative liaison between all engaged services
- Budget oversight, staffing, and recruitment
- Long-term clinic development
- Responsible for all nonclinical patient-related issues
- Identify necessary preparation for all aspects of typical clinic visit
- Develop structure for ongoing education for all staff
- Develop internal feedback system to measure implementation success
- Responsible for quality protocols and documentation
- Advance the implementation of multidisciplinary care pathways to ensure high reliability
- Financial performance; examine all aspects of cost structure
- Optimize labor as discussed earlier and reevaluate, reduce, supply discretionary funds

Visit Volumes and Space

Predicting present and future patient visit numbers in the preoperative clinic depends on the chosen model for care. As noted previously, preoperative clinics range in the number of in-person visits and virtual visits (electronic screening and phone calls). For those preoperative clinics with in-person provider visits, the type of provider also varies between systems. An acceptable method of determining how many patients each provider will see is based on the percentage of the surgical volume in each ASA classification. For instance, **Table 1** shows an example of a preoperative

Table 1					
Estimating visit volumes in a preoperative clinic					
	Virtual Preoperative Evaluation	**Anesthesiology**	**Internal Medicine**	**Advanced Practice Provider**	**Total**
Operating Room Patients					
ASA 1	1000	—	—	—	1000
ASA 2	2000	—	—	—	2000
ASA 3	—	3500	2100	1400	7000
ASA 4	—	800	200	—	1000
Subtotal	3000	4300	2300	1400	11,000
Procedural patients requiring anesthesia	500	500	—	—	1000
Surgery Center					
ASA 1	5000	—	—	—	5000
ASA 2	3000	—	—	—	3000
ASA 3	—	—	—	—	—
ASA 4	—	—	—	—	—
Subtotal	8000	—	—	—	8000
Total	11,000	4800	2300	1400	20,000

clinic that includes both virtual visits and in-person visits with multiple provider types. Total volumes are determined by surgical volume, out-of-operating-room procedures, and ASA classification.

This model assumes that all preoperative patients are seen in the preoperative clinic. In most health care systems, this is unrealistic and a percentage of this number based on demand may need to be taken into account. Predicting the volume of future patients to be seen can be based on current surgical growth at the facility and the size and growth targets of the preoperative program. If future surgical growth is undetermined, it may helpful to use national statistics and consider that hospital-based procedural growth throughout the United States has been fairly sluggish, whereas ambulatory surgical procedures have continued to increase.[3,4] The model in **Tables 1** and **2** assumes this type of surgical growth with staggered volumes accommodating expansion.

As part of the operational plan, physical space for delivering preoperative services may vary. Programs may choose to deliver care in a large, centralized clinic, whereas

Table 2				
Predicting future volumes in a preoperative clinic				
	2016	**2017**	**2018**	**2019**
Virtual evaluations	11,500	11,845	12,200	12,566
Anesthesiology	4800	4837	4874	4911
Internal medicine	2300	2312	2323	2335
Advanced practice provider	1400	1407	1414	1421
Total	20,000	20,400	20,811	21,233

Calculations estimate 3% increase in ambulatory surgical volume and 0.5% in inpatient surgical volume.

others may have multiple satellite clinics geographically associated with surgeon offices. Each strategy has advantages and disadvantages.

Financial Resources

A significant aspect of developing or expanding a preoperative program is the dependence on financial resources to secure staff, space, and capital needs. Partnering with a financial expert to write a business plan and advise as necessary throughout the planning process is recommended. Funding resources vary between facilities, particularly between community and academic models. Making the financial case for a preoperative program may be challenging, in part because preoperative programs generally rely on funds saved rather than generation of revenue, so value and return on investment are difficult to demonstrate. When justifying resource use in a preoperative program, it is gainful to emphasize that preoperative evaluations have historically been performed within the system before the implementation of the preoperative clinic. This evaluation is usually done in a piecemeal, inefficient manner and development of a preoperative clinic simply shifts the use of resources already in play. The advantage of the preoperative program is that the resources are managed centrally by experts in perioperative care with gains in efficiency noted. Relocating preoperative care to a centralized clinic can also improve resource use in surgical clinics and improve the efficiency of surgical teams that generate financial margin in the operating room.

Performance Management/Quality Improvement

A successful preoperative program includes a quality improvement process to drive reliable, standardized patient care, developing an error-resistant system. Trackable metrics are often defined at the stage of developing specific goals for a preoperative program. These metrics are often refined to some degree when creating a financial model. Conceptually, perioperative metrics may be plentiful but, realistically, these qualitative metrics are difficult to track in an automated manner. A creative approach to goals and metrics helps to show the value of a program because data are difficult to produce and measure. For example, metrics such as postoperative length of stay and mortality may be easily obtained but difficult to directly attribute to preoperative care. Surgical delay and cancellation rates may be more easily attributed to delivery of preoperative care but can be equally challenging to track.[46] It may be useful to consider metrics that are unique to the specific program (eg, blood use relative to preoperative anemia, surgical case start times and turnover times with reasons for delay, staff overtime in the operating room, surgeon productivity). Commonly followed metrics used to justify developing preoperative programs include[9,43,50]:

- Surgical delays and cancellations
- Unindicated diagnostic testing
- Postoperative length of stay
- Postoperative complication rates and mortality
- Cost savings
- Patient satisfaction
- Preoperative preparation time

SUMMARY

Preoperative clinics are uniquely positioned as the entry points for patients to the surgical continuum of care. As the gatekeepers to the perioperative period, preoperative clinics begin the process of identifying and managing undiagnosed or poorly controlled comorbidities in order to optimize each patient's medical condition. Effective preoperative clinics provide patients with the best opportunity to avoid perioperative complications, minimize morbidity and mortality risks, minimize length of hospital stay, and participate in shared decision making during the initial surgical consultation. Within the context of preoperative evaluation, clinicians must be knowledgeable and adept at assessing patients of highly variable medical complexity. Preoperative clinicians must also be familiar with the impact of a broad range of chronic and acute medical conditions on patients' risks for anesthesia and surgery and remain aware of multiple practice guidelines, regulatory requirements, and approaches for efficient management. Despite the evolution in preoperative care, the primary purpose of preoperative clinic evaluation is to guide perioperative medical management with the goal of reducing perioperative morbidity and enhancing patient outcomes.

REFERENCES

1. Weiser TG, Regenbogen SE, Thompson KD, et al. An estimation of the global volume of surgery: a modeling strategy based on available data. Lancet 2008; 372(9633):139–44.
2. Levinson DR. Department of Health and Human Services, Office of the Inspector General. Adverse events in hospitals: national incidence among Medicare beneficiaries. 2010. OEI-06-09-00090. Available at: https://oig.hhs.gov/oei/reports/oei-06-09-00090.pdf. Accessed August 12, 2015.
3. Cullen KA, Hall MJ, Golosinskiy A. Ambulatory surgery in the United States 2006. National Health Statistics Reports; 2009. Available at: http://www.cdc.gov/nchs/data/nhsr/nhsr011.pdf. Accessed August 12, 2015.
4. DeFrances C, Lucas CA, Buie VC, et al. 2006 national discharge summary. National Health Statistics Reports; 2008. Available at: http://www.cdc.gov/nchs/data/nhsr/nhsr005.pdf. Accessed August 12, 2015.
5. Hobson and Co. The case for a perioperative- focused anesthesia solution: multiple benefits from a single solution. An ROI white paper. 2008. Available at: http://www.sisfirst.com/pdf/articles/100220.pdf. Accessed August 12, 2015.
6. Vaghadia H, Fowler C. Can nurses screen all outpatients? Performance of a nurse based model. Can J Anaesth 1999;46:1117–21.
7. van Klei WA, Hennis PJ, Moen J, et al. The accuracy of trained nurses in preoperative health assessment: results of the OPEN study. Anaesthesia 2004;59: 971–8.
8. Bader A, Sweitzer B, Kumar A. Nuts and Bolts of preoperative clinics: the view from three institutions. Cleve Clin J Med 2009;76(Suppl 4):S104–11.
9. Yen C, Tsai M, Macario A. Preoperative evaluation clinics. Curr Opin Anaesthesiol 2010;23:167–72.
10. Lee JA. The anesthetic out-patient clinic. Anaesthesia 1949;4:169–74.
11. Chase CR, Merz BA, Mazuzan JE. Computer assisted patient evaluation (CAPE): a multipurpose computer system for an anesthesia service. Anesth Analg 1983; 62:198–206.
12. Edward GM, Biervliet JD, Hollmann MW, et al. Comparing the organizational structure of the preoperative assessment clinic at eight university hospitals. Act Anaesthesiol Belg 2008;59:33–7.
13. Macario A, Roizen MF, Thisted RA, et al. Reassessment of preoperative laboratory testing has changed the test-ordering patterns of physicians. Surg Gynecol Obstet 1992;175:539–47.

14. Yuan H, Chung F, Wong D, et al. Current preoperative testing practices in ambulatory surgery are widely disparate: a survey of CAS members. Can J Anesth 2005;52:675–9.
15. Chung F, Yuan H, Yin L, et al. Elimination of preoperative testing in ambulatory surgery. Anesth Analg 2009;108:467–75.
16. Kaplan EB, Sheiner LB, Boeckmann AJ, et al. The usefulness of preoperative laboratory screening. JAMA 1985;253:3576–81.
17. Roizen MF, Kaplan EB, Schreider BD, et al. The relative roles of the history and physical examination and laboratory testing in preoperative evaluation for outpatient surgery: the 'Starling' curve for preoperative laboratory testing. Anesthesiol Clin North America 1987;5:5–34.
18. Roizen MF. More preoperative assessment by physicians and less by lab tests. N Engl J Med 2000;342:204–5.
19. Fischer SP. Development and effectiveness of an anesthesia preoperative evaluation clinic in a teaching hospital. Anesthesiology 1996;85:196–206.
20. Badner NH, Craen RA, Paul TL, et al. Anesthesia preadmission: a new approach through use of a screening questionnaire. Can J Anaesth 1998;45:87–92.
21. Digner M. At your convenience: preoperative assessment by telephone. J Perioper Pract 2007;17:294–301.
22. Law TT, Suen DT, Tam YF, et al. Telephone preanesthesia assessment for ambulatory breast surgery. Hong Kong Med J 2009;15:179–82.
23. Harnett MJ, Correll DJ, Hurwitz S, et al. Improving efficiency and patient satisfaction in a tertiary teaching hospital preoperative clinic. Anesthesiology 2010;112:66–72.
24. Hepner DL, Bader AM, Hurwitz S, et al. Patient satisfaction with preoperative assessment in a preoperative assessment testing clinic. Anesth Analg 2004;98:1099–105.
25. Bouamrane MM, Mair FS. Implementation of an integrated preoperative care pathway and regional electronic clinical portal for preoperative assessment. BMC Med Inform Decis Mak 2014;14:93.
26. Bouamrane MM, Mair FS. A study of clinical and information management processes in the surgical pre-assessment clinic. BMC Med Inform Decis Mak 2014;14:22.
27. Flamm M, Fritsch G, Hysek M, et al. Quality improvement in preoperative assessment by implementation of an electronic decision support tool. J Am Med Inform Assoc 2013;20:e91–6.
28. Wong DT, Kamming D, Salenieks ME, et al. Preadmission anesthesia consultation using telemedicine technology: a pilot study. Anesthesiology 2004;100:1605–7.
29. Tsen LC, Segal S, Pothier M, et al. The effect of alterations in a preoperative assessment clinic on reducing the number and improving the yield of cardiology consultations. Anesth Analg 2002;95:1563–8.
30. Halaszynski TM, Juda R, Silverman DG. Optimizing postoperative outcomes with efficient preoperative assessment and management. Crit Care Med 2004;32:S76–86.
31. Davenport DL, Henderson WG, Khuri SF, et al. Preoperative risk factors and surgical complexity are more predictive of costs than postoperative complications: a case study using the National Surgical Quality Improvement Program (NSQIP) database. Ann Surg 2005;242:463–71.
32. Ferschl MB, Tung A, Sweitzer B, et al. Preoperative clinic visits reduce operating room cancellations and delays. Anesthesiology 2005;103:855–9.
33. Dexter F, Marcon E, Epstein RH, et al. Validation of statistical methods to compare cancellation rates on the day of surgery. Anesth Analg 2005;101:465–73.

34. Strum DP, Vargas LG, May JH. Surgical subspecialty block utilization and capacity planning: a minimal cost analysis model. Anesthesiology 1999;90:1176–85.
35. Correll D, Bader AM, Tsen LC. Value of preoperative clinic visits in identifying issues with potential impact on operating room efficiency. Anesthesiology 2006; 105:1254–9.
36. Gibby GL. How preoperative assessment programs can be justified financially to hospital administrators. Int Anesthesiol Clin 2002;40:17–30.
37. Issa MRN, Isoni NFC, Soares AM, et al. Preanesthesia evaluation and reduction of preoperative care costs. Rev Bras Anestesiol 2011;61:60–71.
38. Power LM, Thackray NM. Reduction of preoperative investigations with the introduction of an anaesthetist-led preoperative assessment clinic. Anaesth Intensive Care 1999;27:481–8.
39. Starsnic MA, Guarnieri DM, Norris MC. Efficacy and financial benefit of an anesthesiologist-directed university preadmission evaluation center. J Clin Anesth 1997;9:299–305.
40. Klopfenstein CE, Forster A, Van Gessel E. Anesthetic assessment in an outpatient consultation clinic reduces preoperative anxiety. Can J Anaesth 2000;47:511–5.
41. van Klei WA, Moons KG, Rutten CL, et al. The effect of outpatient preoperative evaluation of hospital inpatients on cancellation of surgery and length of hospital stay. Anesth Analg 2002;94:644–9.
42. Wijeysundera DN, Austin PC, Beattie WS, et al. A population-based study of anesthesia consultation before major non-cardiac surgery. Arch Intern Med 2009;169:595–602.
43. Vazirani S, Lankarani-Fard A, Liang LJ, et al. Perioperative processes and outcomes after implementation of a hospitalist-run perioperative clinic. J Hosp Med 2012;7(9):697–701.
44. Vetter TR, Goeddel LA, Boudreaux AM, et al. The perioperative surgical home: how can it make the case so everyone wins? BMC Anesthesiol 2013;13:6.
45. Gupta SK, Kant S, Chanderashekar R. Modern trends in planning and designing hospitals. In: Principles and practice. 1st edition. Delhi (India): Jaypee; 2007. p. 18–25.
46. Bader A, Hepner Dl. The role of the preoperative clinic in perioperative risk reduction. Int Anesthesiol Clin 2009;47:151–60.
47. Joint Commission medical record documentation requirements. 2011. Available at: http://www.srhcc.org/workfiles/Joint%20Commission%20Medical%20Record %20Documentation%20Requirements%202011.pdf. Accessed August 12, 2015.
48. Fleischer LA, Fleischmann KE, Auerbach AD, et al. 2014 ACC/AHA guidelines on perioperative cardiovascular evaluation and management of patients undergoing noncardiac surgery: a report of the American College of Cardiology/American Heart Association Task Force on Practice Guidelines. J Am Coll Cardiol 2014; 64(22):e77–137.
49. Gupta A, Gupta N. Setting up and functioning of a preoperative clinic. Indian J Anaesth 2010;54(6):504–7.
50. Varughese AM, Byczkowski TL, Wittkugel FP, et al. Impact of a nurse practitioner-assisted preoperative assessment program on quality. Paediatr Anaesth 2006;16: 723–33.

Preoperative Consultations

Stephan R. Thilen, MD, MS[a],*, Duminda N. Wijeysundera, MD, PhD, FRCPC[b,c], Miriam M. Treggiari, MD, PhD, MPH[d,e]

KEYWORDS

- Preoperative care • Preoperative period • Perioperative care • Perioperative period
- Referral and consultation • Delivery of health care • Physician's practice pattern
- Organization and administration

KEY POINTS

- Medical consultations outside the scope of the routine preanesthesia evaluation by anesthesiologists and surgeons are separately billed and have been increasing in frequency.
- Preoperative consultations are often not driven by patient medical or surgical risk factors, and show unwarranted geographic variation.
- There is substantial variation between surgical specialties in the frequency of use of preoperative consultation.
- There are no studies guiding the indication for preoperative consultation or definitively determining the role of preoperative consultation on patients' outcomes.
- Future payment models may facilitate improved coordination of consultations with other aspects of preoperative care.

INTRODUCTION

Although all surgical patients undergo routine preoperative evaluations by surgeons and anesthesiologists, many are further referred for preoperative medical consultation. Such medical consultations are distinct from routine preoperative visits and are separately billed. Most preoperative medical consultations are provided by specialists

[a] Department of Anesthesiology & Pain Medicine, 325 Ninth Avenue, Box 359724, Seattle, WA 98104, USA; [b] Li Ka Shing Knowledge Institute of St. Michael's Hospital, 30 Bond Street, Toronto, Ontario M5B 1W8, Canada; [c] Department of Anesthesia, Toronto General Hospital, University of Toronto, Eaton Wing 3-450, 200 Elizabeth Street, Toronto, Ontario M5G 2C4, Canada; [d] Department of Anesthesiology and Perioperative Medicine, Oregon Health and Science University, 3181 Southwest Sam Jackson Park Road, Mail Code UHN-2, Portland, OR 97239, USA; [e] Department of Public Health and Preventive Medicine, Oregon Health and Science University, 3181 Southwest Sam Jackson Park Road, Mail Code UHN-2, Portland, OR 97239, USA
* Corresponding author.
E-mail address: sthilen@yahoo.com

Anesthesiology Clin 34 (2016) 17–33
http://dx.doi.org/10.1016/j.anclin.2015.10.003
1932-2275/16/$ – see front matter © 2016 Elsevier Inc. All rights reserved.
anesthesiology.theclinics.com

in internal medicine, cardiology, and family practice but they may be provided by other medical subspecialists. The volume of preoperative consultations has increased[1] in recent years, and these consultations now consume substantial resources. This article reviews the current role and practice patterns of preoperative medical consultations and provides a framework for how the use of consultations could reasonably be improved.

THE PURPOSE OF CONSULTATION

Ultimately, the purpose of preoperative medical consultations is to improve value-based, patient-centered surgical outcomes. In addition to a good surgical result per se, there are several different outcomes that are important and relevant to patients. Examples of desirable perioperative outcomes include reduced anxiety, satisfactory pain control, rapid recovery, and ability to return to a normal living situation, including return to work. Nonetheless, avoiding complications is an overarching goal. The most frequent complications, as reported by the National Surgical Quality Improvement Program, are listed in **Box 1**.

Prevention of perioperative complications is a major focus of surgeons' and anesthesiologists' training and practice. Although complications can be related to patient, provider, or system factors, they can be thought of as surgical or medical. There is a paucity of data on how preoperative medical consultations affect the complications listed in **Box 1** and other complications; however, it is plausible that consultants' services are more likely to positively affect nonsurgical (ie, medical) complications. For example, deep vein thrombosis would be affected by the medical consultant if this area of care is delegated to the consultant. The typical consultant services are listed in **Box 2**.

Previous studies have documented that specific questions are rarely asked by the surgeon requesting a preoperative consultation. In a retrospective analysis of 202 cardiology consultations, 108 were requested for an evaluation, 79 for clearance, and 9 did not specifically request to address any concerns.[2] The most common problem leading to a request for consultation was an abnormal electrocardiogram. Another study reported that referral dynamics was a reason for referral.[3]

Box 1	
Perioperative complications, National Surgical Quality Improvement Program 2005 to 2013	
Complications	**Frequency (%)**
Bleeding requiring transfusion of >4 units of blood	5.0
Superficial wound infection	2.2
Sepsis within 30 d postoperatively	1.7
Urinary tract infection	1.6
Postoperative pneumonia	1.4
Organ/space surgical site infection	1.2
Unplanned intubation	1.2
Ventilator dependent >48 h after surgery	1.2
Septic shock within 30 d postoperatively	0.9
Deep incisional surgical site infection	0.7
Deep vein thrombosis/thrombophlebitis	0.7
Wound disruption	0.5
Acute renal failure requiring dialysis	0.4
Cardiac arrest	0.4
Q-wave myocardial infarction within 30 d postoperatively	0.3
Pulmonary embolism	0.3

Box 2
Most common services provided by preoperative medical consultants

Preoperative medical consultants can:

- Complete documentation of History and Physical Examination
- Assess/stratify risk
- Order additional investigations
- Optimize comorbidities
- Discuss perioperative care
- Delay or cancel surgery
- Arrange for comanagement

Katz and colleagues[4] surveyed surgeons, anesthesiologists, and cardiologists to determine the intended indications and perceived utility of preoperative cardiology consultations. They found substantial disagreement among the specialties as to the reason for consultations being obtained. The study also included chart review of 55 cardiology consultations. Although there was agreement that optimizing an inadequately treated cardiac condition before surgery was important, only 11% of patients (6 of 55) required intervention for new findings. The most commonly confirmed reason for a referral for consultation was preoperative clearance; however, surgeons, anesthesiologists, and cardiologists did not agree on the meaning of this term. Furthermore, for most consultations, there was no clear reason for the referral.

In a survey of Canadian surgeons, PausJenssen and colleagues[5] found that almost half of the respondents indicated that the reason for a preoperative consultation was to clear a patient, but 33% disagreed with this statement. Cardiac risk stratification was a common reason for referral. There was controversy among the surgeons with regard to whether the surgeon or the medical consultant should discuss operative risk with the patient.

Even when patients are referred for preoperative medical consultations without specific questions, it is frequently reported that new or undertreated conditions are found.[6–8] Uncontrolled hypertension and impaired fasting glucose were common findings in a cohort of patients scheduled for ophthalmic surgery.[9] It has been proposed that finding such conditions makes preoperative medical consultations valuable and that it is justified to refer many patients for preoperative general medical examinations. However, a well-organized and coordinated routine preoperative assessment process should effectively identify common conditions, such as poorly controlled hypertension, and should facilitate selective referral of patients with these conditions.[10] Moreover, there is no evidence that the perioperative context is an exception from the otherwise applicable finding that general health checks do not reduce morbidity or mortality.[11]

CURRENT USE OF PREOPERATIVE MEDICAL CONSULTATIONS

The use of preoperative medical consultations has increased over the past 2 decades. A study was conducted by Thilen and colleagues[1] to assess the prevalence and trends of preoperative consultations and preoperative office visits in the Medicare population. The largest increase in consultations was associated with ophthalmologic procedures. Compared with 1995, patients undergoing ophthalmic surgery in 2006 were

66% more likely to have a preoperative consultation. The second largest increase in consultations was observed in orthopedic surgery; the increase was 56% comparing 2006 with 1995 (**Fig. 1**).

In the United States, most preoperative consultations are provided within a few weeks of the day of surgery.[12,13] **Fig. 2** is based on data from an integrated health care system (ie, health maintenance organization) and shows the frequency distribution of preoperative consultations in the 42 days preceding the date of surgery, with peaks on preoperative days 7 and 14. About 75% of all consultations were provided within 14 days of surgery.[12] The same pattern was found in a study using Medicare data.[13] In Canada, many preoperative consultations are provided earlier in the preoperative course and may occur as early as 90 days preoperatively.[14] This difference may, in part, be caused by differences in usual waiting times for elective surgical procedures between Canada and the United States.

Several studies have found substantial practice variation with regard to the use of preoperative medical consultations. In an analysis of perioperative data for patients undergoing major surgery at 79 acute care hospitals in Ontario, Canada, patient-level and surgery-level factors were weak predictors of consultation use, and the individual hospital was the major determinant of whether patients underwent preoperative medical consultation.[15] Differences in rates of consultations across hospitals were large (range, 10–897 per 1000 procedures). **Fig. 3** shows these rates with 95% confidence intervals. Such practice variation may reflect uncertainty about when preoperative consultations are useful.

In a study on preoperative consultation for Medicare beneficiaries undergoing cataract surgery, with the exception of patient age, nonmedical factors drove the use of preoperative consultations. Consultations were associated with nonblack race, urban residence, type of facility where the procedure was performed (hospital outpatient vs ambulatory surgery center), and involvement of an anesthesiologist (vs nurse

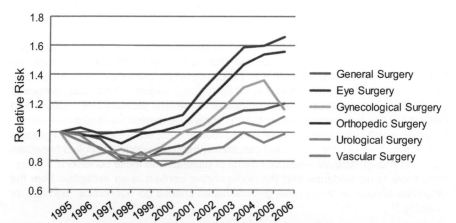

Fig. 1. Relative frequency of receiving a preoperative consultation. Data based on analysis of Medicare data for patients undergoing 20 common procedures in 6 different specialties. Over the 12-year period, there was a significant increase in the proportion of patients who had preoperative consultation for all specialties except vascular surgery. The largest increase in consultations was in ophthalmology. Compared with 1995, patients undergoing surgery in 2006 were 66% more likely to have a preoperative consultation. The adjusted relative risk was 1.66 and the 95% confidence interval (CI) 1.59 to 1.72. The second largest increase in consultations was observed in orthopedic surgery: 56% comparing 2006 with 1995.

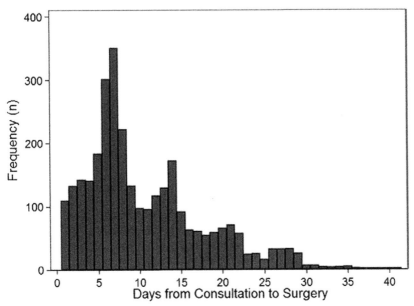

Fig. 2. Frequency distribution of preoperative consultations in the 42 days preceding surgery. The data show a bimodal distribution with peaks on preoperative days 7 and 14. (*From* Thilen SR, Bryson CL, Reid RJ, et al. Patterns of preoperative consultation and surgical specialty in an integrated healthcare system. Anesthesiology 2013;118:1032; with permission.)

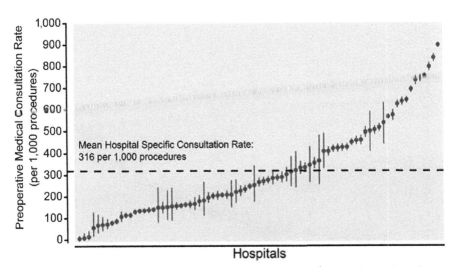

Fig. 3. Hospital-specific rates of preoperative medical consultation for major elective noncardiac surgery. Rates of preoperative medical consultation (per 1000 procedures) for major elective noncardiac surgery at 79 individual Ontario hospitals in Ontario between April 1, 2004, and February 28, 2009. The circles are point estimates, whereas the lines are exact binomial 95% CIs. The dashed horizontal line is the mean hospital-specific consultation rate. (*From* Wijeysundera DN, Austin PC, Beattie WS, et al. Variation in the practice of preoperative medical consultation for major elective noncardiac surgery: a population-based study. Anesthesiology 2012;116:30; with permission.)

anesthetist). An important source of variability was in the geographic referral regions in the United States where the procedures were performed. The range of consultation rates varied from 0 to 692 per 1000 cataract procedures. **Fig. 4** shows these rates by hospital referral region with 95% confidence intervals. **Figs. 3** and **4** show comparable patterns, although 1 study was based on major inpatient surgeries in Canada and the other was based on a low-risk outpatient procedure in the United States.

The use of preoperative consultation also varies depending on the surgical specialty referring the patient. In a cohort of 13,673 patients enrolled in a single health maintenance organization system, patients having ophthalmic, orthopedic, or urologic surgery were more likely to have consultations compared with those having general surgery. For each of these specialties, patients were 2-fold to 4-fold more likely to be evaluated with a preoperative consultation compared with general surgery. This variation exists despite the Accreditation Council for Graduate Medical Education requiring that all surgeons, regardless of specialty, be trained to perform a general medical preoperative assessment.[16] The variation between specialties might be explained by differences in their approaches to the care of patients and the degree of collaboration with consultants.

Several studies have reported a high rate of referral of low-risk patients for preoperative medical consultations.[2,3,12,13,17] Thilen and colleagues[12], in their study of preoperative medical consultations in an integrated health care system, found that lower-risk patients were most likely to be referred for consultations. **Fig. 5** shows the frequency of referral for patients with low versus high Revised Cardiac Risk Index.

Preoperative medical consultations may be both overused and underused. Although consultations are almost certainly overused for low-risk patients,[18] there

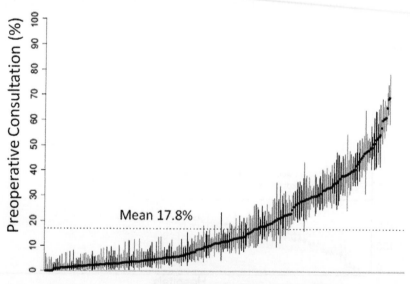

Fig. 4. Points represent unadjusted proportions of individuals undergoing consultation before cataract surgery across 306 hospital referral regions (HRRs) during 2005 to 2006. Vertical lines represent exact binomial 95% CIs. The dotted horizontal line denotes the overall proportion undergoing consultation (17.8%). The HRRs are ordered along the X axis from lowest to highest frequency of consultations. (*From* Thilen SR, Treggiari MM, Lange JM, et al. Preoperative consultations for Medicare patients undergoing cataract surgery. JAMA Intern Med 2014;174:387; with permission.)

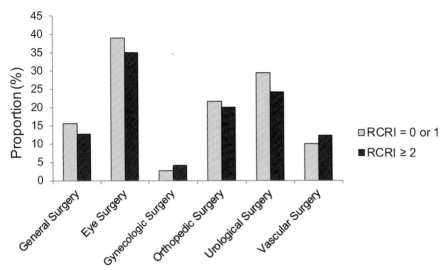

Fig. 5. Frequency of preoperative medical consultation by surgical specialty and cardiac risk. Patients having ophthalmic, orthopedic, or urologic surgery were more likely to have consultations compared with those having general surgery. Patients with Revised Cardiac Risk Index scores of 0 or 1 were more likely to be referred for preoperative medical consultations than patients with higher Revised Cardiac Risk Index scores. RCRI, Revised Cardiac Risk Index.

are also patients who undergo procedures with suboptimally controlled medical conditions. Thus, there is a need for improved ways of identifying patients who are the most likely to benefit from a preoperative medical consultation.

THE COST OF PREOPERATIVE MEDICAL CONSULTATIONS

For low-risk patients undergoing low risk and intermediate-risk procedures, the cost of consultations may exceed the cost of preoperative testing. Two recent studies indicate that the cost of preoperative consultations for Medicare patients undergoing cataract surgery is higher than the cost for preoperative testing. Thilen and colleagues[19] used 2006 Medicare data to estimate the relative cost of common preoperative interventions, including common tests (ie, chest radiographs, electrocardiograms, common laboratory tests) and preoperative medical consultations provided by family practitioners, internists, pulmonologists, cardiologists, or endocrinologists, that occurred within 42 days preoperatively. Consultations also included office visits provided by the same specialties that far exceeded the usual rate of such visits. The study sample included only low-risk patients with Revised Cardiac Risk Index scores of 0 or 1. The partition of the average preoperative evaluation cost per Medicare patient undergoing cataract surgery in this study is shown in **Fig. 6**.

Chen and colleagues[20] reported consistent findings in a study that used 2011 Medicare data and focused on patients with cataracts.

Preoperative medical consultations have been found to be associated with increased preoperative testing.[21] This relationship also held true in a subgroup analysis of patients undergoing knee arthroscopy as well as in Medicare patients undergoing cataract surgery. Both of these procedures carry low risk and are usually performed in the ambulatory setting.[20,22]

Cataract $58.19

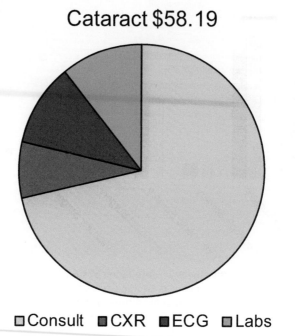

☐Consult ■CXR ■ECG ☐Labs

Fig. 6. The breakdown of average cost spent for the preoperative evaluation of patients with Revised Cardiac Risk Index of 0 or 1 undergoing a first cataract operation, based on analysis of 2006 Medicare data. The average total cost of preoperative medical consultation and common preoperative testing is $58.19 per patient. For consultations (Consult), chest radiographs (CXR), electrocardiograms (ECG), and laboratory studies (Labs), the costs were $41.54, $4.20, $6.16, and $6.29, respectively. The chart shows the relative costs for consultations versus testing.

It has been suggested that financial pressures and changes in reimbursement systems, such as bundled payments for entire surgical episodes, may lead to reorganization of preoperative evaluations by surgeons and anesthesiologists.[18] A previous study was conducted in light of anticipated reimbursement changes to analyze the cost/benefit ratio of routine preoperative and postoperative medical evaluation of surgical patients at a large teaching hospital.[3] The investigators concluded that preoperative medical consultations for low-risk patients were of limited benefit and estimated that the annual cost of routine preoperative medical consultations would be $1 billion. These data, combined with the changes in financial incentives, may lead to increased performance of routine patient screenings via chart review and, if the patient's condition seems stable, the obtaining of a simple history and medication list from the primary care provider.

COORDINATION OF PERIOPERATIVE CARE

The US health care system is fragmented and economically costly. An estimated 20% to 34% of health care dollars are spent on ineffective measures, so identification and reduction of these costs are now of particular interest.[23–25] Perioperative care is no exception from the pattern of fragmented care. An element of poor coordination is inherent in the preoperative consultation process because, although there are at least 3 key providers involved in the preoperative care of patients with consultations, by definition only 2 are immediately involved in the consultation process; namely the referring physician and the consultant. The partially overlapping roles of the physicians in the preoperative team are illustrated in **Fig. 7**.

Although the anesthesiologist is arguably the primary user of the information derived from the consult,[26] the consultation report is naturally prepared for the requester of the consultation, who is usually the referring surgeon. As discussed earlier, it has been reported that surgeons and anesthesiologists have substantially disparate perceptions of preoperative consultations. Specialists in cardiology, internal medicine, and family medicine, who provide most preoperative medical consultations, usually have limited direct exposure to anesthesiology during their training, and may have limited awareness of the training, competencies, and role of anesthesiologists. Perhaps this explains why in many published studies on preoperative medical consultations, anesthesiologists are not discussed as having a role in perioperative care and the words anesthesia, anesthesiologist, or anesthesiology do not appear.[3,7,8,27–33] Many studies on cohorts of patients who received consultations also report that it was not possible to determine the reason for a referral, presumably because it was made verbally and the reason was not explicitly noted in the consultation report. It is likely that the dissemination of the consultation report to all members of the perioperative care team has improved with the increased use of electronic medical records (EMRs); however, it is also clear that this problem is not completely resolved. It is often the case that consultants who are external to an ambulatory surgery center or hospital submit reports directly to the surgeon and they are not always entered into the surgical facility's EMR in a timely manner.

MEDICOLEGAL ASPECTS

It is unclear to what extent medicolegal considerations influence the decision to refer for preoperative medical consultation. In a survey of Canadian surgeons,

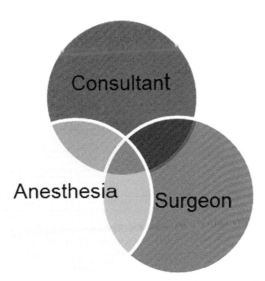

Fig. 7. The preoperative team. Preoperative management is an area of medical care that encompasses surgeons, preoperative medical consultants, and anesthesiologists. There is overlap in the roles of these providers. The Venn diagram shows the unique role of the consultant as represented by the red area that lies outside the yellow and blue circles.

69% disagreed that consultations are requested for medicolegal reasons.[5] It is not clear that referral for preoperative medical consultations decreases medicolegal risk. Poorly written consults may be a substantial liability, and it is preferred that the consultant never gives absolute instructions. The surgeon and/or anesthesiologist may have good reasons to not follow a consultant's recommendations. Recommendations regarding anesthetic choice and technique and intraoperative management, including types of monitoring, are inappropriate and unnecessary because these areas are within the core area of expertise of anesthesiologists. Such recommendations could theoretically increase liability because of how they can be presented to a jury by a malpractice attorney. In addition, it has been pointed out that routine test results that are not recognized preoperatively only increase liability, and the same applies to consultation reports. Therefore, it is critical that the full consultation report be made available in a timely manner to the entire perioperative team, including both surgeon and anesthesiologist. As an example, a consultation report containing important information on myocardial ischemia, such as the heart rate threshold from a stress test or which electrocardiogram leads showed ischemic changes, can become a liability if not made available to the anesthesiologist.

Current guidelines on cardiovascular evaluation before noncardiac surgery do not recommend routine preoperative cardiology consultation for patients with established coronary artery disease, or routine consultation for patients with risk factors for coronary artery disease. Specifically, current guidelines do not recommend testing for patients with established and stable coronary artery disease unless the results could change perioperative management.[34] It is understood that these patients are at increased risk for perioperative myocardial infarction and other major adverse cardiac events compared with patients without coronary artery disease or risk factors, but this risk is not reduced by additional testing or preoperative revascularization.[35] Appropriate adherence to current guidelines and a thoughtful explanation of the current recommendations to the patient and family members are likely to offer better medicolegal protection than referral for additional testing that is not indicated.

Further research, using qualitative methods, is needed to better determine the role of medicolegal concerns as a factor motivating referral.

OUTCOMES AND PREOPERATIVE MEDICAL CONSULTATIONS

Most published studies on preoperative consultation have not included outcomes such as length of stay, surgical site infection, urinary tract infection, sepsis, wound dehiscence, acute renal failure, deep vein thrombosis, major adverse cardiac events (eg, myocardial infarction, cardiac arrest), in-hospital stroke, mortality, and patient satisfaction. Several studies have reported ostensibly less significant outcomes, such as the reason for the request, which recommendations were made, quality of the consultation, compliance with recommendations, and effect on care processes.[3,5,7,29–31,33,36] These studies were small (60–530 patients) single-center studies and did not use comparison groups. They often reported finding 10% to 15% new or undertreated conditions in consulted patients, and 10% to 25% of those had a change in management.[13]

There are no published randomized controlled trials that compare perioperative outcomes of patients who underwent preoperative medical consultation with the outcomes of patients who did not. Nonetheless, there are 4 nonrandomized comparative studies. All are retrospective cohort studies, with 3 of them using historical controls.

Wijeysundera and colleagues[21] used population-based administrative databases and included all patients who underwent major surgery in Ontario, Canada, over a period of 10 years. Propensity score methods were used to assemble a 1:1 matched cohort. The primary end point was 30-day mortality. Despite the adjustment, preoperative medical consultation was associated with significant, albeit small, increases in mortality. The increased mortality may be explained by initiation of β-blocker therapy, which was significantly more common among patients who had undergone consultation. This practice may have inadvertently led to increased mortality and stroke. Hospital length of stay was also increased for patients with consultations. Although their administrative data did not include data on severity of illness or on obesity and smoking, a sensitivity analysis that included the number of recent acute care hospitalization in the propensity score did not change the main findings.

Faggiano and colleagues[37] conducted a retrospective review of the medical records for 622 consecutive patients who underwent open repair of abdominal aortic aneurysms. They compared the patients in a historical cohort undergoing surgery in the years 2000 to 2002 with those in a recent cohort undergoing surgery between 2003 and 2008. Patients in the recent cohort had preoperative cardiology consultations if they had any risk factor for cardiac disease, which can be assumed to have applied to most of the patients. The primary outcome was in-hospital mortality. The number of major cardiac perioperative complications decreased over time, and the in-hospital mortality was 0.9% in the recent cohort, compared with 3.4% in the historic cohort. Also, the long-term mortality was significantly reduced in patients operated on in the recent compared with the historical cohort. An important limitation of this study, which is related to the use of historical controls, is that the recent cohort had a higher proportion of patients who presented on guideline-consistent pharmacologic therapy including β-blockers, statins, and antiplatelet drugs.

Vazirani and colleagues[38] conducted a single-center study evaluating the effect of a change in directorship of the preoperative clinic at a Veterans' Affairs (VA) Medical Center. After the change, hospitalists were available to direct all evaluations, including ordering of cardiac studies. When the preoperative clinic changed from being run by anesthesiologists to being run by hospitalists, length of postoperative stay decreased. In-hospital mortality, which was a secondary outcome, also improved. Similar to the previous report, this study has the limitations inherent in the use of historical controls. Certain preoperative evaluation processes that were not related to the direct involvement of hospitalists were also changed between the two periods; for example, poorly controlled diabetics (hemoglobin A1C level >9%) were referred to primary care before they were accepted to the preoperative clinic.

Ohrlander and colleagues[39] conducted a retrospective analysis of 2 historical cohorts, both of which included consecutive patients undergoing elective endovascular aneurysm repair for infrarenal abdominal aortic aneurysm. Unlike the historical cohort (years 1998–2006), the recent cohort (years 2007–2011) was seen in preoperative consultation by an internal medicine physician with a subspecialty focus on vascular diseases. Again, the recent cohort had a higher proportion of patients who presented on guideline-consistent pharmacologic therapy, which is an important potential confounding factor. The 30-day mortality was not different between the two compared groups.

An important study was conducted by Auerbach and colleagues[40] on perioperative medical consultations, which were defined as any consultation within 1 day before or after surgery. In this single-center cohort study of 1282 patients undergoing inpatient surgery, 117 received perioperative medical consultation. Consulted patients were of a similar age, sex, and race, but more frequently had an American Society of Anesthesiologists score of 4 or higher, diabetes, vascular disease, and chronic renal failure. Processes of care were not improved in consulted patients, even after adjusting for differences in severity of illness. Patients receiving consultations were no more likely to have a serum glucose level of less than 200 mg/dL, receive perioperative β-blockers (which were widely recommended at the time of this study), or receive venous thromboembolism prophylaxis. Despite no improvement in these measures, consultations were associated with increased hospital stay and costs. An important difference between these and previous historical data is in the restriction of the definition of consultation to a narrow perioperative window, with likely limited opportunity for preoperative and perioperative care optimization.

It is evident that meaningful data on outcomes associated with preoperative medical consultations are very limited. Given how consultations are requested and provided, it is not surprising that they have not been found to have a positive effect on outcomes. In the large cohort study by Wijeysundera and colleagues[21], the investigators pointed out that their findings "should not be interpreted as a justification for abandoning preoperative consultation but rather as a stimulus to examine it more closely and conduct more high-quality research to establish which aspects of perioperative care do more good than harm." Nevertheless, the lack of data has hampered development of a comprehensive guideline for indications and appropriateness criteria for preoperative medical consultations.

RECOMMENDATIONS

The American College of Surgeons has no guideline or statement on preoperative medical consultations and neither does any other national professional society of which these authors are aware. Even the American Society of Anesthesiologists has advised only these nonspecific criteria for consultations: "Any evaluations, tests, and consultations required for a patient are done with the reasonable expectation that such activities will result in benefits that exceed the potential adverse effects. Potential benefits may include a change in the content or timing of anesthetic management or perioperative resource use that may improve the safety and effectiveness of anesthetic processes involved with perioperative care. Potential adverse effects may include interventions that result in injury, discomfort, inconvenience, delays, or costs that are not commensurate with the anticipated benefits."[41]

More research is needed to enable standardization of criteria determining which patients are referred for preoperative consultation. Despite a lack of data to guide a comprehensive guideline for indications for preoperative medical consultations, there are reasons to think that improvements can be made so that a greater value is achieved from the resources now devoted to preoperative medical consultations.

- Preoperative medical consultations should be ordered based on medical indications.
- Low-risk patients undergoing low-risk procedures are unlikely to benefit and should not be referred for preoperative medical consultation.
- In hospitals and ambulatory surgery centers with a preoperative assessment clinic (PAC), requests for preoperative medical consultations and associated testing or other interventions should be coordinated and made in conjunction with the assessment in the PAC. It is understood that the need for consultation depends on the capabilities offered by the PAC. For example, proficiency with electrocardiogram interpretation is likely to avoid many unnecessary

consultation requests and the PAC should be able to provide a common risk assessment, such as one based on the Revised Cardiac Risk Index. Referral based on the PAC assessment should improve coordination with the preoperative process and mitigate variation between different surgical specialties as well as between individual surgeons. This approach should also help to ensure that the consultation is obtained to address specific issues.

- Consult requests should be documented and clearly state the reason for the request (ie, what issues need to be addressed by the consultant). The term "clearance" should not be used.
- Consultants should be knowledgeable about, and committed to implement, current guidelines, such as the American College of Cardiology (ACC)/American Heart Association (AHA) guideline on perioperative cardiovascular evaluation and management of patients undergoing noncardiac surgery.
- Summary information regarding a patient's diagnoses and current medications and so forth should be obtainable from the patient's primary care provider without the inconvenience and expense of a formal consultation and office visit. Likewise, basic information regarding coronary stents and cardiovascular implantable electronic devices should be available from a cardiologist's office.
- Incentives under new payment models (eg bundled payments) should be carefully calibrated so that they do not amount to a disincentive to obtain needed consultations.

The many significant benefits of PACs have been outlined (See Edwards A, Slawski B: Preoperative Clinics, in the issue). The establishment of a PAC may be viewed as a first step in any effort to provide excellent preoperative care. Typically, patients have seen the surgeon before the PAC evaluation. All patients must have a preanesthesia assessment by an anesthesiologist (or a Certified Registered Nurse Anesthesiologist), and there is an advantage if this assessment can be performed in the PAC. In this manner, it is usually evident at the time of the PAC assessment whether the unique expertise of a medical consultant is needed in addition to the services provided by the surgeon and the anesthesiologist. Our recommendations, given earlier, are based on the assumption that a timely preanesthesia assessment is provided in the PAC. The American Society of Anesthesiologists Practice Advisory for Preanesthesia Evaluation states that an evaluation should be performed before the day of surgery for patients with high severity of disease as well as for patients undergoing procedures with high surgical invasiveness. Ideally, the PAC staff should include providers who are knowledgeable about current guidelines such as the ACC/AHA guideline on perioperative cardiovascular evaluation and management of patients undergoing noncardiac surgery.[34] If this is not the case, then referral for consultation is required more frequently; for example, patients with cardiac disease often need to be referred to a consultant who is knowledgeable about the current guideline. However, little is gained by referring to a cardiologist or other consultant who is not familiar with the guideline.

According to a report by Fischer,[42] there was a 73% decrease in preoperative consultations when an anesthesiologist-directed PAC was established in a teaching hospital. Notwithstanding the seminal report by Fischer,[42] it is not clear at this time whether a particular specialty is best prepared to assume the role of directing the several aspects of preoperative care, including ordering of preoperative medical consultations. It has been suggested that perioperative medicine, including preoperative care, is an important area for anesthesiology training and practice,[43] and the American

Society of Anesthesiologists has recently presented the vision of the perioperative surgical home. A survey published in 2002 reported that many academic anesthesiology departments seemed reluctant to allocate resources to residency training in preoperative evaluation.[44] Since that time, a modest requirement for training in this area has been added.

As noted earlier, outcomes improved when a hospitalist-managed medical preoperative clinic was established at a VA hospital. Internal medicine specialists, and especially hospitalists, have embraced this concept and shown a substantial commitment to this area of medicine. Hospitalists have seen an extraordinary increase of their workforce and have steadily increased their involvement with perioperative care. Internal medicine training requirements now include perioperative care, and many important contributions to the relevant literature have been made by hospitalists. The leading United States conferences on perioperative medicine, such as the Perioperative Medicine Summit and Overview of Perioperative Medicine, have been largely led by hospitalists. A recent study compared board certification requirements in anesthesiology, internal medicine, family medicine, and surgery, and found that internal medicine had the highest number of matches between board certification requirements and key elements of preoperative care.[45] Other studies have reported that anesthesiologists are well prepared to order preoperative tests and perform well on testing of knowledge in perioperative medicine. However, these studies did not compare all specialties and did not specifically investigate the question of referral for preoperative medical consultations.[46,47]

SUMMARY

In the changing landscape of health care resource use and increasing financial constraints, perioperative medicine is likely to undergo major changes. The role of preoperative consultation should evolve as a rational approach, based on the best science available, and emerge as a value-based service.

Preoperative medical consultation is an important intervention that currently is not ordered in a rational manner and there is evidence of unwarranted variation in its use. Consultations should be available within a well-organized and coordinated process of preoperative assessment. In our opinion, consultations are most likely to benefit patients undergoing the highest-risk surgical procedures and patients with high medical risk undergoing high-risk and intermediate-risk surgical procedures. Importantly, the patients who are most likely to benefit from preoperative medical consultations should be identified days to weeks before surgery to allow preoperative optimization to be adequately addressed. Patient referrals should include clearly articulated questions and adequate clinical information. The preoperative consult should be readily accessible to the anesthesia and surgical team involved in the procedure as well as to the providers involved in the postoperative care. It is likely that new payment methodologies, with changing financial incentives, will facilitate a more appropriate use of this important resource.

REFERENCES

1. Thilen SR, Treggiari MM, Weaver EM. Trends of preoperative consultations in the Medicare population 1995-2006. Abstract presented at the Annual Meeting of the American society of Anesthesiologists. Chicago, October 16, 2011.
2. Kleinman B, Czinn E, Shah K, et al. The value to the anesthesia-surgical care team of the preoperative cardiac consultation. J Cardiothorac Anesth 1989;3: 682-7.

3. Gluck R, Muñoz E, Wise L. Preoperative and postoperative medical evaluation of surgical patients. Am J Surg 1988;155:730–4.
4. Katz R, Barnhart J, Ho G, et al. A survey on the intended purposes and perceived utility of preoperative cardiology consultations. Anesth Analg 1998;87:830–6.
5. PausJenssen L, Ward H, Card S. An internist's role in perioperative medicine: a survey of surgeons' opinions. BMC Fam Pract 2008;9:4.
6. Levinson W. Preoperative evaluations by an internist–are they worthwhile? West J Med 1984;141:395–8.
7. Ferguson RP, Rubinstien E. Preoperative medical consultations in a community hospital. J Gen Intern Med 1987;2:89–92.
8. Clelland C, Worland RL, Jessup DE, et al. Preoperative medical evaluation in patients having joint replacement surgery: added benefits. South Med J 1996;89:958–61.
9. Phillips MB, Bendel RE, Crook JE, et al. Global health implications of preanesthesia medical examination for ophthalmic surgery. Anesthesiology 2013;118(5): 1038–45.
10. Schonberger RB, Burg MM, Holt N, et al. The relationship between preoperative and primary care blood pressure among veterans presenting from home for surgery: is there evidence for anesthesiologist-initiated blood pressure referral? Anesth Analg 2012;114:205–14.
11. Krogsboll LT, Jørgensen KJ, Grønhøj Larsen C, et al. General health checks in adults for reducing morbidity and mortality from disease: Cochrane systematic review and meta-analysis. BMJ 2012;345:e7191.
12. Thilen SR, Bryson CL, Reid RJ, et al. Patterns of preoperative consultation and surgical specialty in an integrated healthcare system. Anesthesiology 2013; 118(5):1028–37.
13. Thilen SR, Treggiari MM, Lange JM, et al. Preoperative consultations for Medicare patients undergoing cataract surgery. JAMA Intern Med 2014;174:380–8.
14. Wijeysundera D, Austin P, Hux J, et al. Development of an algorithm to identify preoperative medical consultations using administrative data. Med Care 2009; 47:1258–64.
15. Wijeysundera DN, Austin PC, Beattie WS, et al. Variation in the practice of preoperative medical consultation for major elective noncardiac surgery: a population-based study. Anesthesiology 2012;116:25–34.
16. Available at: www.acgme.org. Accessed July 30, 2015.
17. Devereaux PJ, Ghali WA, Gibson NE, et al. Physician estimates of perioperative cardiac risk in patients undergoing noncardiac surgery. Arch Intern Med 1999; 159:713–7.
18. Fleisher LA. Preoperative consultation before cataract surgery: are we choosing wisely or is this simply low-value care? JAMA Intern Med 2014;174:389–90.
19. Thilen SR, Treggiari MM, Weaver EM. The Cost of Preoperative Consultations and Testing in Low Risk Medicare Surgical Patients. Abstract presented at the 7th annual meeting of the Society for Perioperative Assessment and Quality Improvement. Miami Beach (FL), March 8, 2013.
20. Chen CL, Lin GA, Bardach NS, et al. Preoperative medical testing in Medicare patients undergoing cataract surgery. N Engl J Med 2015;372:1530–8.
21. Wijeysundera DN, Austin PC, Beattie WS, et al. Outcomes and processes of care related to preoperative medical consultation. Arch Intern Med 2010;170:1365–74.
22. Cornea AM, Thilen SR, Weaver EM, et al. Preoperative consultation and use of testing for orthopedic surgery patients covered under a commercial insurance plan. Abstract presented at the 9th Annual Perioperative Medicine Summit. Scottsdale, February 21, 2014.

23. Berwick DM, Hackbarth AD. Eliminating waste in US health care. JAMA 2012; 307:1513–6.
24. Kuehn BM. Movement to promote good stewardship of medical resources gains momentum. JAMA 2012;307(895):902–3.
25. Qaseem A, Alguire P, Dallas P, et al. Appropriate use of screening and diagnostic tests to foster high-value, cost-conscious care. Ann Intern Med 2012;156:147–9.
26. Lubarsky D, Candiotti K. Giving anesthesiologists what they want: how to write a useful preoperative consult. Cleve Clin J Med 2009;76(Suppl 4):S32–6.
27. Mackenzie TB, Popkin MK, Callies AL, et al. The effectiveness of cardiology consultation. Concordance with diagnostic and drug recommendations. Chest 1981;79:16–22.
28. Klein L, Levine D, Moore R, et al. The preoperative consultation. Response to internists' recommendations. Arch Intern Med 1983;143:743–4.
29. Pupa LE, Coventry JA, Hanley JF, et al. Factors affecting compliance for general medicine consultations to non-internists. Am J Med 1986;81:508–14.
30. Ballard WP, Gold JP, Charlson ME. Compliance with the recommendations of medical consultants. J Gen Intern Med 1986;1:220–4.
31. Golden WE, Lavender RC. Preoperative cardiac consultations in a teaching hospital. South Med J 1989;82:292–5.
32. Macpherson DS, Lofgren RP. Outpatient internal medicine preoperative evaluation: a randomized clinical trial. Med Care 1994;32:498–507.
33. Mollema R, Berger P, Girbes AR. The value of peri-operative consultation on a general surgical ward by the internist. Neth J Med 2000;56:7–11.
34. Fleisher LA, Fleischmann KE, Auerbach AD, et al, American College of Cardiology, American Heart Association. 2014 ACC/AHA guideline on perioperative cardiovascular evaluation and management of patients undergoing noncardiac surgery: a report of the American College of Cardiology/American Heart Association Task Force on practice guidelines. J Am Coll Cardiol 2014;64:e77–137.
35. McFalls EO, Ward HB, Moritz TE, et al. Coronary-artery revascularization before elective major vascular surgery. N Engl J Med 2004;351:2795–804.
36. Dudley JC, Brandenburg JA, Hartley LH, et al. Last-minute preoperative cardiology consultations: epidemiology and impact. Am Heart J 1996;131:245–9.
37. Faggiano P, Bonardelli S, De Feo S, et al. Preoperative cardiac evaluation and perioperative cardiac therapy in patients undergoing open surgery for abdominal aortic aneurysms: Effects on cardiovascular outcome. Annals of Vascular Surgery 2012;26:156–65.
38. Vazirani S, Lankarani-Fard A, Liang LJ, et al. Perioperative processes and outcomes after implementation of a hospitalist-run preoperative clinic. J Hosp Med 2012;7:697–701.
39. Ohrlander T, Nessvi S, Gottsater A, et al. Influence of preoperative medical assessment prior to elective endovascular aneurysm repair for abdominal aortic aneurysm. Int Angiol 2012;31:368–75.
40. Auerbach AD, Rasic MA, Sehgal N, et al. Opportunity missed: medical consultation, resource use, and quality of care of patients undergoing major surgery. Arch Intern Med 2007;167:2338–44.
41. Committee on Standards and Practice Parameters, Apfelbaum JL, Connis RT, et al. Practice advisory for preanesthesia evaluation: an updated report by the American Society of Anesthesiologists Task Force on Preanesthesia Evaluation. Anesthesiology 2012;116:522–38.
42. Fischer SP. Development and effectiveness of an anesthesia preoperative evaluation clinic in a teaching hospital. Anesthesiology 1996;85:196–206.

43. Grocott MP, Pearse RM. Perioperative medicine: the future of anaesthesia? Br J Anaesth 2012;108:723–6.
44. Tsen LC, Segal S, Pothier M, et al. Survey of residency training in preoperative evaluation. Anesthesiology 2000;93:1134–7.
45. Cline KM, Roopani R, Kash BA, et al. Residency board certification requirements and preoperative surgical home activities in the United States: comparing anesthesiology, family medicine, internal medicine, and surgery. Anesth Analg 2015; 120:1420–5.
46. Katz RI, Dexter F, Rosenfeld K, et al. Survey study of anesthesiologists' and surgeons' ordering of unnecessary preoperative laboratory tests. Anesth Analg 2011;112:207–12.
47. Adesanya A, Joshi G. Comparison of knowledge of perioperative care in primary care residents versus anesthesiology residents. Proc (Bayl Univ Med Cent) 2006; 19:216–20.

Perioperative Ethical Issues

Arvind Chandrakantan, MD, MBA*, Tracie Saunders, MD, MDiv

KEYWORDS

- Shared decision-making • Do Not Resuscitate • Medical ethics
- Affordable Care Act • Operating room

KEY POINTS

- Shared decision-making is an important emerging paradigm in clinical medicine.
- Physicians must respect the basic tenets of patient autonomy and present options to patients without regard to incentivization.
- Shared decision-making can be useful in the preoperative evaluation of higher-risk surgical candidates.
- Do-Not-Resuscitate (DNR) orders should be evaluated on a case-by-case basis. There should be no uniform suspension of orders for the Operating Room.
- Preoperative discussion about DNR should be initiated as early as possible.

SHARED DECISION-MAKING

Introduction

Shared decision-making (SDM) is an emerging paradigm in medical ethics. It involves the reconciliation of 2 views: (1) the physician as the medical expert, and (2) the patient, with their individual values and viewpoints about present and future medical therapies. Despite its increased acceptance, SDM is hardly new. Several ancient cultures accepted and practiced this, including India and Japan.[1,2] In the United States, SDM was introduced in 1998, in the Presidential Advisory on Consumer Quality in the Healthcare Industry. Although definitions have some variability, Charles and colleagues[3] suggested the key characteristics should include the following: (1) that at least 2 participants, the patient and physician, are involved; (2) that both parties share information; (3) that both parties take steps to build a consensus about preferred treatment; and (4) that an agreement is reached on treatment to implement.

There is some disagreement on this definition, that is, that there can be an agreement to disagree.[4] The same investigators, however, also note shrinking consultation

Neither author has any conflicts of interest/disclosures.
Department of Anesthesiology, Institutional Ethics Committee, Stony Brook University Medical Center, HSC Level 4, Room # 060, Stony Brook, NY 11794, USA
* Corresponding author.
E-mail address: Arvind.Chandrakantan@stonybrookmedicine.edu

Anesthesiology Clin 34 (2016) 35–42
http://dx.doi.org/10.1016/j.anclin.2015.10.004
1932-2275/16/$ – see front matter
anesthesiology.theclinics.com

times and external pressures may have led to a decrease in patient engagement in the SDM process. A recent Cochrane study attempted to elucidate the value of SDM in the clinical setting; however, it was found lacking in high-grade evidence.[5]

Ethical Issues

As noted previously, SDM attempts to reconcile 2 views that are sometimes diametrically opposed and sometimes aligned. Physicians (and all health care professionals by default) are under the obligation to provide treatment for the benefit of the patient, known as beneficence. They are also obligated to not provide treatment that may harm a patient or may cause the least possible harm out of all possible alternatives, known as nonmaleficence. Using these 2 synonymous ethical guiding principles, physicians use a rubric called "best judgment" or "best practice" in order to offer optimal therapy to the patient. Patients, however, may have very different perceptions of the offered treatment. This viewpoint is fashioned by a variety of factors, including social, linguistic, cultural, and religious practice.[6] The patient's right to their health care decision-making without undue influence or coercion from their provider is known as patient autonomy. The crux of medical ethics with regards to SDM is whether ambiguous or reduced patient engagement reduces patient autonomy.

The uncertainty of patient autonomy led the legal community to obtain informed consent. Although a detailed discussion of informed consent is beyond the scope of this article, most states use 1 of 3 standards: (1) the reasonable physician standard, (2) the reasonable patient standard, and (3) the subjective standard. The first 2 are more intuitive, that is, stating what a similar physician or patient would want to know under a similar set of circumstances. The subjective standard is more complex, because it requires the physician to tailor the consent to the individual patient.[7] Several authors have attempted to elucidate this standard, by creating risk and certainty axes.[8] The higher the risk and the higher the uncertainty, the more detailed the consent. The converse is also true: with lower risk and only one viable option, the consent process can be simpler.

One routinely overlooked phenomenon is not the patient value axis, but the physician incentive axis. There are egregious differences in procedure reimbursement all over the country, and there are abundant data to indicate that physician recommendation is at least partly aligned with this incentive.[9] Although there is no governing body that scrutinizes this issue purely outside of the ethical issues, the Centers for Medicare and Medicaid Services (CMS) recently released a list of physicians who receive the highest reimbursement. All data can be accessed by the public on their website.[7] CMS has hoped that with this transparency physicians can better align themselves to their patients' values without being tied to adverse incentivization.

Affordable Care Act

Section 3506 of the Affordable Care Act mandates that the Department of Health and Human Services establish an independent entity to formulate and implement standards for educational tools for "preference-sensitive" patient care needs. In essence, this mandates gubernatorial funding entities to assist and fund decision-making tools to help patients understand interventions with regard to cost and evidence base.[10] To date, this program has been appropriated and not funded. Regardless, it represents a greater shift toward a model of consumer-based pricing, which is probably the way of the future.[11]

Evidence for Shared Decision-Making Preoperatively

The evidence for SDM is robust in some areas and indeterminate in others. A systematic Cochrane Review in 2011 analyzed the effect of SDM in 31 studies. Decision aids clearly involved patient's involvement and improved knowledge and realistic perception of outcomes. They reduced the incidence of discretionary surgery, without any apparent adverse health care outcome.[12] Whether this improves adherence, especially in low socioeconomic and non-English-speaking groups is yet to be elucidated.

There are multiple studies demonstrating that there is value in SDM. For example, in orthopedic and adult cardiac surgery, where there are frail, elderly patients with multiple comorbidities making them higher-risk surgical candidates, there is a real perceived value in SDM.[13] With value-based purchasing, with an emphasis on cost-based outcomes, there is a greater need to engage patients in formulating a proper decision. Approximately 1% to 2% of diagnosis-related group (DRG) payments will be withheld and paid to hospitals based on outcomes.[14] Despite this, there is still a large variability in the published literature in this area, and standardized approaches are yet to be developed that can impact SDM on a large scale.[15] This large variability has been attributed to continuity of care, the expectations of the individual patient, as well as the oversimplification of the medical encounter process.[16] There is also a need to identify so-called vulnerable populations, which may have incomplete knowledge of the perioperative process due to linguistic, cultural, or other barriers.[17]

Barriers and Motivators

A systematic review from 2008 identified 38 studies in the literature identifying the various factors in SDM. The most frequent reported barriers included time constraints, lack of applicability due to patient characteristics, and clinical situation. The most positive facilitators of SDM included provider motivation, positive impact on the clinical process, and patient outcomes.[18]

Barriers to Shared Decision-Making

Time is the most frequently cited constraint to the SDM model. Multiple authors have aptly pointed out that SDM is a practice improvement. Therefore, appropriate utilization of SDM may paradoxically solve some of the time encounter issues by introducing a greater degree of responsibility to the patient.[10] Lack of applicability of SDM to the clinical scenario is slightly more complex and difficult to delineate; this demands more individualization of care to a given patient than the uniform application of a framework.[3,19] The chronic clinical situation lends itself better to SDM, because it demands greater participation and adherence from the patient. The multiplicity of treatment pathways allows for a greater health care provider-patient interaction.[20]

Motivators for Shared Decision-Making

Although provider education is probably the single most important determination of adoption of SDM, the area remains poorly studied. A recent *Cochrane Review* suggests that the economic benefits must outweigh the costs associated with training. However, it also suggests that some training is better than none, and that all stakeholders should be part of the training process.[5] Although the data are still emerging about the value of SDM in improving health care outcomes, there are studies demonstrating positive outcomes.[21] More studies with larger sample sizes are needed to demonstrate larger effect.

Summary

SDM is a valuable tool for helping to facilitate the provider-patient interaction. There is a greater push for using SDM in the current health care environment under the Affordable Care Act. Although more study is needed, there are data to support the utilization of SDM in the clinical setting with regard to patient satisfaction, clinical outcomes, and greater patient-provider interaction.

DO NOT RESUSCITATE IN THE OPERATING ROOM
Introduction

To the anesthesiologist, the phrase Do Not Resuscitate (DNR) is hard to grasp when preparing to anesthetize a patient. By definition, that is what anesthesiologists do. They resuscitate all the time: before, during, and after surgery. In fact, anesthesia without resuscitation could lead to death; this is what it means to "get a patient through surgery," the basic premise of perioperative medicine. At the same time, there is a growing population of patients with severe illnesses who may benefit from surgical procedures that require anesthesia, but they do not want cardiopulmonary resuscitation (CPR) done to them or they do not want to be intubated and on a ventilator for any length of time.

How Does One Reconcile These Two Perspectives?

Reportedly 15% of patients with DNR orders find themselves in the perioperative arena to undergo procedures that require anesthesia with the expectation of improving the patient's quality of life.[22] The presence of a DNR order for patients who undergo emergency surgery is an independent risk factor for poor surgical outcome and postoperative mortality.[23,24] Nevertheless, CPR is most successful in returning patients to their prior level of functioning when performed in the perioperative period compared with any other time.[25]

The patient has the right to refuse resuscitation, and the anesthesiologist has the right to refuse to provide anesthesia that they believe is unsafe and may cause harm, including the death of their patient. Both perspectives are allowed and honored. The difficulty comes in communicating these perspectives on a case-by-case basis.

This is the 21st century, and there are numerous ways of communicating. The face-to-face way is the best way to communicate end-of-life decisions between direct health care providers and patients and or their families and legal agents. The electronic medical record (EMR) is a great way to document these communications, but it is not a good way to make day-to-day clinical decisions. Making decisions based on reading the EMR in isolation of evaluating the current status of a specific person's clinical condition has the potential for dangerous medical errors and misunderstandings.

Humans are living longer and surviving better with chronic diseases, and the outlook is even brighter for the future. With this in mind, the culture in the medical community that avoids speaking about death until it is imminent is unacceptable.

- The decisions made at the end of life do not seem to get the same attention as those made at the beginning of life; this is fraught with error and delusion.
- DNR has no age limitation. It should be discussed for the entire age spectrum, from very young to very old, depending on the clinical diagnosis and prognosis.
- Discussion early in the course of disease is ideal.
- Resources and training aimed at improving clinician knowledge and skills in advance care discussions must be developed and implemented.
- Shifting paradigm focus to the concept of goals of care, such as pain management, preventing and treating nausea, vomiting, and diarrhea, living at home, and so on, is preferable.
- The anesthesiologist may have to introduce the idea of discussing advance directives during the preoperative evaluation for scheduled surgery in a patient with severe illness.[26]

Biomedical ethical principles and Do Not Resuscitate
Health care ethics is traditionally organized and discussed around the moral principles of autonomy, beneficence, nonmaleficence, and justice/fairness.

Autonomy A fundamental principle in biomedical ethics that undergirds the DNR order is autonomy. Respect for individual autonomy is paramount and must be maintained as much as possible in the perioperative period. Autonomy requires that patients be informed about their condition and the options available. Educating patients about the medical and surgical options for managing a clinical problem is complex. This situation is difficult for both the patient and the health care team. There is not enough time allotted to educate patients properly. Some patients may have no basic knowledge of surgery and anesthesia. Patients have different levels of medical knowledge, and acute or chronic illness may interfere with understanding. Patients' cultural, religious, and spiritual backgrounds need to be considered as well. Where does the surgeon find time to relay all of this information? Health care providers must be aware of their own biases when presenting information to their vulnerable patients.

Beneficence Beneficence is another ethical principle that helps guide the decision to offer medical treatment, including making the DNR order. Autonomy is always the primary ethical principle that guides medical decision-making, but beneficence is very important as well. Beneficence is centered on the idea of doing good; medical treatment must be of some benefit to the patient. It must be a realistic calculation and not an idealistic one. A surgeon must not offer a dying patient a procedure just because it can be done or because there is an indication when it has no chance of prolonging life or mitigating suffering. Too often dying patients undergo surgical procedures that offer no benefit.

Nonmaleficence It is one thing for a trauma patient to die in the operating room during life-saving efforts. It is quite another thing for a terminally ill patient to die in the operating room. Did the anesthesia hasten the patient's death? Did the anesthesiologist's care actually result in more pain and suffering for an already dying patient? Physicians must operate under the principle of Do No Harm. Not doing anything is better than causing a person pain and suffering.

Justice/fairness Unfortunately, health care resources in the world are limited, and choices are made every day about who benefits from which treatment, medication, procedure, physician, and hospital. It is also unfortunate that individual hospitals typically do not consider justice in the daily operations. "Decrease turnover time" is heard ad nauseam but never "increase justice."

> *Of all the forms of inequality, injustice in health is the most shocking and the most inhumane. In 1965, Martin Luther King Jr spoke these words in Montgomery, Alabama, at the end of the Selma to Montgomery march that had been attended by the black and white physicians of the Medical Committee for Human Rights.*[27]

All too often health outcomes can be determined by access to health care and associated costs, which in too many cases explains the worldwide health care disparities among people of color. Attention to the DNR order potentially saves money and reserves precious resources for more viable clinical scenarios, but who decides? Is it ethical for a physician to base clinical care decisions on ability to pay?

In 1990, the Patient Self-Determination Act was passed in response to variable patterns of DNR ordering and the disregard for ethical principles in end-of-life care.[28]

A more plain and forthright way to sort out the clinical data, patient characteristics, and values in a systematic manner is by means of 4 topics. The 4 topics are

1. Medical indications
2. Patient preferences
3. Quality of life
4. Contextual features

The perioperative 4 topics chart provides a framework for careful ethical analysis of every clinical case, including and especially perioperative cases.

Guidelines for perioperative physician-patient conversation:

1. Provide information, options, data, and prognosis in writing.
2. Make sure the patient has an advocate present when delivering important and pertinent information. Patients may not hear what is said, let alone understand it.
3. Allow enough time for the patient to digest the diagnosis.
4. Be prepared to provide a list of physicians that can provide a second opinion.
5. Health Care Proxy document must be on the chart before elective surgery.
6. Every effort must be made to identify health care advocate/agent in urgent and emergent situations.
7. There is no automatic suspension of DNR orders during the perioperative period.
8. Advance directives should be discussed at the preoperative evaluation and immediately preoperatively with the anesthesiology team for clarification because anesthesiology team members may not be comfortable providing anesthesia to patients with DNR orders.

It is never ethically permissible to automatically suspend DNR orders for surgery. Giving patients the option of having their DNR orders suspended for surgery preserves their right to make decisions consistent with their values and health care goals.

Who Is Responsible to Discuss and Clarify Do-Not-Resuscitate Orders During the Perioperative Period?

According to the American College of Surgeons' 2014 Statement on Advance Directives by Patients: "Do Not Resuscitate" in the Operating Room,

> It is generally expected that the surgeon will assume primary responsibility for advising patients regarding risks, benefits, and alternatives when discussing a potential operation. This policy focuses on patients who accept a surgeon's recommendation to have surgery and who already have in place an advance directive, specifically, a "Do Not Resuscitate" (DNR) order. The best approach for these patients is a policy of "required reconsideration" of the existing DNR orders. Required reconsideration means that the patient or designated surrogate and the physicians who will be responsible for the patient's care should, when possible, discuss the new intraoperative and perioperative risks associated with the surgical procedure, the patient's treatment goals, and an approach for potentially life-threatening problems consistent with the patient's values and preferences.[29]

How do you discuss DNR with the patient and family at the preoperative evaluation visit with the anesthesiologist?

1. Ask permission
2. Start with what they know
3. Speak in short sentences
4. Allow silence

5. Expect any emotion
6. Prepare for the next steps

(*Adapted from* Morrison WE. Telling him. Anesthesiology 2015;123:226–8.)

Summary

Perioperative patients have the right to make decisions regarding their surgical and anesthesia care, including the right to refuse treatment or to issue DNR orders as part of an Advance Directive. Health care providers must comply with the patient's wishes regarding care. If an anesthesiologist is uncomfortable providing anesthesia care to a patient with a DNR order on the chart, this must be discussed with the surgeon/patient and reconciled. Automatic suspension or continuation of a DNR order for a patient undergoing surgery cannot be justified. Perioperative team members should consult with the patient and, if necessary, with an ethics expert or committee to determine whether the DNR order is to be maintained or completely or partially suspended during the perioperative period.

REFERENCES

1. Sharma A. A guide to Hindu spirituality. Bloomington (IL): World Wisdom; 2006.
2. Asai A, Aizawa K. Death with dignity is impossible in contemporary Japan: considering patient peace of mind in end-of-life care. Eubios J Asian Int Bioeth 2012;22(2):49–53.
3. Charles C, Gafni A, Whelan T. Shared decision-making in the medical encounter: what does it mean? (or it takes at least two to tango). Soc Sci Med 1997;44(5):681–92.
4. Elwyn G, Edwards A, Kinnersley P. Shared decision-making in primary care: the neglected second half of the consultation. Br J Gen Pract 1999;49(443):477–82.
5. Legare F, Stacey D, Turcotte S, et al. Interventions for improving the adoption of shared decision making by healthcare professionals. Cochrane Database Syst Rev 2014;(9):CD006732.
6. Gravel K, Legare F, Graham ID. Barriers and facilitators to implementing shared decision-making in clinical practice: a systematic review of health professionals' perceptions. Implementation Sci 2006;1:16.
7. Available at: https://depts.washington.edu/bioethx/topics/consent.html.
8. Whitney SN, McGuire AL, McCullough LB. A typology of shared decision making, informed consent, and simple consent. Ann Intern Med 2004;140(1):54–9.
9. Sada MJ, French WJ, Carlisle DM, et al. Influence of payor on use of invasive cardiac procedures and patient outcome after myocardial infarction in the United States. J Am Coll Cardiol 1998;31(7):1474–80.
10. Fowler FJ, Levin CA, Sepucha KR. Informing and involving patients to improve the quality of medical decisions. Health Aff 2011;30(4):699–706.
11. Lee EO, Emanuel EJ. Shared decision making to improve care and reduce costs. N Engl J Med 2013;368(1):6–8.
12. Stacey D, Legare F, Col NF, et al. Decision aids for people facing health treatment or screening decisions. Cochrane Database Syst Rev 2014;(1):CD001431.
13. Gainer R, Buth K, Legare J, et al. The changing face of cardiac surgery: frailty, age, and adverse outcomes create a mandate for shared decision making. Can J Cardiol 2013;29(10).
14. Youm J, Chenok K, Belkora J, et al. The emerging case for shared decision making in orthopaedics. J Bone Joint Surg Am 2012;94A(20):1907–12.
15. Slover J, Shue J, Koenig K. Shared decision-making in orthopaedic surgery. Clin Orthop Relat Res 2012;470(4):1046–53.

16. Katz SJ, Hawley S. The value of sharing treatment decision making with patients expecting too much? JAMA 2013;310(15):1559–60.
17. Ankuda CK, Block SD, Cooper Z, et al. Measuring critical deficits in shared decision making before elective surgery. Patient Educ Couns 2014;94(3):328–33.
18. Legare F, Ratte S, Gravel K, et al. Barriers and facilitators to implementing shared decision-making in clinical practice: update of a systematic review of health professionals' perceptions. Patient Educ Couns 2008;73(3):526–35.
19. Col N, Bozzuto L, Kirkegaard P, et al. Interprofessional education about shared decision making for patients in primary care settings. J Interprof Care 2011;25(6):409–15.
20. Montori VM, Gafni A, Charles C. A shared treatment decision-making approach between patients with chronic conditions and their clinicians: the case of diabetes. Health Expect 2006;9(1):25–36.
21. Wilson SR, Strub P, Buist AS, et al. Shared treatment decision making improves adherence and outcomes in poorly controlled asthma. Am J Respir Crit Care Med 2010;181(6):566–77.
22. Lapuma J, Silverstein MD, Stocking CB, et al. Life-sustaining treatment. A prospective-study of patients with DNR orders in a teaching hospital. Arch Intern Med 1988;148(10):2193–8.
23. Kazaure H, Roman S, Sosa JA. High mortality in surgical patients with do-not-resuscitate orders analysis of 8256 patients. Arch Surg 2011;146(8):922–8.
24. Speicher PJ, Lagoo-Deenadayalan SA, Galanos AN, et al. Expectations and outcomes in geriatric patients with do-not-resuscitate orders undergoing emergency surgical management of bowel obstruction. JAMA Surg 2013;148(1):23–8.
25. Peatfield RC, Taylor D, Sillett RW, et al. Survival after cardiac arrest in hospital. Lancet 1977;1(8024):1223–5.
26. Sanderson A, Zurakowski D, Wolfe J. Clinician perspectives regarding the do-not-resuscitate order. JAMA Pediatr 2013;167(10):954–8.
27. Washington HA. 'Medical apartheid' (Harriet A. Washington). New York Times Book Review 2007;6.
28. Koch K. Patient self-determination act. J Fla Med Assoc 1992;79(4):240–3.
29. Available at: https://www.facs.org/about-acs/statements/19-advance-directives#.

Preoperative Laboratory Testing

Matthias Bock, MD, Priv-Doz[a,b], Gerhard Fritsch, MD, Priv-Doz[b,c],
David L. Hepner, MD, MPH[d],*

KEYWORDS

- Preoperative testing • Preprocedure testing • Choosing wisely • Electrocardiograms
- Pregnancy testing • Coagulation studies • Patient safety • Complication

KEY POINTS

- Preoperative testing should be based on the patient's history, review of medical records, physical examination, and type of procedure.
- It is important to avoid testing in healthy patients and in those having minimally invasive procedures. Furthermore, it is not necessary to repeat recent testing if there is no change in the patient's condition.
- Preoperative electrocardiograms (ECGs) should not be ordered in asymptomatic persons undergoing low-risk surgical procedures regardless of age. Preoperative ECGs can be considered in patients with coronary heart disease, significant arrhythmia, peripheral arterial disease, cerebrovascular disease, or other significant structural heart disease.
- In institutions that do not require preoperative pregnancy testing, obtaining an accurate menstrual history is essential, and testing should be ordered if there is any doubt. It is appropriate to consider pregnancy testing in any woman of childbearing age.
- Coagulation studies identify clotting factor deficiencies in vitro and are not predictive of clinical bleeding. Therefore, routine coagulation studies are not recommended.

Preoperative Assessment Testing Clinics coordinate preoperative surgical, anesthesia, nursing, and laboratory care.[1] The prior history, medical records, previous tests, and consultations are reviewed, and a medical history and physical examination are conducted. Laboratory testing and electrocardiogram (ECG) should only be ordered if necessary.

Decades ago, advances in technology with the introduction of a multiphasic battery of laboratory tests led to an increase in the number of tests ordered with the

[a] Department of Anesthesia and Intensive Care Medicine, Central Hospital, Via Lorenz Boehler 5, Bolzano 39100, Italy; [b] Department of Anesthesiology, Perioperative Medicine and Intensive Care, Paracelsus Medical University, Muellner Hauptrstrasse 48, Salzburg 5020, Austria; [c] Department of Anesthesiology and Intensive Care, UKH Lorenz Boehler, Donaueschingerstrasse 3, Vienna 1220, Austria; [d] Department of Anesthesiology, Perioperative, and Pain Medicine, Brigham and Women's Hospital, Harvard Medical School, 75 Francis Street, Boston, MA 02459, USA
* Corresponding author.
E-mail address: dhepner@partners.org

Anesthesiology Clin 34 (2016) 43–58
http://dx.doi.org/10.1016/j.anclin.2015.10.005 anesthesiology.theclinics.com
1932-2275/16/$ – see front matter © 2016 Elsevier Inc. All rights reserved.

assumption that early presymptomatic diagnosis will optimize care and reduce medical costs.[2] However, more testing is likely to lead to an increased number of abnormal results, leading to further unnecessary workup with an increase in medical costs and the possibility of increased morbidity from more medical interventions. Further workup is likely to lead to delays or cancellations of a surgical procedure that may be medically necessary and is likely to provoke anxiety and be very inconvenient for the patient. In addition, the medicolegal risk is greater if a test is ordered and not followed than if a test is not ordered based on the patient's history. Preoperative testing should be based on a targeted history and physical examination, on the patient's comorbidities, and on the type of surgery. It is important to avoid repetition of prior testing if there is no change in the patient's condition, and to avoid testing in healthy patients having minimally invasive procedures. Routine testing does not increase safety or the possibility of surgery cancellation, even in elderly patients with multiple comorbidities, for minimally invasive procedures such as cataract surgery.[3] Goal-oriented preoperative testing must first take into account the surgical procedure and a thorough history and physical examination (**Fig. 1**).

The American Board of Internal Medicine Foundation launched the Choosing Wisely campaign back in 2012 with a goal of advancing a national dialogue on avoiding unnecessary medical tests, treatments, and procedures.[4] The American Society of Anesthesiologists (ASA) is a partner in the Choosing Wisely Campaign and is encouraging ongoing dialogue between patients and anesthesiologists to eliminate unnecessary tests and procedures.[5] The final "Top-Five" list of common low-value activities to question in the field of anesthesiology includes baseline laboratory studies and diagnostic cardiac testing. Baseline laboratory studies, such as complete blood count, basic or complete metabolic panel, and coagulation studies, are not necessary in healthy patients without significant systemic disease, when blood loss is expected to be minimal.[6] Baseline diagnostic cardiac testing, such as transthoracic or transesophageal echocardiogram or cardiac stress test, is not necessary in asymptomatic stable patients with known cardiac disease undergoing low- or moderate-risk noncardiac surgery.[6] These tests were chosen based on how frequently they were ordered (very often), the impact on quality and cost of care (little benefit and expensive), and the evidence for its recommendation (weak).[6] Interestingly, other baseline studies, such as the ECG and chest radiography (CXR), were not included in this list. In addition, baseline pregnancy testing in premenopausal women of childbearing age did not make the list.

In a recent large Canadian retrospective cohort study of preoperative testing before low-risk procedures, Kirkham and colleagues[7] found that ECG was performed before nearly a third of procedures and a CXR before 10.8% of low-risk surgeries. There was a significant regional and institution level variation present, with as much as a 30-fold difference between institutions. Older age, procedure type, and preoperative medicine and anesthesia consultation were associated with routine ECG ordering. Cardiac comorbidities (eg, coronary artery disease, atrial fibrillation) were associated with preoperative ECG and CXR, but the effect sizes were smaller than those mentioned above. The investigators noticed a decrease in testing since 2010, which coincides with the elimination of reimbursement for routine preoperative CXR and ECG before cataract surgery.[7]

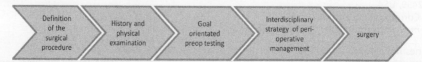

Fig. 1. Goal-orientated interdisciplinary process-flow of surgical patients.

In another population-based study, the same investigators evaluated preoperative blood work before low-risk surgeries.[8] They demonstrated that routine blood work was done before nearly a third of these surgeries. They demonstrated that comorbidities (eg, atrial fibrillation, venous thromboembolism, congestive heart failure, liver disease), cardiac risk factors (eg, diabetes, hypertension), age, and preoperative medical consultation were associated with routine blood testing. Furthermore, they also found that there was significant variation between institutions. It is important to note that preoperative medical consultation but not anesthesia consultation was associated with increased testing. Even more so than comorbidities, patient-independent factor, such as location of surgery, was one of the strongest predictors for preoperative laboratory testing.[8] Chen and colleagues[9] also recently demonstrated that preoperative laboratory testing before cataract surgery was more likely to be associated with provider practice patterns (eg, ophthalmologist, preoperative visit) rather than with patient characteristics. Fifty-three percent of patients underwent a preoperative test, despite evidence against routine preoperative testing[3,10] and guidelines that reflect this evidence.[11]

The information from these recent studies is very important, given that there has been an increase in medical consultations before cataract surgery over the past decade.[12] Cataract surgery is also the surgical procedure that has been associated with the highest probability of having patients being seen for a preoperative consult[13]; this is likely a result of the demographics of patients scheduled to have a cataract surgery being older and having more comorbidities than the average surgical patient.[10] However, given that complications following cataract surgery are extremely low and the lack of benefit of preoperative testing before cataract surgery, an evaluation by an anesthesiologist in a preoperative clinic is more likely to be cost-effective without an increased in perioperative risk. Numerous medical societies discourage testing in patients having low-risk surgical procedures, such as cataract surgeries, and have published guidelines or advisories stating so.[11] Unfortunately, a recent study demonstrated that over a 14-year period, during which many societies released statements against preoperative testing, there was no significant overall changes in the preoperative ordering of CXR, hematocrit, urine analysis, or cardiac stress testing.[14] This lack of significant overall changes may be partly explained by the temporal increase of preoperative visits during the same time period. There was a decrease in the ordering of preoperative ECGs during this time period. This decrease is likely a result of the recommendation from the American College of Cardiology/American Heart Association (ACC/AHA) to avoid ECG in all patients undergoing low-risk surgery.[15,16] The ACC/AHA perioperative guidelines are widely accepted and were first published in 1996.[17] The Centers for Medicare and Medicaid do not cover routine preoperative ECGs or those ordered based on age.[18]

TEST GRID STUDIES

Contrary to recommendations by the ASA[19] and by the European Society of Anaesthesiology,[20] many patients still undergo a priori defined test grids before surgery. A large randomized controlled trial (RCT) and a Cochrane meta-analysis demonstrated the lack of effectiveness of preoperative test grids for cataract surgery.[3,10] A recent outcome analysis after vitreoretinal surgery provides further evidence against preoperative test grids before ophthalmologic surgery.[21] Comorbidity and type of anesthesia, but not preoperative tests, determined the risk of postoperative adverse events.[21]

In a prospective European cohort analysis of patients undergoing noncardiac surgery, medical history and age, but not laboratory tests, had a predictive value for postoperative complications.[22] The omission of preoperative test grids did not affect postoperative outcome after ambulatory surgery in a Canadian RCT.[23] Furthermore, routine testing and abnormal results of unindicated tests were not associated with postoperative complications. Fairly good evidence exists that preoperative test grids do not affect outcome after low-risk surgery.[24] There are no data on the effectiveness of preoperative test grids before high-risk surgery.

ROLE OF AGE

Controversy exists whether age should be criteria for ordering preoperative laboratory workup. Dzankic and colleagues[25] demonstrated that although there is an increased incidence of abnormal creatinine, hemoglobin, and serum glucose in elderly patients, only the ASA classification and the type of surgical procedures were predictive of postoperative complications. However, age was a predictive factor for postoperative complications in another European analysis.[22]

ELECTROCARDIOGRAM

Screening ECGs are frequently ordered preoperatively, yet their prognostic value is unclear. Many institutions use an age-based guideline for deciding when to begin ECG screening. These age-based ECG guidelines evolved because of the increasing incidence of heart disease with age, such that by age 60, about 25% of patients will have ECGs that show abnormalities.[26] The prognostic value of this test is extremely limited, and there is no clear guidance from the literature on when this test should be ordered or for what period before surgery a particular ECG is valid. In addition, anesthesiologists may vary in decisions regarding which particular ECG abnormalities warrant further investigation in the preprocedure setting. Surgeons and anesthesiologists may be reluctant to proceed with even minor surgery in older patients without review of a baseline ECG despite the lack of prognostic evidence. Some think there is value in having a preoperative ECG to demonstrate a baseline should ECG abnormalities occur postoperatively. However, there is no study that validates the impact of having a baseline ECG on postoperative management. There is evidence that ECGs are unlikely to be useful prognostic indicators in lower-risk surgery.[27] This work suggests that routine preoperative ECG screening should not be done in these low-risk cases unless patients have specific established cardiovascular disease, and that ECG testing should be performed mainly in patients who undergo higher risk surgery.

The practice advisory issued by the ASA in March of 2012 summarizes current evidence and expert opinion on the value of preoperative testing. It notes that 100% of both consultants and ASA members surveyed thought that ECGs were indicated in selected but not all patients preoperatively.[19] The Task Force recognized that although age alone may not be an indication for an ECG, ECG abnormalities may be higher in older patients and in patients with multiple cardiac risk factors. Important factors to consider include presence of cardiac disease, respiratory disease, and invasiveness of surgery. Current studies regarding age as a factor in preoperative ECG ordering are difficult to interpret. It is challenging to look at the impact of age alone in the absence of all other related comorbidities, invasiveness of surgery, and outcomes. One observational study reported that the presence of ischemic episodes on the preoperative ECG was correlated with perioperative myocardial infarction (MI) for older patients undergoing coronary bypass surgery.[28] In summary, the Task Force did not reach consensus on a specific minimum age for ordering preoperative ECGs in patients without specific risk factors. An ECG may be indicated for patients with known cardiovascular risk factors or with risk factors identified in the course of preprocedure assessment.

The recommendations listed above relate to appropriate ordering of preoperative ECGs; there may be wide variation in whether the anesthesiologist decides to act on an abnormal result. There are many reasons that an ECG can be read as abnormal; part of the difficulty with preoperative ECG ordering is that many abnormalities do not require additional investigation or cardiology consultation before proceeding with surgery. The risk/benefit of further workup of any specific ECG abnormality needs to be carefully considered. The question that needs to be asked is whether there is a substantial probability that further workup of a specific ECG abnormality will result in a change in perioperative management. Understanding which abnormalities have a significant association with undiagnosed concerning cardiac issues is essential to decrease unnecessary further testing and consultation.

Correll and colleagues[29] attempted to determine whether it was possible to target ECG ordering to patient risk factors. The hypothesis was that perhaps a set of triggers could be identified to target patients with a significant likelihood of having ECG abnormalities that when viewed by consultant anesthesiologists and cardiologists would result in further evaluation. This set of triggers could then be used to reduce the number of preoperative ECGs ordered that have no impact on further management. A group of anesthesiologists and cardiologists with expertise in preoperative assessment defined a group of abnormalities on a preoperative ECG that would result in further assessment before the patient could proceed to surgery: major Q waves, major ST junction/segment depression, major T-wave changes, ST segment elevation, Mobitz type II or higher blockade, left bundle branch block, and atrial fibrillation. The consensus of the cardiologists and anesthesiologists involved in this study was that the presence of any of these abnormalities on an ECG would warrant further evaluation regardless of whether the patient was having surgery or not. This evaluation could range from simply obtaining a previous ECG for comparison, obtaining existing cardiac testing results, performing a new stress test, or obtaining a cardiology consultation. Patients in this study were analyzed to determine the impact of specific patient risk factors on the presence of significant abnormalities on a preoperative ECG. Patients at risk of having a significant ECG abnormality included those who were greater than 65 years of age, had a history of heart failure, high cholesterol, angina, MI, or severe valvular disease. Interestingly, age greater than 65 years alone, in the absence of other cardiac risk factors, was significantly associated with the presence of significant ECG abnormalities. Therefore, it may be reasonable to obtain an ECG in those older than 65 undergoing high-risk surgical procedures. Of note, this study was not powered to detect differences in postoperative outcomes, and only differences in preoperative management were analyzed.

The first set of Perioperative Guidelines on Cardiovascular Evaluation for Noncardiac Surgery was published in 1996[17] and claimed that intervention was almost never necessary just to lower the risk of surgery. It further stated that the goal was the reasonable use of testing in a cost containment era, and that the final clinical judgment be made by the health care provider and patient, based on the clinical history. The second set of guidelines was published in 2002,[30] the third set in 2007,[15] and the most recent iteration, in 2014.[16] The ACC/AHA 2014 guidelines on perioperative cardiovascular evaluation and care for noncardiac surgery discourage preoperative ECGs in asymptomatic persons undergoing low-risk surgical procedures regardless of age.[16] Even though ECG abnormalities are more common in older patients,[31] there is contradictory evidence on their predictive value for perioperative complications.[22,27] Therefore, a preoperative ECG ordered routinely in those older than 50 to 60 years does not seem to add any value in predicting postoperative complications beyond cardiac risk factors. The ACC/AHA 2014 perioperative guidelines state that preoperative resting 12-lead ECG is reasonable for patients with known coronary heart disease, significant arrhythmia, peripheral arterial disease, cerebrovascular disease, or other significant structural heart disease. Furthermore, they state that a preoperative resting 12-lead ECG may be considered for asymptomatic patients, except for low-risk surgery.[16]

HIGHLY SENSITIVE TROPONIN

Various clinical features and the effects of pain therapy obscure the diagnosis of myocardial ischemia and MI during the perioperative period. Both American and European authorities[16,32] recommend the revised cardiac risk index (RCRI) by Lee and colleagues[33] for preoperative cardiac risk stratification. Risk factors incorporated within the RCRI include coronary artery disease, congestive heart failure, cerebrovascular disease, insulin-dependent diabetes mellitus, risk associated with the surgical procedure, and preoperative serum creatinine level greater than 2 mg/dL. The question arises as to whether specific markers for myocardial damage might improve preoperative risk assessment and detect risk factors for negative cardiac outcomes such as silent myocardial ischemia.

Increases in serum cardiac troponin concentrations reflect cardiac injury and improve the prediction of cardiac outcomes by adding information to clinical scores.[34] Patients scheduled for major surgery had a significantly higher in-hospital mortality (6.9%) in the case of elevated preoperative highly sensitive troponin (hs-TnT; >14 ng/L) when compared with control (1.2%).[35] However, the clinical usefulness of troponin for preoperative risk stratification has been questioned because of the low specificity of the test.[34,36]

A recent prospective observational trial of 455 patients scheduled for open vascular surgery demonstrated that 38.0% of the cohort had a preoperative hs-TnT greater than the 99th percentile for a healthy population (14 ng/L) in the absence of clinical signs for cardiac conditions.[37] Preoperative hs-TnT levels 17.8 ng/L or greater and an absolute perioperative hs-TnT change 6.3 ng/L or greater 24 hours after surgery were associated with the occurrence of postoperative major cardiac events in this investigation. A combination of the RCRI and preoperative hs-TnT or the absolute change in hs-TnT increased the predictive value of the clinical score. Elevated preoperative and postoperative hs-TnT levels were also common among patients undergoing abdominal surgery.[38] However, under these circumstances, the peak hs-TnT concentration was not associated with a composite outcome of 30-day major cardiac events or 180-day mortality.

Both the ACC/AHA and the European Society of Cardiology/European Society of Anaesthesiology do not recommend routine preoperative testing for cardiac troponins.[16,32] According to the European societies, physicians may consider the use of preoperative cardiac biomarkers in high-risk patients, such as patients suffering from severe coronary artery disease.[32] The ACC/AHA recommends the measurement of troponin in the case of signs or symptoms suggestive of myocardial ischemia or MI.[16]

NATRIURETIC PEPTIDES

Ventricular wall stress triggers the secretion of B-type natriuretic peptide (BNP), which induces vasodilation, natriuresis, and diuresis.[39] BNP is cleaved together with biologically inactive N-terminal proBNP (NT-proBNP) from a common precursor in a 1:1 ratio. Both peptides have to be analyzed and interpreted separately because they own different half-times. The increase of plasma concentrations of BNP and NT-proBNP is a nonspecific marker of myocardial damage and may occur at any stage of heart failure during myocardial ischemia, atrial fibrillation, pulmonary diseases, pulmonary embolism, or high-output states. Furthermore, these markers are also elevated during renal failure and in older patients.[39] Preoperative concentrations of BNP depend on patients' general condition and on the type of procedure with its associated cardiac morbidity, which also explains the high prevalence of elevated BNP and NT-proBNP concentrations in vascular surgery patients.[36] In addition, there is a lack of a clear-cut definition of a pathologic range of natriuretic peptide (NP) concentrations.[39] Januzzi and colleagues[40] proposed an NT-proBNP cutoff point of 300 pg/mL for ruling out heart failure as the cause of dyspnea in the emergency department. On the other hand, the diagnostic threshold of NT-proBNP for the risk stratification of a composite of nonfatal MI, acute heart failure, or death between index surgery and 3-year follow-up among patients undergoing non-cardiac emergency surgery was 725 pg/mL or greater.[41]

A recent review on the effectiveness of preoperative NPs for risk stratification suggests various thresholds of BNP for predicting the composite outcome of 30-day mortality and nonfatal MI, depending on the type of surgery.[36] Two meta-analyses studying patients scheduled for vascular surgery and for intermediate and major noncardiac surgery[42,43] found that analyzing NPs improved preoperative risk classification. The latter trial did not distinguish between the types of NPs, even though the methodology is very important for the determination of the prognostic value of cardiac biomarkers. Systematic reviews using study-specific diagnostic thresholds tend to overestimate the predictive power compared with systematic reviews, which identify a single diagnostic threshold for the entire cohort.[44] NP concentrations are dynamic values reflecting the magnitude of myocardial damage. Additional NP determination after the surgical procedure enhanced the prognostic value of a composite of cardiac outcome when compared with preoperative NP measurement alone.[43]

Preoperative BNP and NT-proBNP levels provide additional prognostic value for cardiac complications and mortality among high-risk vascular surgery patients. However, useful risk thresholds and cutoff points are still lacking. According to the European Society of Cardiology and the European Society of Anaesthesiology,[32] the use of preoperative BNP and NT-proBNP levels might be considered in high-risk patients undergoing major surgical procedures. The ACC/AHA state that measurement of NPs may be helpful in assessing patients with heart failure and in diagnosing heart failure during the postoperative period in patients at high risk for heart failure.[16]

RENAL FUNCTION TESTING

Physiologic functions of the kidneys are manifold. Besides water balance and elimination of waste, many other important systems, such as erythropoiesis, hormonal regulations, acid-base system, and cardiocirculatory functions, are included in the complex network of renal function. Diabetes, arteriosclerosis, chronic heart failure, and coronary heart disease are the major diseases commonly associated with impaired renal function influencing outcomes after surgery.

Laboratory assessment of serum markers for preoperative renal function is in widespread use. The most common parameters in use are serum creatinine, blood urea nitrogen, estimated glomerular filtration rate (eGFR), and calculated creatinine clearance.[24,45,46] Besides these well-known tests, new parameters, such as cystatin C and neutrophil gelatinase associated lipocalin (NGAL) are making their way into clinical use.[47] Plasma-cystatin C represents a functional damage biomarker and NGAL correlates with tubular damage. Existing data cannot yet define the exact role of these newer laboratory parameters.

Renal function tests are not only incorporated in various perioperative risk scores but also mentioned in numerous preoperative guidelines and practice advisories.[16,19,33,48,49] Renal function parameters have been shown to predict adverse outcome in various surgical settings when being pathologic. In a large epidemiologic study, Bishop and colleagues[49] demonstrated that elevated creatinine values were associated with unexpected perioperative death. Odds ratios for death range between 1.2 and 8.1 when comparing normal with pathologic test results.[50,51] This range is mainly determined by the severity of the surgical procedure. However, in patients undergoing low-risk procedures and ambulatory surgery, renal function parameters show no correlation to complications and thus cannot be recommended as a routine.[23,24] Serum creatinine, a waste product of metabolism, has several disadvantages in the prediction of renal function. Its level directly depends on muscle mass, gender, and age. Therefore, it seems to be reasonable to use parameters that eliminate these confounding factors. eGFR calculates renal function by eliminating the influence of body mass, gender, and age.[52,53] A reduction of eGFR (<60 mL/min/1.73 m^2) has been associated with a 3-fold increase in postoperative 30-day mortality after vascular and cardiac surgery.[54] This increase in mortality has even been accentuated at lower eGFRs. In patients undergoing major vascular or cardiac surgery, eGFR represents a reasonable test for detecting subclinical renal failure.[55]

PREOPERATIVE URINE ANALYSES

There is no evidence supporting routine urine analysis in asymptomatic patients without clinical suspicion. A recent study of orthopedic, cardiothoracic, and vascular patients at a Veterans Administration medical center demonstrated that a urine culture was obtained before 25% of procedures. Asymptomatic bacteriuria was detected in 11% of these patients. Although postoperative urinary tract infection was more frequent among patients with bacteriuria than those without, surgical site infection was similar in both groups. Furthermore, bacteriuria was rarely treated. When treated, it was associated with no benefit. The authors conclude that preoperative urinalysis and treatment of asymptomatic bacteriuria should be avoided in these patients.[56]

The ASA Task Force does not recommend routine preanesthesia urinalysis except for specific procedures including prosthesis implantation and urologic procedures, or in the presence of urinary tract symptoms.[19] Therefore, the decision to obtain a urinalysis should be made on a case-by-case basis based on patient and procedure risk factors.

PREOPERATIVE PREGNANCY TESTING

The detection of a pregnancy in a woman undergoing nonobstetric surgery will very likely alter management. The patient may decide to cancel the procedure; the surgeon may change the nature of the procedure, and the anesthesiologist may alter the anesthetic plan or cancel the procedure. Although the ASA Task Force thinks that the literature is inadequate to inform patients or physicians on whether anesthesia causes harmful effects in early pregnancy, it recommends that pregnancy testing be considered in female patients of childbearing age if the results would change the patient's management.[19]

Institutions vary in guidelines regarding preprocedure pregnancy testing. In all women of childbearing age in whom the history may be unreliable, routine pregnancy testing should be considered. In institutions that do not mandate preprocedure pregnancy testing, obtaining an accurate menstrual history is critical, and pregnancy testing should be offered where appropriate. The threshold should be low for ordering this test in pediatric patients who are menstruating, in women who are poor historians, in women actively trying to become pregnant, or in women with histories of irregular menses.

The sensitivity and specificity will depend on the type of testing used and the point during the menstrual cycle at which the test is obtained. The pregnancy test will be positive when the upper limits of the threshold for measurement of human chorionic gonadotropin (hCG) are exceeded. For serum pregnancy tests, this is usually in the range of 1 to 5 mIU/mL of hCG. A higher threshold is set for urine pregnancy tests; it is generally within the range of 20 to 50 mIU/mL. Therefore, if the test is obtained very early after implantation, a serum pregnancy test can be positive even though the urine pregnancy test is negative. There are ultrasensitive urine hCG assays that can detect hCG levels as low as 0.5 mIU/mL; these can potentially detect pregnancy on the day of implantation. The anesthesiologist should be familiar with the specific test used at his/her institution, because the standard urine tests used in clinical practice are generally not ultrasensitive. If the urine test is not ultrasensitive, it may not be reliably positive until a week or 2 after a missed period.[57]

TESTING FOR BLOOD GLUCOSE AND GLYCATED HEMOGLOBIN

There are no data from high-quality studies supporting routine testing for preoperative glucose parameters in healthy patients. Diabetes mellitus is an important risk factor for long-term outcomes after surgery. Postoperative in-hospital mortality was 3.5% in diabetic patients and 0.9% in a nondiabetic control group matched by surgical procedures.[58] The key question therefore is whether preoperative routine testing for blood glucose parameters predicts negative outcomes in selected patient populations.

Due to the lack of RCTs, there is only a low level of evidence for the impact of routine preoperative testing for blood glucose or glycated hemoglobin (HbA$_{1c}$) on the perioperative management of surgical patients and on postoperative outcome. Two systematic reviews summarize the effect of preoperative testing. The National Institute for Health and Clinical Excellence (NICE) review analyzed studies published between 1966 and 2002,[59] whereas a recent systematic review included trials published between 2001 and March 2013.[60] Neither of these systematic reviews recommends routine preoperative testing for blood glucose or HbA$_{1c}$ in otherwise healthy patients. Almost all the studies published did not distinguish between patients with already diagnosed diabetes mellitus and patients without preoperative diagnosis of diabetes.

Blood glucose tests should be performed if there is clinical suspicion of disturbances in glucose metabolism. There is a correlation between elevated blood glucose levels and abnormal postoperative values and worsening of postoperative outcomes.[61] Hence, in certain high-risk groups, such as patients undergoing vascular surgery, orthopedic surgery, and spine surgery, routine testing for blood glucose might be justified. Elevated preoperative blood glucose concentrations have been associated with increased risk of infectious complications among patients scheduled for spine surgery, knee or hip replacement, and orthopedic trauma surgery.[62–64] Vascular surgery patients with elevated blood glucose concentrations are at risk for myocardial ischemia and infarction, release of markers for myocardial damage, and cerebrovascular ischemic events.[65,66] Moreover, preoperative hyperglycemia is a risk factor for increased 30-day mortality in patients undergoing noncardiac, nonvascular surgery and for increased long-term mortality in vascular surgery patients.[65,67] Vascular surgery patients are particularly prone to preoperatively undiagnosed diabetes mellitus, because more than a third of these patients without history or signs of impaired glucose tolerance or diabetes presented with impaired glucose tolerance or newly diagnosed diabetes mellitus.[68] Preoperative glucose levels significantly predicted the risk of myocardial ischemia up to 2 days after surgery among this well-defined risk group.[68] Moreover, these patients presented with an increased incidence of cardiovascular events and a higher mortality even in a long-term follow-up.[69] Preoperative blood glucose concentration was a risk factor for 1-year mortality, but not for in-hospital complications after noncardiac surgery in a recent retrospective study.[70] Interestingly, hyperglycemic patients with undiagnosed diabetes had a higher rate of mortality at 1 year and a higher risk of composite negative outcomes than those with known diabetes.[70,71]

HbA$_{1c}$ reflects intermediate-term glucose control and plays an important role in the preparation of diabetic patients for elective surgery. Preoperative HbA$_{1c}$ greater than 53 mmol/mol was a predictor of postoperative hyperglycemia in patients with diabetes undergoing elective noncardiac surgery.[72] Neither the NICE review[59] nor its update[60] detected an impact of elevated levels of HbA$_{1c}$ on postoperative outcomes in unselected patients undergoing elective surgery. In patients scheduled for colorectal surgery, elevated levels of HbA$_{1c}$ predicted a prolonged recovery, increased postoperative blood glucose levels, and an increased risk of infectious complications.[73] Elevated preoperative values of HbA$_{1c}$ were further associated with an increased risk of infectious complications after joint replacement surgery,[62] and of cardiac complications after vascular surgery.[65] Even slightly elevated values for HbA$_{1c}$ (43–53 mmol/mol) were associated with increased cardiac morbidity after both elective and urgent vascular surgery in patients with undiagnosed prediabetes.[74] Elevated concentrations of HbA$_{1c}$ did not predict increased postoperative 30-day mortality in patients scheduled for cardiac and major surgery.[75] However, HbA$_{1c}$ is a risk factor for increased long-term mortality in vascular surgery patients.[76] Further research is required to clarify the impact of testing for HbA$_{1c}$ on postoperative mortality.

HEMATOCRIT

Routine hematocrit is not indicated. Rather, a targeted history and physical examination should determine whether a preoperative hematocrit should be done.[59] Highly invasive surgeries with the potential for significant blood loss may be an indication for a preoperative hematocrit.[60] The Anesthesia Task Force recommends that type and invasiveness of procedure, extremes of age, and history of liver disease, anemia, bleeding, and other hematologic disorders be considered in determining the need for a preprocedure hematocrit.[19]

COAGULATION STUDIES

A good preoperative bleeding history is the first step that needs to be taken before considering ordering coagulation studies, because unexpected coagulation defects are uncommon. A systematic review of the literature recommended avoiding routine coagulation screening before procedures to predict bleeding risk.[77] A good history looking for bleeding abnormalities is more important and includes a family history of coagulation issues, history of increased bleeding with previous surgical procedures, and use of anticoagulants. Clinical conditions that predispose patients to bleeding, such as liver and renal dysfunction, should also be noted. A study of neurosurgery patients compared an assessment of patient history with preoperative hemostasis screening and demonstrated that patient history had a higher sensitivity for the detection of bleeding.[78]

The partial thromboplastin time (PTT) and prothrombin time were developed to identify clotting factor deficiencies in vitro and are not predictive of clinical bleeding.[79] The results of these tests must be put in context of the patient's current status, past bleeding challenges, and family history. It is important to note that the presence of lupus anticoagulant will prolong the PTT results and is not predictive of increased bleeding.[77] Other investigators have demonstrated no relationship between an incidental elevation of coagulation studies and predictability of postoperative bleeding.[80]

GENETIC TESTING

Patients demonstrate a high interindividual and interracial variability in their response to various drugs, especially opioids. The detection of opioid plasma concentrations does not necessarily predict the level of analgesia,[81] due to the huge variability in the minimum effective plasma level of opioids.[82] There is increasing evidence that genetic variations also have a major impact on both the pharmacokinetics and the pharmodynamics of warfarin, nonsteroidal anti-inflammatory drugs, benzodiazepines, antiemetics, and proton pump inhibitors.[83]

There are numerous genetic variations of the cytochrome (CYP) 450 enzyme system, a microsomal drug metabolism superfamily involved in the biotransformation of most drugs like analgesics, antibiotics, antiarrhythmic agents, antiplatelet drugs, and psychiatric agents. The CYP enzymes CYP3A4 and CYP2D6 are highly prone to genetic variability,[83] leading to either hypermetabolism of prodrugs inducing toxic levels of analgesics or other agents, or reduced metabolism of already biologically effective drugs. Many physicians are still unaware of a US Food and Drug Administration–approved genetic test for CYP2D6 available since 2006.[84] This test should only be considered if the family or the patient's history gives clues to genetic variability of the CYP status. The test may only be reasonable for patients undergoing elective major surgery because it takes a week to perform.

SUMMARY

In conclusion, preoperative evaluation relies on information from multiple sources, including the medical record, history, and physical examination, and findings from medical tests, including ECG. Because risk assessment relies on a medical history and physical examination, it is important to be more selective in the ordering of tests and consults. A test is likely to be indicated if it can identify abnormalities and change the diagnosis and management plan, or the patient's outcome.

Additional factors to be considered include coexisting medical disease, clinical risk factors, the type and invasiveness of the surgery, and the patient's functional capacity. Additional tests, evaluations, and consultations should only be done if the information to be obtained will result in changes in the perioperative management of the patient.

Routine testing must be avoided, because unexpected results will probably not be clinically significant for the surgery and will only lead to more needless testing, unnecessary anxiety for the patient, and delays in proceeding to the operating room. Excessive testing is expensive, and it may delay the operation and place the patient at risk for unnecessary interventions.

REFERENCES

1. Correll DJ, Bader AM, Hull MW, et al. The value of preoperative clinic visits in identifying issues with potential impact on operating room efficiency. Anesthesiology 2006;105(6):1254–9.
2. Roizen MF. More preoperative assessment by physicians and less by laboratory tests (editorial). N Engl J Med 2000;342:204–5.
3. Schein OD, Katz J, Bass EB, et al. The value of routine preoperative medical testing before cataract surgery. N Engl J Med 2000;342:168–75.
4. Cassel CK, Guest JA. Choosing wisely: helping physicians and patients make smart decisions about their care. JAMA 2012;307:1801–2.
5. Available at: http://www.choosingwisely.org/societies/american-society-of-anesthesiologists. Accessed November 6, 2015.
6. Onuoha OC, Arkoosh VA, Fleisher LA. Choosing wisely in anesthesiology: the gap between evidence and practice. JAMA Intern Med 2014;174:1391–5.
7. Kirkham KR, Wijeysundera DN, Pendrith C, et al. Preoperative testing before low-risk surgical procedures. CMAJ 2015;187(11):E349–58.
8. Kirkham KR, Wijeysundera DN, Pendrith C, et al. Preoperative laboratory investigations: rates and variability prior to low-risk surgical procedures. Anesthesiology, in press.
9. Chen CL, Lin GA, Bardach NS, et al. Preoperative medical testing in Medicare patients undergoing cataract surgery. N Engl J Med 2015;372:1530–8.
10. Keay L, Lindsley K, Tielsch J, et al. Routine preoperative medical testing for cataract surgery. Cochrane Database Syst Rev 2012;3:CD007293.
11. American Academy of Ophthalmology. Routine pre-operative laboratory testing for patients scheduled for cataract surgery: clinical statement. 2014. Available at: http://www.aao.org/clinical-statement/routine-preoperative-laboratory-testing-patients-s. Accessed November 6, 2015.
12. Thilen SR, Treggiari MM, Lange JM, et al. Preoperative consultations for Medicare patients undergoing cataract surgery. JAMA Intern Med 2014;174:380–8.
13. Thilen SR, Bryson CL, Reid RJ, et al. Patterns of preoperative consultation and surgical specialty in an integrated healthcare system. Anesthesiology 2013;118:1028–37.
14. Sigmund AE, Stevens ER, Blitz JD, et al. Use of preoperative testing and physicians' response to professional society guidance. JAMA Intern Med 2015;175:1352–9.
15. Fleisher LA, Beckman JA, Brown KA, et al. ACC/AHA 2007 Guidelines on perioperative cardiovascular evaluation and care for noncardiac surgery: executive summary: a report of the American College of Cardiology/American Heart Association Task Force on Practice Guidelines (Writing Committee to Revise the 2002 Guidelines on Perioperative Cardiovascular Evaluation for Noncardiac Surgery). Circulation 2007;116:1971–96.
16. Fleisher LA, Fleischmann KE, Auerbach AD, et al. 2014 ACC/AHA guideline on perioperative cardiovascular evaluation and management of patients undergoing noncardiac surgery: executive summary: a report of the American College of

Cardiology/American Heart Association Task Force on Practice Guidelines. J Am Coll Cardiol 2014;64:2373–405.

17. Eagle KA, Brundage BH, Chaitman BR, et al. Guidelines for perioperative cardiovascular evaluation for noncardiac surgery: report of the American College of Cardiology/American Heart Association Task Force on Practice Guidelines (Committee on Perioperative Cardiovascular Evaluation for Noncardiac Surgery). Circulation 1996;93:1278–317.

18. Hepner DL. The role of testing in the preoperative evaluation. Cleve Clin J Med 2009;76(Suppl 4):S22–7.

19. Pasternak LR, Arens JF, Caplan RA, et al. Practice advisory for preanesthesia evaluation. An updated report by the American Society of Anesthesiologists Task Force on Preanesthesia Evaluation. Anesthesiology 2012;116:522–38.

20. De Hert S, Imberger G, Carlisle J, et al, Task Force on Preoperative Evaluation of the Adult Noncardiac Surgery Patient of the European Society of Anaesthesiology. Preoperative evaluation of the adult patient undergoing non-cardiac surgery: guidelines from the European Society of Anaesthesiology. Eur J Anaesthesiol 2011;28:684–722.

21. Shalwala A, Hwang RY, Tabing A, et al. The value of preoperative medical testing for vitreoretinal surgery. Retina 2015;35:319–25.

22. Fritsch G, Flamm M, Hepner DL, et al. Abnormal pre-operative tests, pathologic findings of medical history, and their predictive value for perioperative complications. Acta Anaesthesiol Scand 2012;56:339–50.

23. Chung F, Yuan H, Yin L, et al. Elimination of preoperative testing in ambulatory surgery. Anesth Analg 2009;108:467–75.

24. Johansson T, Fritsch G, Flamm M, et al. Effectiveness of non-cardiac preoperative testing in non-cardiac elective surgery: a systematic review. Br J Anaesth 2013;110:926–39.

25. Dzankic S, Pastor D, Gonzalez C, et al. The prevalence and predictive value of abnormal laboratory tests in elderly surgical patients. Anesth Analg 2001;93:301–8.

26. Goldberger AL, O'Konski M. Utility of the routine electrocardiogram before surgery and on general hospital admission. Ann Intern Med 1986;105:552–7.

27. Noordzij PG, Boersma E, Bax JJ, et al. Prognostic value of routine preoperative electrocardiography in patients undergoing noncardiac surgery. Am J Cardiol 2006;97:1103–6.

28. Knight AA, Hollenberg M, London MJ, et al. Perioperative myocardial ischemia: importance of the preoperative ischemic pattern. Anesthesiology 1988;68:681–8.

29. Correll DJ, Hepner DL, Chang C, et al. Preoperative electrocardiograms: patient factors predictive of abnormalities. Anesthesiology 2009;110:1217–22.

30. Eagle KA, Berger PB, Calkins H, et al. ACC/AHA guideline update for perioperative cardiovascular evaluation for noncardiac surgery: executive summary: a report of the American College of Cardiology/American Heart Association Task Force on Practice Guidelines (Committee to Update the 1996 Guidelines on Perioperative Cardiovascular Evaluation for Noncardiac Surgery). J Am Coll Cardiol 2002;39:542–53.

31. Liu LL, Dzankic S, Leung JM. Preoperative electrocardiogram abnormalities do not predict postoperative cardiac complications in geriatric surgical patients. J Am Geriatr Soc 2002;50:1186–91.

32. Kristensen SD, Knuuti J, Saraste A, et al. The Joint Task Force on non-cardiac surgery: cardiovascular assessment and management of the European Society of Cardiology (ESC) and the European Society of Anaesthesiology (ESA). 2014

ESC/ESA Guidelines on non-cardiac surgery: cardiovascular assessment and management. Eur Heart J 2014;35:2383–431.

33. Lee TH, Marcantonio ER, Mangione CM, et al. Derivation and prospective validation of a simple index for prediction of cardiac risk of major noncardiac surgery. Circulation 1999;100:1043–9.

34. Biccard BM, Naidoo P, de Vasconcellos K. What is the best pre-operative risk stratification tool for major adverse cardiac events following elective vascular surgery? A prospective observational cohort study evaluating pre-operative myocardial ischaemia monitoring and biomarker analysis. Anaesthesia 2012; 67:389–95.

35. Weber M, Luchner A, Seeberger M, et al. Incremental value of high-sensitive troponin T in addition to the revised cardiac index for peri-operative risk stratification in non-cardiac surgery. Eur Heart J 2013;34:853–62.

36. Biccard BM, Devereaux PJ, Rodseth RN. Cardiac biomarkers in the prediction of risk in the non-cardiac surgery setting. Anaesthesia 2014;69:484–93.

37. Gillmann H-J, Meinders A, Groshennig A, et al. Perioperative levels and changes of high-sensitivity troponin T are associated with cardiovascular events in vascular surgery patients. Crit Care Med 2014;42:1498–506.

38. Gillies MA, Shah ASV, Mullenheim J, et al. Perioperative myocardial injury in patients receiving cardiac output-guided haemodynamic therapy: a substudy of the OPTIMISE Trial. Br J Anaesth 2015;115:227–33.

39. Daniels LB, Maisel AS. Natriuretic peptides. J Am Coll Cardiol 2007;50:2357–68.

40. Januzzi JL Jr, Camargo CA, Anwaruddin S, et al. The N-terminal Pro-BNP investigation of dyspnea in the emergency department (PRIDE) study. Am J Cardiol 2005;95:948–54.

41. Farzi S, Stojakovic T, Marko TH, et al. Role of N-terminal pro B-type natriuretic peptide in identifying patients at high risk for adverse outcome after emergent non-cardiac surgery. Br J Anaesth 2013;110:554–60.

42. Rodseth RN, Padayachee L, Biccard BM. A meta-analysis of the utility of preoperative brain natriuretic peptide in predicting early and intermediate-term mortality and major adverse cardiac events in vascular surgical patients. Anaesthesia 2008;63:1226–33.

43. Rodseth RN, Biccard BM, Le Manach Y, et al. The prognostic value of preoperative and post-operative B-type natriuretic peptides in patients undergoing noncardiac surgery. B-type natriuretic peptide and N-terminal fragment of pro-B-type natriuretic peptide: a systematic review and individual patient data meta-analysis. J Am Coll Cardiol 2014;63:170–80.

44. Potgieter D, Simmers D, Ryan L, et al. N-terminal pro-B-type natriuretic peptides' prognostic utility is overestimated in meta-analyses using study-specific optimal diagnostic thresholds. Anesthesiology 2015;123:264–71.

45. Shavit L, Dolgoker I, Ivgi H, et al. Neutrophil gelatinase-associated lipocalin as a predictor of complications and mortality in patients undergoing non-cardiac major surgery. Kidney Blood Press Res 2011;34:116–24.

46. Cho E, Kim SC, Kim MG, et al. The incidence and risk factors of acute kidney injury after hepatobiliary surgery: a prospective observational study. BMC Nephrol 2014;15:169.

47. Martensson J, Martling CR, Bell M. Novel biomarkers of acute kidney injury and failure: clinical applicability. Br J Anaesth 2012;109(6):843–50.

48. Hoste EA, Clermont G, Kersten A, et al. RIFLE criteria for acute kidney injury are associated with hospital mortality in critically ill patients: a cohort analysis. Crit Care 2006;10(3):R73.

49. Bishop MJ, Souders JE, Peterson CM, et al. Factors associated with unanticipated day of surgery deaths in Department of Veterans Affairs hospitals. Anesth Analg 2008;107:1924–35.
50. Bicknell CD, Cowan AR, Kerle MI, et al. Renal dysfunction and prolonged visceral ischaemia increase mortality rate after suprarenal aneurysm repair. Br J Surg 2003;90:1142–6.
51. Kertai MD, Boersma E, Bax JJ, et al. Comparison between serum creatinine and creatinine clearance for the prediction of postoperative mortality in patients undergoing major vascular surgery. Clin Nephrol 2003;59(1):17–23.
52. Cockcroft DW, Gault MH. Prediction of creatinine clearance from serum creatinine. Nephron 1976;16:31–41.
53. Levey AS, Bosch JP, Lewis JB, et al. A more accurate method to estimate glomerular filtration rate from serum creatinine: a new prediction equation. Modification of Diet in Renal Disease Study Group. Ann Intern Med 1999;130: 461–70.
54. Mooney JF, Ranasinghe I, Chow CK, et al. Preoperative estimates of glomerular filtration rate as predictors of outcome after surgery: a systematic review and meta-analysis. Anesthesiology 2013;118:809–24.
55. Huynh TT, van Eps RG, Miller CC 3rd, et al. Glomerular filtration rate is superior to serum creatinine for prediction of mortality after thoracoabdominal aortic surgery. J Vasc Surg 2005;42(2):206–12.
56. Drekonja DM, Zarmbinski B, Johnson JR. Preoperative urine cultures at a veterans affairs medical center. JAMA Intern Med 2013;173:71–2.
57. Davies S, Byrn F, Cole LA. Human chorionic gonadotropin testing for early pregnancy viability and complications. Clin Lab Med 2003;23:257–64.
58. Krolikowska M, Kataja M, Poyhia R, et al. Mortality in diabetic patients undergoing non-cardiac surgery: a 7-year follow-up study. Acta Anaesthesiol Scand 2009; 53(6):749–58.
59. National Institute for Health and Care Excellence. Preoperative tests for elective surgery. NICE guidelines [CG3] Published date: June 2003. Available at: https://www.nice.org.uk/guidance/cg3. Accessed November 6, 2015.
60. Bock M, Johansson T, Fritsch G, et al. The impact of preoperative testing for blood glucose concentration and haemoglobin A1c on mortality, changes in management and complications in noncardiac elective surgery. Eur J Anaesthesiol 2015;32:152–9.
61. Akhtar S, Barash PG, Inzucchi SE, et al. Scientific principles and clinical implications of perioperative glucose regulation and control. Anesth Analg 2010;110: 478–97.
62. Jamsen E, Nevalainen P, Kalliovalkama J, et al. Preoperative hyperglycemia predicts infected total knee replacement. Eur J Intern Med 2010;21:196–201.
63. Olsen MA, Nepple JJ, Riew KD, et al. Risk factors for surgical site infection following orthopaedic spinal operations. J Bone Joint Surg Am 2008;90:62–9.
64. Richards JE, Kauffmann RM, Zuckerman SL, et al. Relationship of hyperglycemia and surgical-site infection in orthopaedic surgery. J Bone Joint Surg Am 2012;94: 1181–0.
65. Feringa HH, Vidakovic R, Karagiannis SE, et al. Impaired glucose regulation, elevated glycated haemoglobin and cardiac ischaemic events in vascular surgery patients. Diabet Med 2008;25:314–9.
66. McGirt MJ, Woodworth GF, Brooke BS, et al. Hyperglycemia independently increases the risk of perioperative stroke, myocardial infarction, and death after carotid endarterectomy. Neurosurgery 2006;58:1066–72.

67. Noordzij PG, Boersma E, Schreiner F, et al. Increased preoperative glucose levels are associated with perioperative mortality in patients undergoing noncardiac, nonvascular surgery. Eur J Endocrinol 2007;156:137–42.
68. Dunkelgrun M, Schreiner F, Schockman DB, et al. Usefulness of preoperative oral glucose tolerance testing for perioperative risk stratification in patients scheduled for elective vascular surgery. Am J Cardiol 2008;101:526–9.
69. van Kuijk JP, Dunkelgrun M, Schreiner F, et al. Preoperative oral glucose tolerance testing in vascular surgery patients: long-term cardiovascular outcome. Am Heart J 2009;157:919–25.
70. Abdelmalak BB, Knittel J, Abdelmalak JB, et al. Preoperative blood glucose concentrations and postoperative outcomes after elective non-cardiac surgery: an observational study. Br J Anaesth 2014;112:79–88.
71. Kotagal M, Symons RG, Hirsch IB, et al, SCOAP-CERTAIN Collaborative. Perioperative hyperglycemia and risk of adverse events among patients with and without diabetes. Ann Surg 2015;261:97–103.
72. Moitra VK, Greenberg J, Arunajadai S, et al. The relationship between glycosylated hemoglobin and perioperative glucose control in patients with diabetes. Can J Anaesth 2010;57:322–9.
73. Gustafsson UO, Thorell A, Soop M, et al. Haemoglobin A1c as a predictor of postoperative hyperglycaemia and complications after major colorectal surgery. Br J Surg 2009;96:1358–64.
74. O'Sullivan CJ, Hynes N, Mahendran B, et al. Haemoglobin A1c (HbA1C) in non-diabetic and diabetic vascular patients. Is HbA1C an independent risk factor and predictor of adverse outcome? Eur J Vasc Endovasc Surg 2006;32:188–97.
75. Acott AA, Theus SA, Kim LT, et al. Long-term glucose control and risk of perioperative complications. Am J Surg 2009;198:596–9.
76. McFalls EO, Ward HB, Moritz TE, et al. Predictors and outcomes of a perioperative myocardial infarction following elective vascular surgery in patients with documented coronary artery disease: results of the CARP trial. Eur Heart J 2008;29: 394–401.
77. Chee YL, Crawford JC, Watson HG, et al. Guidelines on the assessment of bleeding risk prior to surgery or invasive procedures. Br J Haematol 2008;140: 496–504.
78. Seicean A, Schiltz NK, Seicean S, et al. Use and utility of preoperative hemostatic screening and patient history in adult neurosurgical patients. J Neurosurg 2012; 116:1097–105.
79. Available at: https://www.aacc.org/publications/cln/articles/2012/january/coagulation-tests. Accessed November 6, 2015.
80. Burk CD, Miller L, Handler SD, et al. Preoperative history and coagulation screening in children undergoing tonsillectomy. Pediatrics 1992;89:691–5.
81. Klepstad P, Kaasa S, Skauge M, et al. Pain intensity and side effects during titration of morphine to cancer patients using a fixed schedule dose escalation. Acta Anaesthesiol Scand 2000;44:656–64.
82. Mather LE, Glynn CJ. The minimum effective analgetic blood concentration of pethidine in patients with intractable pain. Br J Clin Pharmacol 1982;14:385–90.
83. Trescot AM. Genetics and implications in perioperative analgesia. Best Pract Res Clin Anaesthesiol 2014;28:153–66.
84. Kitzmiller JP, Groen DK, Phelps MA, et al. Pharmacogenomic testing: relevance in medical practice: why drugs work in some patients but not in others. Cleve Clin J Med 2011;78:243–57.

Evaluation of Major Organ Systems

Preoperative Assessment of the Patient with Cardiac Disease Undergoing Noncardiac Surgery

Lee A. Fleisher, MD

KEYWORDS

- Preoperative • Cardiac • Myocardial infarction • Stress testing
- Coronary revascularization

KEY POINTS

- New guidelines have been published by the American Heart Association/American College of Cardiology and the European Society of Cardiology to define the evidence surrounding preoperative cardiovascular management.
- Preoperative cardiovascular testing should only be performed if it affects the management of patients with increased risk and poor exercise capacity.
- Coronary revascularization before noncardiac surgery is indicated only in patients in whom it is warranted, independent of noncardiac surgery.
- Guidelines for perioperative antiplatelet management in patients with coronary stents is currently undergoing revision.
- Indications for perioperative beta-blockade are restricted to those already taking these agents with a class IIb indication for initiation allowing for sufficient time for titration.

The past several years has seen a dramatic increase in the number and quality of randomized and prospective studies to define the optimal and most cost-effective approach for preoperative cardiovascular evaluation and management for noncardiac surgery, including studies evaluating the role of coronary revascularization before noncardiac surgery and perioperative beta-blockers. In 2014, the American Heart Association/American College of Cardiology (AHA/ACC) Guidelines on Perioperative Cardiovascular Evaluation before Noncardiac Surgery were updated, which included a new algorithm and new recommendations regarding perioperative beta-blockade usage.[1] In addition, the European Society of Cardiology has also published guidelines for preoperative cardiac risk assessment and perioperative cardiac management in noncardiac surgery.[2] These recommendations are similar to the AHA/ACC

Department of Anesthesiology and Critical Care, Perelman School of Medicine at the University of Pennsylvania, 3400 Spruce Street, Philadelphia, PA 19437, USA
E-mail address: Lee.fleisher@uphs.upenn.edu

Anesthesiology Clin 34 (2016) 59–70
http://dx.doi.org/10.1016/j.anclin.2015.10.006   anesthesiology.theclinics.com
1932-2275/16/$ – see front matter © 2016 Elsevier Inc. All rights reserved.

recommendations with an algorithm, and the AHA/ACC and European Society of Cardiology discussed their recommendations before simultaneous publication to ensure that any differences in recommendations were fully vetted. Part of the rationale for updating the guidelines from both groups was the recent concerns regarding the publications by Poldermans and his group. After extensive discussion, the ACC/AHA Writing Committee determined the approach outlined in **Box 1**.

The basic tenet in preoperative evaluation remains that information regarding the extent and stability of disease will affect patient management and lead to improved outcome (**Box 2**). In the case of cardiovascular disease, preoperative evaluation seeks to define the extent of coronary artery disease and left ventricular function.

CLINICAL ASSESSMENT

Since the original manuscript by Goldman and colleagues[3] in 1977 describing a Cardiac Risk Index, multiple investigators have validated various clinical risk indices for their ability to predict perioperative cardiac complications. The Revised Cardiac Risk Index (RCRI) was developed in a study of 4315 patients aged 50 years or older undergoing elective major noncardiac procedures in a tertiary care teaching hospital. Six independent predictors of complications were identified and included in the RCRI: high-risk type of surgery, history of ischemic heart disease, history of congestive heart failure, history of cerebrovascular disease, preoperative treatment with insulin, and preoperative serum creatinine of greater than 2.0 mg/d, with increasing cardiac complication rates noted with increasing number of risk factors.[4] The RCRI has become the standard tool in the literature in assessing the prior probability of perioperative cardiac risk in a given individual and has been used to direct the decision to perform cardiovascular testing and implement perioperative management protocols, and has recently been validated for both short- and long-term outcomes.[5]

More recently, a risk calculator was developed using data from the American College of Surgeons National Surgical Quality Improvement Project (ACS-NSQIP; **Fig. 1**; available from: http://site.acsnsqip.org).[6] It is based on 1,414,006 patients encompassing 1557 unique surgical codes. The authors found that the ACS NSQIP surgical risk calculator was a decision support tool that can be used to estimate the risks of most operations. The advantage of the ACS-NSQIP risk calculator is that it incorporates both clinical and surgical risk. Additionally, age is incorporated into the risk

---

Box 1
Approach to publications from Poldermans

1. The Evidence Review Committee will include the DECREASE trials in the sensitivity analysis, but the systematic review report will be based on the published data on perioperative beta-blockade, with data from all DECREASE trials excluded.

2. The DECREASE trials and other derivative studies by Poldermans should not be included in the clinical practice guideline data supplements and evidence tables.

3. If nonretracted DECREASE publications and/or other derivative studies by Poldermans are relevant to the topic, they can only be cited in the text with a comment about the finding compared with the current recommendation, but should not form the basis of that recommendation or be used as a reference for the recommendation.

From Fleisher LA, Fleischmann KE, Auerbach AD, et al. 2014 ACC/AHA guideline on perioperative cardiovascular evaluation and management of patients undergoing noncardiac surgery: a report of the American College of Cardiology/American Heart Association Task Force on practice guidelines. J Am Coll Cardiol 2014;64(22):e83; with permission.

> **Box 2**
> **Perioperative interventions based on preoperative cardiac evaluation**
>
> Decision to forego surgery
>
> Modification of the surgical procedure
>
> Delay case for treatment of unstable symptoms
>
> Modification of perioperative medical therapy
>
> Initiation of beta-blockers, statins, α-2 agonists
>
> Modification of postoperative monitoring (eg, intensive care unit)
>
> Coronary revascularization before noncardiac surgery
>
> Modification of location of care
>
> Consideration of palliative care
>
> Appropriate allocation of transplant organs

calculator. A primary issue with all of these indices from the anesthesiologist's perspective is that a simple estimate of risk does not help in refining perioperative management, and therefore it is important that the anesthesiologist determine the extent and stability of the patient's coronary artery disease by obtaining information from the primary caregiver or cardiologist or through a thorough history or physical examination.

A thorough history should focus on cardiovascular risk factors and symptoms or signs of unstable cardiac disease states, such as myocardial ischemia with minimal exertion, active congestive heart failure, symptomatic valvular heart disease, and significant cardiac arrhythmias. In patients with symptomatic coronary disease, the preoperative evaluation may lead to the recognition of a change in the frequency or pattern of anginal symptoms. In virtually all studies, the presence of active congestive heart failure preoperatively has been associated with an increased incidence of perioperative cardiac morbidity.[7] Stabilization of ventricular function and treatment for pulmonary congestion is prudent before elective surgery. Also, it is important to determine the etiology of the left heart failure because the type of perioperative monitoring and treatments would be different.

Patients with a prior myocardial infarction (MI) have coronary artery disease, although a small group of patients may sustain an MI from a nonatherosclerotic mechanism. Since the publication of the original guidelines in 1996, there has been a consensus that the traditional recommendation to wait 6 months for elective surgery should be modified.[8] Instead, patients should be evaluated from the perspective of their risk for ongoing ischemia. A recent analysis using Medicare claims data suggests that the risk of reinfarction remains high for at least 2 months after a MI, and that coronary artery bypass grafting may decrease that risk, and coronary stent placement soon after an MI does not.[9,10] The current guidelines have adopted the 60-day recommendation.

For those patients without overt symptoms or history, the probability of coronary artery disease varies with the type and number of atherosclerotic risk factors present. Diabetes mellitus is common in the elderly and represents a disease that impacts on multiple organ systems. Diabetes accelerates the progression of atherosclerosis, which can frequently be silent in nature, leading many clinicians to assume coronary artery disease in this population and treating them as such. Diabetes is an independent risk factor for perioperative cardiac morbidity and the preoperative treatment with insulin has been included in the RCRI. In attempting to determine the degree of this increased probability, the treatment

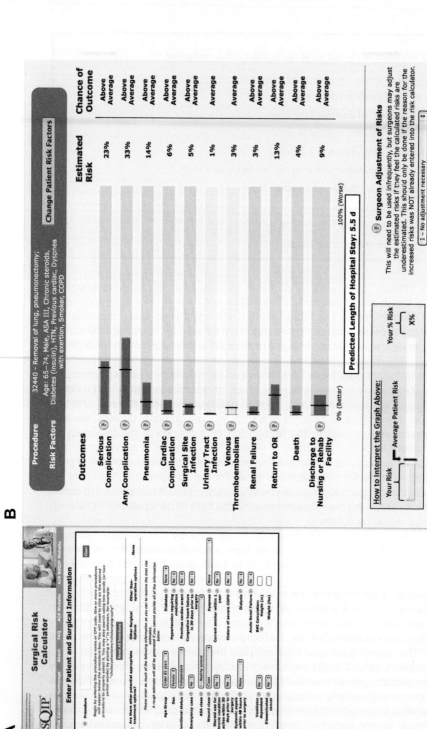

Fig. 1. National Surgical Quality Improvement Program (NSQIP) risk calculator. (A) The online site display where patient and surgical features may be input into the data calculator. (B) As an example, the surgical risk calculation has been performed for a patient undergoing a pneumonectomy with specific risk factors. The resulting surgical risk calculation, including negative outcomes, percent risk of these outcomes occurring, as well as the chance of the outcome (eg, average, above average) are displayed. Note in the lower right hand corner that the surgeon may adjust this risk calculation. In this example, no adjustment has been made. (*Courtesy of* American College of Surgeons; with permission.)

modality, duration of the disease, and other associated end-organ dysfunction should be taken into account, including autonomic neuropathy. Hypertension has also been associated with an increased incidence of silent myocardial ischemia and infarction. Those hypertensive patients with left ventricular hypertrophy and who are undergoing noncardiac surgery are at a greater perioperative risk than nonhypertensive patients.[11] There is a great deal of debate regarding a trigger to delay or cancel an operative procedure in a patient with poorly or untreated hypertension. In the absence of end-organ changes, such as renal insufficiency or left ventricular hypertrophy with strain, it would seem appropriate to proceed with the operation. A randomized trial of treated hypertensive patients without known coronary artery disease who presented the morning of surgery with an elevated diastolic blood pressure was unable to demonstrate any difference in outcome between those who were actively treated versus those in whom surgery was delayed.[12] In contrast, a patient with a markedly elevated blood pressure and the new onset of a headache should have surgery delayed for further evaluation and potential treatment. For the purpose of the guidelines, a list of active cardiac conditions and clinical risk factors were defined.

IMPORTANCE OF THE OPERATIVE PROCEDURE

The operative procedure influences the extent of the preoperative evaluation required by determining the potential range of changes in perioperative management. There are few hard data to define the surgery-specific incidence of complications, and the rate may be very institution dependent. Eagle and colleagues[13] published data on the incidence of perioperative MI and mortality by procedure for patients enrolled in the Coronary Artery Surgery Study (CASS). Higher risk procedures for which coronary artery bypass grafting reduced the risk of noncardiac surgery compared with medical therapy include major vascular, abdominal, thoracic, and orthopedic operations. Ambulatory procedures denote low risk. Vascular surgery represents a unique group of patients in whom there is extensive evidence regarding preoperative testing and perioperative interventions. Endovascular stent placement is associated with lower perioperative risk, particularly the risk of death, but similar long-term mortality compared with open procedures. The current guidelines combined the previous high and intermediate surgical risk categories. The ACS-NSQIP risk calculator incorporates surgical specific risk and therefore has more discriminatory ability. There is evidence to suggest that the rate of surgical mortality is correlated with hospital surgery-specific volume and therefore higher volume hospitals may have better outcomes, which can impact the decision to perform preoperative testing. Locations with less intensive resources, for example, smaller hospitals, may actually perform testing to determine which patients need to be referred to larger centers.

IMPORTANCE OF EXERCISE TOLERANCE

Exercise tolerance is one of the most important determinants of perioperative risk and the need for invasive monitoring. If a patient can walk a mile without becoming short of breath, then the probability of extensive coronary artery disease is small. Alternatively, if patients become dyspneic associated with chest pain during minimal exertion, then the probability of extensive coronary artery disease is high. Reilly and colleagues[14] demonstrated that the likelihood of a serious complication occurring was inversely related to the number of blocks that could be walked or flights of stairs that could be climbed. Exercise tolerance can be assessed with formal treadmill testing or with a questionnaire that assesses activities of daily living (**Table 1**). There is some suggestion that cardiopulmonary testing is useful for predicting risk more accurately.

Table 1
Duke Activity Status Index

Activity	Weight (in METs)
Can you...	
1. Take care of yourself, that is, eating, dressing, bathing, or using the toilet?	2.75
2. Walk indoors, such as around your house?	1.75
3. Walk a block or 2 on level ground?	2.75
4. Climb a flight of stairs or walk up a hill?	5.50
5. Run a short distance?	8.00
6. Do light work around the house like dusting or washing dishes?	2.70
7. Do moderate work around the house like vacuuming, sweeping floors, or carrying groceries?	3.50
8. Do heavy work around the house like scrubbing floors or lifting or moving heavy furniture?	8.00
9. Do yardwork like raking leaves, weeding, or pushing a power mower?	4.50
10. Have sexual relations?	5.25
11. Participate in moderate recreational activities like golf, bowling, dancing, doubles tennis, or throwing a baseball or football?	6.00
12. Participate in strenuous sports like swimming, singles tennis, football, basketball, or skiing?	7.50

Abbreviation: METs, metabolic equivalents (1 MET is the equivalent of resting oxygen consumption).

From Hlatky MA, Boineau RE, Higginbotham MB, et al. A brief self-administered questionnaire to determine functional capacity (the Duke Activity Status Index). Am J Cardiol 1989;64(10):651–4; with permission.

APPROACH TO THE PATIENT

Fig. 2 presents in algorithmic form a framework for determining which patients are candidates for cardiac testing for ischemic heart disease.[1] Given the availability of this evidence, the AHA/ACC Writing Committee chose to include the level of the recommendations and strength of evidence for many of the pathways. Importantly, the value of adopting the algorithm depends on local factors, such as current perioperative risk and the rate of use of testing.

The new algorithm combines clinical and surgical risk (step 3). Those at low risk (<1% major adverse cardiac events) proceed to surgery. The new approach collapses intermediate and high risk into 1 category of increased risk. If the patient has moderate or greater exercise capacity, then the patient should proceed to surgery. In patients with poor exercise capacity, the key question is whether further testing will change management. A key change in the new algorithm is the incorporation of noninvasive treatment or palliation as one of the potential rationales for testing.

CHOICE OF DIAGNOSTIC TEST

There are multiple noninvasive diagnostic tests that have been proposed to evaluate the extent of coronary artery disease before noncardiac surgery. Although exercise electrocardiogram has been the traditional method of evaluating individuals for the presence of coronary artery disease, patients with a good exercise tolerance rarely benefit from further testing. Therefore, pharmacologic stress testing has become popular, particularly as a preoperative test in vascular surgery patients.

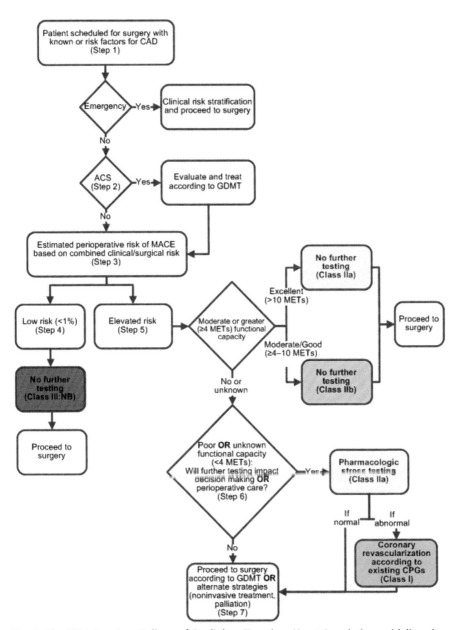

Fig. 2. The 2014 American College of Cardiology/American Heart Association guideline algorithm depicting the stepwise approach to perioperative cardiac assessment for CAD, ACS, acute coronary syndrome, CAD, coronary artery disease; CPG, clinical practice guideline; GDMT, guideline-directed medical therapy; MACE, major adverse cardiac event; MET, metabolic equivalent; NB, no benefit. (*From* Fleisher LA, Fleischmann KE, Auerbach AD, et al. 2014 ACC/AHA guideline on perioperative cardiovascular evaluation and management of patients undergoing noncardiac surgery: a report of the American College of Cardiology/American Heart Association Task Force on practice guidelines. J Am Coll Cardiol 2014;64(22):e94; with permission.)

Several authors have shown that the presence of a redistribution defect on dipyridamole thallium imaging in patients undergoing peripheral vascular surgery is predictive of postoperative cardiac events. To increase the predictive value of the test, several strategies have been suggested. Lung uptake, left ventricular cavity dilation, and redistribution defect size have all been shown to be predictive of subsequent morbidity.[15] The appearance of new or worsened regional wall motion abnormalities is considered a positive test. The advantage of this test is that it is a dynamic assessment of ventricular function. Dobutamine echocardiography has also been studied and was found to have among the best positive and negative predictive values.[16] The presence of 5 or more segments of new regional wall motion abnormalities denotes a high-risk group.

INTERVENTIONS FOR PATIENTS WITH DOCUMENTED CORONARY ARTERY DISEASE

There is increasing evidence that coronary revascularization before noncardiac surgery does not decrease the incidence of perioperative cardiac morbidity. McFalls and colleagues[17] reported the results of a multicenter randomized trail in the Veterans Administration Health System in which patients with documented coronary artery disease on coronary angiography (Coronary Artery Revascularization Prophylaxis [CARP] trial), excluding those with left main disease or severely depressed ejection fraction (<20%), were randomized to coronary artery bypass grafting (59%) or percutaneous coronary interventions (41%) versus routine medical therapy. At 2.7 years after randomization, mortality in the revascularization group was not significantly different (22%) compared with the no revascularization group (23%). Within 30 days after the vascular operation, a postoperative MI, defined by increased troponin levels, occurred in 12% of the revascularization group and 14% of the no revascularization group ($P = .37$). In a follow-up analysis, Ward and colleagues[18] reported improved outcomes in the subset who underwent coronary artery bypass grafting compared with percutaneous coronary intervention. In patients who underwent coronary angiography in both the randomized and nonrandomized portion of the CARP trial, only the subset of patients with unprotected left main disease showed a benefit with preoperative coronary artery revascularization.[19] This finding was supported by that of Poldermans and colleagues,[20] who randomized 770 patients undergoing major vascular operations and considered as having intermediate cardiac risk, defined as the presence of 1 or 2 cardiac risk factors to either undergo further risk stratification with stress imaging or proceed right to surgery. All patients received preoperative bisoprolol with a targeted heart rate of 60 to 65 bpm initiated before and continued after surgery. The 30 day incidence of cardiac death and nonfatal MI was similar in both groups (1.8% in the no testing group vs 2.3% in the tested group).

The current evidence does not support the use of percutaneous transluminal coronary angioplasty beyond established indications for nonoperative patients, because the incidence of perioperative complications does not seem to be decreased in those patients in whom percutaneous transluminal coronary angioplasty was performed less than 90 days before surgery.[21,22] Coronary stent placement may be a unique issue and several studies suggest that a minimum of 30 days is required before the rate of perioperative complications is low.[23,24] Several reports suggest that drug-eluting stents may represent an additional risk over a prolonged period (≤12 months), particularly if antiplatelet agents are discontinued.[25] However, newer studies suggest that surgery may be safe in drug-eluting stents if performed within 3 to 6 months of surgery.[26–28] The new guidelines suggest continuing aspirin therapy in all patients with a coronary stent and discontinuing clopidogrel for as short a time interval as possible for patients with bare metal stents for less than 30 days or drug-eluting stents for less than 1 year; however, there is a focused update being finalized at the time of the writing of this review and the readers are urged to review the current guidelines. Based on the nonperioperative literature, there is a suggestion that holding clopidogrel for the traditional 8 days may actually increase the risk associated with a hypercoagulable rebound, suggesting that a shorter period of time may be optimal. A recent cohort study suggests that withdrawal of antiplatelet agents for longer than 5 days is associated with increased major adverse cardiac events.[29]

There is now a great deal of evidence to suggest that perioperative medical therapy can be optimized in those patients with coronary artery disease as a means of reducing perioperative cardiovascular complications. Multiple studies have demonstrated improved outcome in patients given perioperative beta-blockers, especially if the heart rate is controlled, acknowledging the previously discussed concerns regarding the quality of the studies from the Erasmus group.[30,31] Subsequent studies demonstrated that beta-blockers may not be effective if heart rate is not well-controlled, or in lower risk patients.[32–34] The Perioperative Ischemic Evaluation (POISE) trial evaluated 8351 high-risk beta-blocker–naive patients who were randomized to high-dose metoprolol controlled release versus placebo.[35] There was a significant decrease in the primary outcome of cardiovascular events, associated with a 30% reduction in the MI rate, but with a significantly increased rate of 30-day all-cause mortality and stroke. Several recent cohort studies continue to support the fact that high-risk patients on beta-blockers were associated with improved outcome. A Canadian administrative dataset suggests that the perioperative morbidity was higher if beta-blockers were started within 7 days as compared with 8 days or greater.

As part of the update to the current ACC/AHA Guidelines, an Evidence Review Committee was formed to review independently the data on perioperative beta-blockade. Perioperative beta-blockade started within 1 day or less before noncardiac surgery prevents nonfatal MI but increases risks of stroke, death, hypotension, and bradycardia.[36] Without the controversial DECREASE studies, there are insufficient data on beta-blockade started 2 or more days before surgery. Wallace and colleagues[37] reported that perioperative beta-blockade administered according to the Perioperative Cardiac Risk Reduction protocol is associated with a reduction in 30-day and 1-year mortality. Perioperative withdrawal of beta-blockers is associated with increased mortality. The current ACCF/AHA Guidelines on perioperative beta-blockade advocate that perioperative beta-blockade is a class I indication and should be used in patients previously on beta-blockers. The new recommendations changed the recommendation from a class IIa to IIb for patients undergoing vascular surgery who are at high cardiac risk owing to coronary artery disease or the finding of cardiac ischemia on preoperative testing.

Other pharmacologic agents have also been shown to improve perioperative cardiac outcome. In POISE II, alpha-2 agonists were not shown to improve perioperative outcomes.[38] POISE II also evaluated the effectiveness of aspirin therapy in a cohort of patients without a recent stent. Administration of aspirin before surgery and throughout the early postoperative period had no effect on the rate of a composite of death or nonfatal MI but increased the risk of major bleeding.[39] Most recently, perioperative statins have been shown to improve cardiac outcome. Durazzo and colleagues[40] published a randomized trial of 200 vascular surgery patients in which statins were started an average of 30 days before vascular surgery. A significant reduction in cardiovascular complications was demonstrated using this protocol. Le Manach and colleagues[41] demonstrated that statin withdrawal for more than 4 days was associated with a 2.9 odds ratio of increased risk of cardiac morbidity in vascular surgery patients. The guidelines advocate continuing statin therapy in patients currently taking statins as a class I indication. A multimodal approach to medical management should be taken in high-risk patients.

SUMMARY

Preoperative evaluation should focus on identifying patients with symptomatic and asymptomatic coronary artery disease and assessing the exercise capacity of the patient. The decision to perform further diagnostic evaluation depends on the interactions of patient and surgery-specific factors, as well as exercise capacity, and should be reserved for those at increased risk with poor exercise capacity. The indications for coronary interventions are the same in the perioperative period as for the nonoperative setting.

REFERENCES

1. Fleisher LA, Fleischmann KE, Auerbach AD, et al. 2014 ACC/AHA guideline on perioperative cardiovascular evaluation and management of patients undergoing noncardiac surgery: a report of the American College of Cardiology/American Heart Association Task Force on practice guidelines. J Am Coll Cardiol 2014; 64(22):e77–137.
2. Kristensen SD, Knuuti J, Saraste A, et al. 2014 ESC/ESA guidelines on noncardiac surgery: cardiovascular assessment and management: the Joint Task Force on non-cardiac surgery: cardiovascular assessment and management of the European Society of Cardiology (ESC) and the European Society of Anaesthesiology (ESA). Eur Heart J 2014;35(35):2383–431.
3. Goldman L, Caldera DL, Nussbaum SR, et al. Multifactorial index of cardiac risk in noncardiac surgical procedures. N Engl J Med 1977;297:845–50.
4. Lee TH, Marcantonio ER, Mangione CM, et al. Derivation and prospective validation of a simple index for prediction of cardiac risk of major noncardiac surgery. Circulation 1999;100(10):1043–9.
5. Hoeks SE, op Reimer WJ, van Gestel YR, et al. Preoperative cardiac risk index predicts long-term mortality and health status. Am J Med 2009;122(6):559–65.
6. Bilimoria KY, Liu Y, Paruch JL, et al. Development and evaluation of the universal ACS NSQIP surgical risk calculator: a decision aid and informed consent tool for patients and surgeons. J Am Coll Surg 2013;217(5):833–42.e1-e3.
7. Hammill BG, Curtis LH, Bennett-Guerrero E, et al. Impact of heart failure on patients undergoing major noncardiac surgery. Anesthesiology 2008;108(4): 559–67.
8. Eagle KA, Brundage BH, Chaitman BR, et al. Guidelines for perioperative cardiovascular evaluation for noncardiac surgery. Report of the American College of Cardiology/American Heart Association Task Force on practice guidelines (Committee on Perioperative Cardiovascular Evaluation for Noncardiac Surgery). J Am Coll Cardiol 1996;27(4):910–48.
9. Livhits M, Gibbons MM, de Virgilio C, et al. Coronary revascularization after myocardial infarction can reduce risks of noncardiac surgery. J Am Coll Surg 2011;212:1018–26.
10. Livhits M, Ko CY, Leonardi MJ, et al. Risk of surgery following recent myocardial infarction. Ann Surg 2011;253(5):857–64.
11. Hollenberg M, Mangano DT, Browner WS, et al. Predictors of postoperative myocardial ischemia in patients undergoing noncardiac surgery. The Study of Perioperative Ischemia Research. JAMA 1992;268:205–9.

12. Weksler N, Klein M, Szendro G, et al. The dilemma of immediate preoperative hypertension: to treat and operate, or to postpone surgery? J Clin Anesth 2003; 15(3):179–83.
13. Eagle KA, Rihal CS, Mickel MC, et al. Cardiac risk of noncardiac surgery: influence of coronary disease and type of surgery in 3368 operations. CASS Investigators and University of Michigan Heart Care Program. Coronary Artery Surgery Study. Circulation 1997;96(6):1882–7.
14. Reilly DF, McNeely MJ, Doerner D, et al. Self-reported exercise tolerance and the risk of serious perioperative complications. Arch Intern Med 1999;159(18): 2185–92.
15. Fleisher LA, Rosenbaum SH, Nelson AH, et al. Preoperative dipyridamole thallium imaging and Holter monitoring as a predictor of perioperative cardiac events and long tem outcome. Anesthesiology 1995;83:906–17.
16. Mantha S, Roizen MF, Barnard J, et al. Relative effectiveness of four preoperative tests for predicting adverse cardiac outcomes after vascular surgery: a meta-analysis. Anesth Analg 1994;79(3):422–33.
17. McFalls EO, Ward HB, Moritz TE, et al. Coronary-artery revascularization before elective major vascular surgery. N Engl J Med 2004;351(27):2795–804.
18. Ward HB, Kelly RF, Thottapurathu L, et al. Coronary artery bypass grafting is superior to percutaneous coronary intervention in prevention of perioperative myocardial infarctions during subsequent vascular surgery. Ann Thorac Surg 2006;82(3):795–800 [discussion: 800–1].
19. Garcia S, Moritz TE, Ward HB, et al. Usefulness of revascularization of patients with multivessel coronary artery disease before elective vascular surgery for abdominal aortic and peripheral occlusive disease. Am J Cardiol 2008;102(7):809–13.
20. Poldermans D, Bax JJ, Schouten O, et al. Should major vascular surgery be delayed because of preoperative cardiac testing in intermediate-risk patients receiving beta-blocker therapy with tight heart rate control? J Am Coll Cardiol 2006;48(5):964–9.
21. Godet G, Riou B, Bertrand M, et al. Does preoperative coronary angioplasty improve perioperative cardiac outcome? Anesthesiology 2005;102(4):739–46.
22. Posner KL, Van Norman GA, Chan V. Adverse cardiac outcomes after noncardiac surgery in patients with prior percutaneous transluminal coronary angioplasty. Anesth Analg 1999;89(3):553–60.
23. Kaluza GL, Joseph J, Lee JR, et al. Catastrophic outcomes of noncardiac surgery soon after coronary stenting. J Am Coll Cardiol 2000;35(5):1288–94.
24. Wilson SH, Fasseas P, Orford JL, et al. Clinical outcome of patients undergoing non-cardiac surgery in the two months following coronary stenting. J Am Coll Cardiol 2003;42(2):234–40.
25. Schouten O, van Domburg RT, Bax JJ, et al. Noncardiac surgery after coronary stenting: early surgery and interruption of antiplatelet therapy are associated with an increase in major adverse cardiac events. J Am Coll Cardiol 2007;49(1):122–4.
26. Hawn MT, Graham LA, Richman JR, et al. The incidence and timing of noncardiac surgery after cardiac stent implantation. J Am Coll Surg 2012;214(4):658–66 [discussion: 666–7].
27. Hawn MT, Graham LA, Richman JS, et al. Risk of major adverse cardiac events following noncardiac surgery in patients with coronary stents. JAMA 2013; 310(14):1462–72.
28. Wijeysundera DN, Wijeysundera HC, Yun L, et al. Risk of elective major noncardiac surgery after coronary stent insertion: a population-based study. Circulation 2012;126(11):1355–62.

29. Albaladejo P, Marret E, Samama CM, et al. Non-cardiac surgery in patients with coronary stents: the RECO study. Heart 2011;97(19):1566–72.

30. Mangano DT, Layug EL, Wallace A, et al. Effect of atenolol on mortality and cardiovascular morbidity after noncardiac surgery. Multicenter Study of Perioperative Ischemia Research Group. N Engl J Med 1996;335(23):1713–20.

31. Poldermans D, Boersma E, Bax JJ, et al. The effect of bisoprolol on perioperative mortality and myocardial infarction in high-risk patients undergoing vascular surgery. Dutch Echocardiographic Cardiac Risk Evaluation Applying Stress Echocardiography Study Group [see comments]. N Engl J Med 1999;341(24): 1789–94.

32. Juul AB, Wetterslev J, Gluud C, et al. Effect of perioperative beta blockade in patients with diabetes undergoing major non-cardiac surgery: randomised placebo controlled, blinded multicentre trial. BMJ 2006;332(7556):1482.

33. Lindenauer PK, Pekow P, Wang K, et al. Perioperative beta-blocker therapy and mortality after major noncardiac surgery. N Engl J Med 2005;353(4):349–61.

34. Yang H, Raymer K, Butler R, et al. The effects of perioperative beta-blockade: results of the Metoprolol after Vascular Surgery (MaVS) study, a randomized controlled trial. Am Heart J 2006;152(5):983–90.

35. Devereaux PJ, Yang H, Yusuf S, et al. Effects of extended-release metoprolol succinate in patients undergoing non-cardiac surgery (POISE trial): a randomised controlled trial. Lancet 2008;371(9627):1839–47.

36. Wijeysundera DN, Duncan D, Nkonde-Price C, et al. Perioperative beta blockade in noncardiac surgery: a systematic review for the 2014 ACC/AHA guideline on perioperative cardiovascular evaluation and management of patients undergoing noncardiac surgery: a report of the American College of Cardiology/American Heart Association Task Force on practice guidelines. J Am Coll Cardiol 2014; 64(22):2406–25.

37. Wallace AW, Au S, Cason BA. Association of the pattern of use of perioperative beta-blockade and postoperative mortality. Anesthesiology 2010;113(4): 794–805.

38. Devereaux PJ, Sessler DI, Leslie K, et al. Clonidine in patients undergoing noncardiac surgery. N Engl J Med 2014;370(16):1504–13.

39. Devereaux PJ, Mrkobrada M, Sessler DI, et al. Aspirin in patients undergoing noncardiac surgery. N Engl J Med 2014;370(16):1494–503.

40. Durazzo AE, Machado FS, Ikeoka DT, et al. Reduction in cardiovascular events after vascular surgery with atorvastatin: a randomized trial. J Vasc Surg 2004; 39(5):967–75.

41. Le Manach Y, Godet G, Coriat P, et al. The impact of postoperative discontinuation or continuation of chronic statin therapy on cardiac outcome after major vascular surgery. Anesth Analg 2007;104(6):1326–33. Table of contents.

Preoperative Evaluation
Estimation of Pulmonary Risk

Anand Lakshminarasimhachar, MBBS, FRCA[a],*, Gerald W. Smetana, MD[b]

KEYWORDS

- Postoperative pulmonary complication (PPC) • Pulmonary function tests
- Risk indices • Preoperative evaluation • Risk factors

KEY POINTS

- Postoperative pulmonary complications (PPCs) are the second most common postoperative complication; their incidence ranges from 2.0% to 5.6% in the general surgical population.
- PPCs are associated with poor outcomes, longer hospital stays, increased likelihood of rehospitalization, and increased mortality. Surgical, anesthetic, and patient factors contribute to the development of PPCs.
- Reliable predictors include American Society of Anesthesiologist class, functional class, advanced age, surgical site, and prolonged operative time.
- The preoperative evaluation seeks to identify risks for PPCs, change modifiable factors, discuss risks with patients, optimize health before surgery, and plan appropriate perioperative care.
- The overall risk can be predicted using scores that incorporate readily available clinical data. Do not routinely perform pulmonary function tests before high-risk noncardiothoracic surgery.

INTRODUCTION

Postoperative pulmonary complications (PPCs) after major surgery are common and are associated with significant morbidity and high cost of care. In a recent analysis of the National Surgical Quality Improvement Program (NSQIP), of the 165,196 patients who underwent major abdominal surgery, the incidence of PPCs was 5.8%.[1] PPCs have shown to be one of the most significant factors associated with poor patient outcomes, leading to longer durations of hospital stay, increased likelihood of rehospitalization, and increased mortality.[2] Some studies have shown that PPCs predict long-term mortality more accurately than cardiac complications.[3]

[a] Division of Cardiothoracic Anesthesiology, Barnes Jewish Hospital, Washington University School of Medicine in St. Louis, 660, South Euclid Avenue, St Louis, MO 63110, USA; [b] Division of General Medicine and Primary Care, Beth Israel Deaconess Medical Center, Harvard Medical School, Yamins 102C, 330 Brookline Avenue, Boston, MA 02215, USA
* Corresponding author.
E-mail address: lakshmia@anest.wustl.edu

Anesthesiology Clin 34 (2016) 71–88
http://dx.doi.org/10.1016/j.anclin.2015.10.007
1932-2275/16/$ – see front matter © 2016 Elsevier Inc. All rights reserved.

Understanding the potential risk of developing pulmonary complications allows perioperative physicians to choose appropriate anesthetic and surgical care, thereby decreasing the adverse respiratory outcomes. This has become even more relevant with the recent introduction of the concept of the perioperative surgical home.[4] The goals of the perioperative surgical home are to:

- Reduce preoperative testing;
- Reduce day of surgery cancellations;
- Reduce postoperative complications;
- Reduce cost (through reduced testing and reduced perioperative complications); and
- Improve clinical outcomes.

In this article, we review the definition of PPCs, perioperative changes in pulmonary function, risk factors for developing PPCs, the role of preoperative pulmonary function testing, and the role of pulmonary risk indices. The evaluation of patients for lung resection differs substantially and is not discussed in this article.

PULMONARY PATHOPHYSIOLOGY IN THE PERIOPERATIVE PERIOD

The changes in pulmonary function that occur postoperatively are primarily restrictive, with proportional decrease in all lung volumes and no change in airway resistance. The decrease in functional residual capacity (FRC) is the yardstick by which the restrictive defect is gauged. This reduction in lung volumes is generated by the abdominal contents that impinge on and prevent normal movements of the diaphragm and by the abnormal respiratory pattern devoid of sighs and characterized by shallow, rapid respiration (**Fig. 1**).

The decrease in lung volume promotes atelectasis in the dependent areas of the lung; this persists for more than 24 hours in 50% of patients. Arterial hypoxemia occurs from ventilation perfusion (V/Q) mismatch and increased shunt fraction. The vital capacity is reduced by 50% to 60% and the FRC is reduced by about 30% in major upper abdominal and thoracic surgery.[5] Lower abdominal surgery is associated with similar changes, but to a lesser degree. Reduction in lung volume does not occur with surgery on extremities,[6] but most other operative sites, including intracranial, peripheral vascular, and otolaryngeal, have approximately the same modest effect on FRC with reduction of 15% to 20% from preoperative levels. Thus, the operative site is one of the single most important determinants of the degree of pulmonary restriction and risk of PPCs.

Both the residual effects of anesthetic agents and postoperative opioids depress the respiratory drive resulting in diminished response to both hypoxia and hypercarbia. Inhibition of the cough reflex and the impaired mucociliary clearance of pulmonary secretions contribute to risk for postoperative infection.[7] The combination of neuromuscular blockers and anesthetic agents cause diaphragm and chest wall relaxation, which results in the reduction of FRC and thereby thoracic volume.

DEFINITION OF POSTOPERATIVE PULMONARY COMPLICATIONS

A comprehensive list of pulmonary complications includes cough, dyspnea, bronchospasm, hypoxemia, atelectasis, hypercapnia, adverse reaction to pulmonary medication, pleural effusion, pneumonia, pneumothorax, and ventilatory failure.[8] However, this broad definition includes complications that may have no clinical significance. A more reasonable definition is a pulmonary abnormality that produces identifiable disease or dysfunction, is clinically significant, and adversely affects clinical course.[9] This

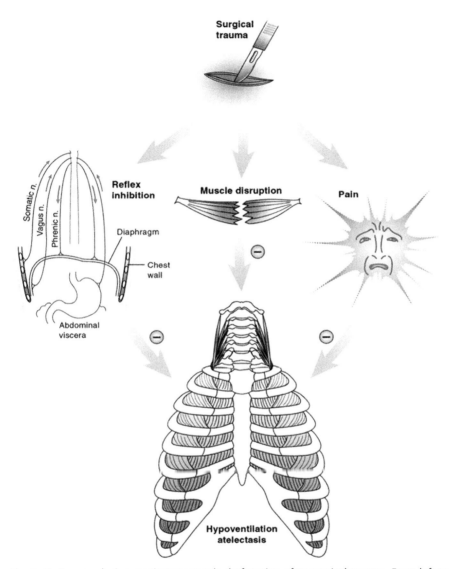

Fig. 1. Factors producing respiratory muscle dysfunction after surgical trauma. From left to right: (1) Surgical trauma stimulates central nervous system reflexes mediated by both visceral and somatic nerves that promote reflex inhibition of the phrenic and other nerves innervating respiratory muscles. (2) Mechanical disruption of the respiratory muscles impairs efficiency. (3) Pain produces voluntary limitation of respiratory motion. These factors tend to reduce lung volumes and can produce hypoventilation and atelectasis. n., nerve. (*From* Warner DO. Preventing postoperative pulmonary complications: the role of the anesthesiologist. Anesthesiology 2000;92(5):1469; with permission.)

list includes several major categories of clinically significant complications,[10,11] including the following:

- Bronchospasm;
- Atelectasis;

- Exacerbation of the underlying chronic lung condition;
- Infection, including bronchitis and pneumonia; and
- Prolonged mechanical ventilation and respiratory failure.

In 1992, Dindo and Clavien proposed a grading system for grading complications, which was modified in 2004[12] (**Box 1**). This serves as a quality assessment tool in patients with postoperative complications from surgery.

PREOPERATIVE RISK ASSESSMENT

A thorough history and physical examination are the most important elements of the preoperative evaluation and risk stratification. A complete history involves assessment of all the risk factors that contribute to the development of PPCs. This evaluation includes an assessment of the general and overall health status and a focused history on pulmonary symptoms including cough, unexplained dyspnea, exercise tolerance, and preexisting lung disease. The risk factors for pulmonary complications can be divided into patient-related risk factors and procedure-related risk factors. **Table 1** summarizes patient-related risk factors.

PULMONARY RISK FACTORS
Smoking

Both a meta-analysis in 2014 and a review of the American College of Surgeons (ACS)-NSQIP database[1] have confirmed that smoking is a significant predictor of PPCs. PCC rates are higher for patients with at least a 20 pack-year smoking history than for those with a lesser pack-year smoking. Smoking cessation for at least 4 weeks before surgery reduces the risk of PPCs, and longer periods of smoking cessation may be even more effective.[13] A lesser duration of preoperative cessation confers less protection against PPCs. In contrast with earlier reports, more recent analyses indicate that briefer durations of cessation do not actually increase PPC risk.

Chronic Obstructive Pulmonary Disease

Chronic obstructive pulmonary disease (COPD) is an important patient-related risk factor for PPCs. In a recent review of patients undergoing major abdominal surgery,

---

Box 1
Examples of grades for postoperative pulmonary complications (Clavien classification)

Grade 1: Atelectasis requiring physiotherapy.

Grade 2: Pneumonia treated with antibiotics.

Grade 3a: Bronchopleural fistula after thoracic surgery requiring surgical closure.

Grade 4a: Respiratory failure needing intubation (single organ dysfunction).

Grade 4b: Respiratory failure needing intubation in combination with renal failure (multiorgan dysfunction).

Grade 5: Death.

Other: 1d for hoarseness after thyroid surgery (the suffix "d" is added for disability for respective grade of complication at discharge).

Adapted from Dindo D, Demartines N, Clavien PA. Classification of surgical complications: a new proposal with evaluation in a cohort of 6336 patients and results of a survey. Ann Surg 2004;240:205; with permission.

Table 1	
Patient-related risk factors for PPCs	
Pulmonary	**Nonpulmonary**
Smoking	Age
Chronic obstructive pulmonary disease	General health status
Asthma	Obesity
Interstitial lung disease	Obstructive sleep apnea
Upper respiratory infection	Pulmonary hypertension
	Heart failure
	Nutritional status
	Dependent functional status
	Neurologic impairment

severe COPD was a significant predictor of PPCs.[1] In patients with severe COPD, the risk of pneumonia carried an odds ratio (OR) of 2.0 (95% CI, 1.8–2.2), unplanned intubation an OR 1.6 (95% CI, 1.4–1.7), and prolonged ventilator dependence (>48 hours) an OR 1.6 (95% CI, 1.4–1.7). In this study, pulmonary history, such as COPD, dyspnea, and smoking, seemed to confer only a moderate risk for developing PPCs. Previous analysis of the NSQIP database[14] showed similar results.

Patients with COPD have an increased risk for PPCs, although there seems to be no prohibitive level of the pulmonary function below which surgery is absolutely contraindicated. Patients with COPD who are particularly high risk based on effort tolerance or spirometric values warrant aggressive preoperative treatment to reduce risk. We describe the specific interventions elsewhere in this article. One must weigh the benefit of surgery against the known risks and even very high-risk patients may proceed to surgery, if the indication is sufficiently compelling.

The onset of an acute pulmonary process or a recent exacerbation of a preexisting lung condition is considered important risk factors for developing PPCs, and their presence is adequate reason to postpone elective surgery. In the NSQIP study, the presence of preexisting pneumonia had an OR of 1.7 for developing postoperative respiratory failure.

Asthma

It is unclear whether a history of asthma is associated with increased rate of clinically significant pulmonary complications. Patient with poorly controlled asthma can have an increased risk of bronchospasm, hypoxemia, hypercapnia, inadequate cough, atelectasis, and pulmonary infection after surgery.[15] Despite early reports indicating that patients with asthma had higher than expected rates of PPCs, more recent studies have found no such complications in patients with well-controlled asthma. In the 2006 guidelines from the American College of Physicians (ACP), the authors suggested that there was good evidence to suggest that asthma is not a risk factor for PPCs.

Interstitial Lung Disease

Patients with pulmonary fibrosis experience a higher rate of morbidity and mortality following resection for lung cancer.[16] There are fewer data about PPCs in patients with interstitial lung disease (ILD) undergoing other types of surgery. In a study involving 336 patients with ILD who underwent major surgery in a tertiary hospital setting, PPCs occurred in 37 patients (11%). Thirteen patients developed pneumonia, the most common PPC, and 11 had acute exacerbation of ILD.[17] Risk factors included lower body mass index (<23 kg/m^2), emergency surgery, and longer duration of anesthesia. The incidence of PPCs after all types of surgery in patients with ILD is not as high as that after lung surgery, but is higher than in the general population.

Upper Respiratory Tract Infection

Few data exist regarding the risk of PPCs in patients with an upper respiratory tract infection. Clinical prudence supports the recommendation of postponing elective surgery during an upper respiratory tract infection, but the evidence supporting this approach is relatively weak. In adults, the risk of bronchospasm, laryngospasm, and desaturation are associated with an upper respiratory tract infection only if symptoms are present or occur within the last 2 weeks before surgery, but this does not increase the morbidity or long-term sequelae.[18]

NONPULMONARY FACTORS
Age

Advanced age is an independent risk factor for PPCs, even after adjusting for comorbidities. In a systematic review prepared for the ACP, advanced age was one of the most important patient-related risk factors.[19] In a more recent review of the ACS-NSQIP database, patients who experienced a PPC were significantly older. When compared with patients less than 60 years old, patients aged 61 to 79 years and 80 years or older had an OR of 1.5 (95% CI, 1.4–1.5) and 2.4 (95% CI, 2.2–2.6), respectively, for developing pulmonary complications. On multivariate analysis age 80 years or older was one of the most important predictors of PPC rates.[1] Therefore, even healthy older patients carry a substantial risk of pulmonary complications after surgery.

General Health Status

The American Society of Anesthesiologist's (ASA) functional status classification (**Table 2**) is a good instrument to evaluate overall physical condition and burden of comorbidities. Higher ASA scores confer higher PPC rates. Advanced ASA score was a significant predictor of PPCs in a recent review that used data from the ACS-NSQIP database. ASA score of greater than 2 was predictive of PPCs. Advanced ASA score increased rates of pneumonia (OR, 4.7; 95% CI, 3.2–6.8), unplanned intubation (OR, 4.4; 95% CI, 3.0–6.7), and prolonged ventilator support for 48 hours or longer (OR, 6.6; 95% CI, 4.3–10.0).[1]

Table 2
American Society of Anesthesiologists (ASA) physical status classification

ASA Class	Class Definition	PPCs Adjusted Odds Ratio (95% CI)
1	A normally healthy patient	Referent
2	A patient with mild systemic disease	1.4 (0.9–2.1)
3	A patient with systemic disease that is not incapacitating	3.3 (2.2–4.9)
4	A patient with an incapacitating systemic disease that is a constant threat to life	6.6 (4.3–10.0)
5	A moribund patient who is not expected to survive for 24 h with or without an operation	NA

Abbreviations: NA, not applicable; PPCs, postoperative pulmonary complications.
Data from Owens WD, Felts JA, Spitznagel EL Jr. ASA physical status classification: a study of consistency of ratings. Anesthesiology 1978;49:239; and Chun KY, Annabelle T, David YL, et al. Pulmonary complications after major abdominal surgery: National Surgical Quality Improvement Program analysis. J Surg Res 2015;198(2):441–9.

Obesity

Obesity was not a significant risk factor for PPC in the 2006 ACP guideline.[19] In a recent review of the ACS-NSQIP database, obesity (body mass index >35 kg/m^2) was not associated with an increase in PPCs. In fact, obesity conferred a slight protective factor against postoperative pneumonia.[1] This confirms previous findings that obesity does not increase the incidence of nosocomial pneumonia.[20] However, body mass index does not take into account individual body types or chest cavity size, for example, that may stratify risk. Obesity is not a significant predictor of PPCs and should not affect patient selection for otherwise high-risk procedures.

Obstructive Sleep Apnea

Obstructive sleep apnea (OSA) is an important risk factor for multiple perioperative complications. OSA may be accompanied by multiple comorbidities and these patients are at increased risk of hypoxemia and hypercapnia in the postoperative period.

In a meta-analysis in 2012, OSA was associated with increased acute respiratory failure (OR, 2.4) and postoperative oxygen desaturation (OR, 2.3).[21] In a database study of more than 6 million operative procedures, OSA was associated with a wide range of increased pulmonary complications. OSA was associated with higher rates of intubation/mechanical ventilation, aspiration pneumonia, and acute respiratory distress syndrome.

OSA is a risk factor for PPCs. In a 2014 practice advisory from the ASA, the authors recommended screening all patients for OSA before surgery.[22] They recommended use of the STOP-BANG tool. Patients with known OSA and patients that are at high risk for OSA should be adequately treated preoperatively with continuous positive airway pressure therapy, which can be continued in the perioperative period.

Pulmonary Hypertension

In a study looking at the impact of pulmonary hypertension on outcomes after noncardiac surgery, patients with pulmonary hypertension experienced a higher morbidity and mortality rate than other high risk historical comparator groups with a higher New York Heart Association class, with other markers of severe pulmonary hypertension being independent risk factors in this cohort.[23] Patients with pulmonary hypertension have an increased risk of congestive heart failure, cardiac arrhythmias, hemodynamic instability, sepsis, and respiratory failure. They had longer duration of intensive care unit and hospital stay and increased readmission rates compared with patients without pulmonary hypertension undergoing noncardiac surgery.

The increased risk of complications in patients with pulmonary hypertension, which may not be modifiable, warrants a careful consideration of the indication for surgery and consideration of canceling surgery or performing a lower risk procedure instead. If the decision is to proceed to surgery, preoperative optimization by personnel skilled in taking care of these patients perioperatively is essential to reduce the potential for adverse outcomes.

Heart Failure

The risk of PPCs may be higher in patients with congestive heart failure than those with COPD. In a systemic review published by the ACCP in 2006, there was good quality evidence that identified congestive heart failure as a significant risk factor for PPCs (OR, 2.93; 95% CI, 1.02–8.43).[19] Congestive heart failure is present in 10% of the individuals over 65 years of age and is a leading cause of postoperative morbidity and mortality for operative procedures.[24]

Chronic Kidney Disease

A serum blood urea nitrogen level of 21 mg/dL or greater was a significant predictor of PPCs in 2 studies by Arozullah and colleagues.[25,26] Increasing levels of blood urea nitrogen increased the risk. In another study by Johnson and colleagues, a preoperative creatinine of 1.5 mg/dL or greater was associated with an increased risk of postoperative respiratory failure (OR, 1.63; 95% CI, 1.49–1.82).

Nutritional Status

Serum albumin concentration is a proxy for nutritional status. In 1 study, a low serum albumin level was the most important predictor of 30-day perioperative morbidity.[14] A serum albumin level of 3.5 g/dL or less was also associated with a higher rate of respiratory failure (OR, 1.485; 95% CI, 1.34–1.64). The 2006 ACP guidelines confirmed the importance of a low albumin level as a predictor of PPCs.[19] A weight loss of greater than 10% in the past 6 months is also an independent risk factor for PPCs.[27]

Dependent Functional Status

In a recent review of the ACS-NSQIP data, dependent functional status (the need for help with daily activities of living) was one of the most important risk factors for PPCs. The OR for pneumonia was 2.6 (95% CI, 2.2–3.1), unplanned intubation OR was 2.3 (95% CI, 1.9–2.9), and prolonged ventilator support (≥48 hours) OR was 2.9 (95% CI, 2.5–3.5).[1] In another study of patients undergoing high-risk surgery, patients who were unable to climb 2 flights of stairs regardless of etiology, had increased cardiopulmonary complications.[28]

Neurologic Impairment

Preoperative neurologic impairment and residual deficits from a previous stroke have been associated with an increased risk of PPCs in more than 1 study.[29] This could probably be because of an increased risk of occurrence of aspiration of gastric or pharyngeal secretions. Altered sensorium is an independent predictor of respiratory failure. Postoperative delirium and confusion increase the risk of pneumonia and respiratory failure.[30]

PROCEDURE-RELATED RISK FACTORS FOR POSTOPERATIVE PULMONARY COMPLICATIONS
Surgical Site

The surgical site is the single most significant factor in predicting the risk of the PPCs.[1] The incidence of the PPCs is inversely related to the distance of the surgical incision from the diaphragm. Major abdominal surgery, particularly upper abdominal procedures results in the diaphragmatic dysfunction, a well-known documented cause of PPCs.[31,32] This is likely to be related to the promotion of low lung volumes and atelectasis. Among the general surgical procedures, the greatest risk factor for PPCs was esophagectomy. The pulmonary complication rate is significantly higher for thoracic and upper abdominal surgery than for lower abdominal and other procedures.[11,33] Major vascular surgery, including abdominal aortic aneurysm repair, head and neck surgery, and neurosurgery, are also associated with a higher risk for PPCs.[27,33]

Duration of Surgery

In the 2015 NSQIP review, the average operating time and the anesthesia times were significantly longer in PPCs present group compared with the PPCs absent group. In the multivariate analyses, prolonged operative time was one of the strongest predictor of pulmonary complications.[1]

In a previous study, patients undergoing procedures longer than 3 to 4 hours had a greater incidence of pulmonary complications (40%) compared with those undergoing surgeries shorter than 2 hours (8%).[34] It is not clear, however, if the duration of the procedure has an effect on PPCs independent of the type and complexity of the procedure itself. Patients in the PPCs present group in the 2015 NSQIP review also experienced more bleeding, cardiac, renal, neurologic, thromboembolic, and infectious complications. Therefore, the duration of the procedure along with its complexity may play a role in the development of PPCs.

Type of Anesthesia and Analgesia

Whether spinal or epidural anesthesia causes fewer PPCs when compared with general anesthesia has been controversial. A study by Rodgers and colleagues[35] reported no difference in patients anesthetized with spinal or general anesthesia for abdominal surgery. This was confirmed in another report of patients undergoing transurethral prostate surgery.[33]

A review of high-risk patients found that the rate of respiratory failure was significantly higher with general anesthesia than with epidural analgesia and light anesthesia.[36] Many other studies have found high rates of respiratory failure in patients undergoing general anesthesia compared with spinal or epidural anesthesia. In another large systematic review of literature looking at 141 trials,[35] there was a reduction in risk of pulmonary complications among patients receiving neuraxial blockade (either spinal or epidural anesthesia) with or without general anesthesia, when compared with those receiving general anesthesia alone. Patients who received epidural analgesia after abdominal aortic aneurysm repair had fewer complications than those receiving parenteral opioids.[37]

Therefore, based on all the studies reviewed, it seems that general anesthesia leads to a higher risk of clinically important pulmonary complications than does epidural or spinal anesthesia, although further research is needed to confirm this. Spinal or epidural anesthesia is safer and should be considered in high-risk patients, when suitable. Regional nerve block is associated with lower risk and can also be considered in high-risk patients.

Neuromuscular Blockade

Residual neuromuscular blockade remains a common and often undetected occurrence in the early postoperative period.[38] Residual neuromuscular blockade results in reduction in forced vital capacity and peak expiratory flow in the immediate postoperative period, indicating impaired respiratory muscle function. It leads to impaired diaphragmatic function, impaired mucociliary clearance owing to poor cough, and ultimately leads to PPCs.

In a study by Berg and colleagues,[39] the use of an intermediate acting neuromuscular blocking agent (atracurium and vecuronium) in comparison with longer acting agents (pancuronium) led to a significantly reduced incidence of residual neuromuscular blockade (5.3% vs 26%; $P<.001$). The patients in the pancuronium group developed more PPCs when compared with the patients in the atracurium/vecuronium group. Thus, it is important to use a neuromuscular blocking agent judiciously with monitoring to minimize the incidence of residual neuromuscular block in the postoperative period.

Open Versus Laparoscopic Surgery

The choice of surgical approach may significantly affect the PPCs. A meta-analysis examining laparoscopic versus open resection of colorectal cancer demonstrated faster postoperative recovery defined by spirometry (3 studies), and 21% shorter hospital duration of stay (9 studies); however, the difference in risk and complications between the 2 surgical methods were not different.[40] Although supported by improvements in duration of stay, postoperative pain, surgical risk, and spirometric data, it is unclear whether clinically important PPCs are minimized with use of laparoscopic procedures.

In another review looking at PPCs after laparoscopic and open procedures, 2 studies reported a reduction in atelectasis after laparoscopic surgery compared with open cholecystectomy (2% vs 4%; $P<.001$), and less frequent PPCs after laparoscopic versus open sigmoid resection (2.5% vs 6%; $P<.001$).[41,42]

Laparoscopic procedures may use small incisions, lead to less postoperative pain, and the reduced manipulation of visceral organs may minimize the adverse effects on respiratory muscle. However, the impact of minimally invasive procedure in predicting significant PPCs is less well-established.

Emergency Surgery

In the ACP report,[19] among the studies reporting multivariate analyses, 6 reported emergency surgery as a significant predictor of PPCs, the OR was 2.21 (95% CI, 1.57–3.11).[21]

PHYSICAL EXAMINATION

A detailed physical examination is an important part of the preoperative evaluation. It may allow detection of unrecognized preexisting lung disease. Clinicians should seek signs suggestive of asthma, COPD, OSA, right heart failure (suggestive of cor pulmonale), pulmonary hypertension, neurologic impairment, neuromuscular weakness, and spinal deformities that might modify PPC risk. Most patients undergoing nonthoracic procedures, regardless of the type, may not benefit from preoperative pulmonary function tests and may proceed to surgery without further evaluation.

PREOPERATIVE PULMONARY TESTS

Preoperative tests would be valuable if they provide information that cannot be obtained from history and physical examination and if it helps to determine the probability of a complication in patients who are known to have risk factors. The commonly available preoperative tests as a part of pulmonary risk assessment include the following:

1. Pulmonary function tests;
2. Arterial blood gas;
3. Chest radiograph (CXR); and
4. Exercise testing.

Pulmonary Function Test

Available pulmonary function tests include spirometry, flow volume loops, diffusion capacity for carbon monoxide, cardiopulmonary exercise testing (CPET), and ventilation–perfusion scan. Spirometry is the most commonly performed test in clinical practice.

It is uncertain in what setting pulmonary function tests should be ordered for risk stratification.[43] In the absence of controlled trails that demonstrate that pulmonary function testing is associated with improved outcome, it is difficult to recommend pulmonary function tests as a prerequisite for any patient or operative procedure. There is also a concern that there is an overuse of preoperative pulmonary function tests. A recent study, however, showed that after the publication of the ACP guidelines regarding assessment for PPCs in 2006, the trends of preoperative pulmonary function tests before elective noncardiothoracic surgery decreased significantly.[44]

Bedside spirometry is readily available and measures of forced expiratory volume in 1 second (FEV_1) and forced vital capacity have been proposed as tests to predict PPCs. In a study by McAlister and colleagues,[45] pulmonary function testing data were significantly associated with the incidence of PPCs, but none of the pulmonary function test variables were found to be independent predictors of PPCs by multivariate analyses. In another study, preoperative pulmonary function tests did not predict the risk of PPCs in patients with severe COPD (FEV_1 <50% predicted), whereas duration of surgery, ASA class, and type of procedure were significant predictors.[34]

More recent and rigorous studies either failed to demonstrate a correlation between pulmonary function tests and the incidence of PPCs or could not confirm by multivariate analyses that pulmonary function tests data are independent predictors of PPCs. In most studies of preoperative pulmonary function tests, the incremental value beyond clinical evaluation has not been reported.

Regarding pulmonary function tests as a preoperative test:

1. The 2006 ACP guidelines recommend that clinicians not use preoperative spirometry routinely for predicting the risk of PPCs before general surgical procedures or other high-risk surgeries.
2. Pulmonary function test results should not be used as a primary factor to deny surgery.
3. Consider pulmonary function tests for patients with dyspnea or exercise intolerance that remains unexplained by clinical examination.
4. Pulmonary function tests may be helpful for patients with COPD or asthma if clinical evaluation cannot determine whether the patient is at their best baseline and that airflow obstruction is optimally reduced.

Chest Radiograph

As a part of a routine preoperative evaluation, many clinicians frequently obtain a CXR in older patients, in patients with known pulmonary diseases, and in patients who smoke. However, clinicians may predict most abnormal preoperative CXRs by history and physical examination alone; the CXR may rarely provide unexpected information that influences preoperative management. Hence, CXRs add little to the clinical evaluation in identifying healthy patients at risk for PPCs.

In a meta-analysis looking at the value of routine CXR, Archer and colleagues[46] found that routine preoperative CXRs were low yield for abnormalities that actually change preoperative management. The prevalence of abnormal CXRs increases with age but it is difficult to determine by any evidence-based approach as to which patients will benefit from a preoperative CXR. According to the ACP review, it is reasonable to obtain a CXR in patients with known cardiopulmonary disease and those older than 50 years of age who are undergoing a high-risk surgical procedure like upper abdominal, esophageal, thoracic, or aortic surgery.

Arterial Blood Gas

Arterial blood gas analysis has been used in the past for the preoperative evaluation of non-thoracic surgery patients despite the lack of strong evidence suggesting their value. Patients with hypercapnia (partial pressure of carbon dioxide in arterial blood [$Paco_2$] >45 mm Hg) have been considered high risk from PPCs and mortality.[47]

However, no data suggest that hypercapnia identifies high-risk patients who would not have otherwise been identified based on established clinical risk factors. Hypercapnia is not an absolute contraindication to major noncardiac surgery.

Arterial hypoxemia has been considered as a risk factor for PPCs and a contraindication for surgery. One study reported an association between preoperative hypoxemia and PPCs in patients undergoing surgery for gastric or esophageal cancer.[48] Neither hypoxemia nor hypercapnia have been identified as significant independent predictors of the risk for PPCs.

Exercise Testing

CPET has been used as a screening test in patients undergoing cardiothoracic and nonthoracic surgery and found to predict mortality. Smith and colleagues[49] looked at the predictive value of maximum oxygen consumption (Vo_2 max) and anaerobic threshold obtained during CPET in calculating the morbidity and mortality. They evaluated 9 studies and concluded that Vo_2 max and to a lesser extent the anaerobic threshold are valid predictors of perioperative morbidity and mortality. The quality of data in this review had multiple limitations, so further studies should be conducted before CPET can be recommended as an independent predictor of PPCs before nonthoracic surgery and to define the impact of CPET on the perioperative management. Simple measurements of exercise capacity like stair climbing capacity and the 6-minute walk test are easy to perform and do not need specialized equipment. They have also shown good accuracy and concordance when compared with Vo_2 max.[50]

Echocardiography

There is no evidence currently to support the routine use of echocardiography to detect pulmonary hypertension in the preoperative evaluation of nonthoracic surgery, even in patients with advanced pulmonary disease. However, it may be reasonable to obtain an echocardiogram in those patients with severe lung disease who have signs and symptoms compatible to right heart dysfunction or who have significantly reduced exercise tolerance, to rule out cardiac issues.

RISK SCORES

Risk scores can be useful if they can provide a clear estimate of the probability of a perioperative complication. This information can then be used to stratify the risk and guide the therapeutic options. It can also be used to advise patients regarding perioperative risks and expectations, optimize patients that are at high risk, and plan the postoperative management appropriately.

Four risk indices provide a numerical estimate of the risk rather than a qualitative category of risk. Most of them are derived from patients in the NSQIP database. They are:

1. ARISCAT (Canet) Risk Index[51] – 2010;
2. Gupta Calculator For Postoperative Respiratory Failure[52] – 2011;
3. Gupta Calculator For Postoperative Pneumonia[53] – 2013; and
4. Arozullah Respiratory Failure Index[25] – 2000.

The Arozullah respiratory failure index (**Tables 3** and **4**) identified 6 factors that predict PPCs after adjustment for confounders into consideration. Point scores are assigned based on the strength of association in the multivariate analysis, and patients are stratified into 5 classes with respiratory failure ranging from 0.5% to 26.6%.[29]

Table 3
Arozullah respiratory failure index

Preoperative Predictor	Point Value
Type of surgery	
Abdominal aortic aneurysm	27
Thoracic	21
Neurosurgery, upper abdominal, peripheral vascular	14
Neck	11
Emergency surgery	11
Albumin <3.0 g/dL	9
BUN >30 mg/dL	8
Partially or fully dependent functional status	7
History of chronic obstructive pulmonary disease	6
Age (y)	
>70	6
60–69	4

Abbreviation: BUN, blood urea nitrogen.

From Arozullah AM, Daley J, Henderson WG, et al. Multifactorial risk index for predicting postoperative respiratory failure in men after major noncardiac surgery. Ann Surg 2000;232(2):250; with permission.

Table 4
Performance of the Arozullah respiratory failure index

Class	Point Total	Percent Respiratory Failure
1	≤10	0.5
2	11–19	1.0
3	20–27	4.2
4	28–40	10.1
5	>40	26.6

Adapted from Arozullah AM, Daley J, Henderson WG, et al. Multifactorial risk index for predicting postoperative respiratory failure in men after major noncardiac surgery. Ann Surg 2000;232(2):250; with permission.

The ARISCAT risk index[51] (**Table 5**) includes 7 independent risk factors of any severity that predict PPC rates. Each factor is assigned a weighted score and patients are stratified as low, intermediate, and high risk for developing pulmonary complications.

The Gupta calculator for postoperative respiratory failure uses multiple preoperative factors to predict risk of failure to wean from mechanical ventilation within 48 hours of surgery or unplanned intubation/reintubation postoperatively.[52] The Gupta calculator for postoperative pneumonia is derived in a similar manner to the respiratory failure calculator. Use of Gupta calculators requires use of downloadable interactive spreadsheets.[53]

Table 5
ARISCAT risk index

Factor	Adjusted Odds Ratio (95% CI)	Risk Score
Age (y)		
≤50	1	—
51–80	1.4 (0.6–3.3)	3
>80	5.1 (1.9–13.3)	16
Preoperative oxygen saturation (%)		
≥96	1	—
91–95	2.2 (1.2–4.2)	8
≤90	10.7 (4.1–28.1)	24
Respiratory infection in the last month	5.5 (2.6–11.5)	17
Preoperative anemia (hemoglobin ≤10 g/dL)	3.0 (1.4–6.5)	11
Surgical incision		
Upper abdominal	4.4 (2.3–8.5)	15
Intrathoracic	11.4 (1.9–26.0)	24
Duration of surgery (h)		
≤2	1	
2–3	4.9 (2.4–10.1)	16
>3	9.7 (2.4–19.9)	23
Emergency surgery	2.2 (1.0–4.5)	8

Risk Class	Number of Points in Risk Score	PPC Rate (Validation Sample), %
Low	<26	1.6
Intermediate	26–44	13.3
High	≥45	42.1

Adapted from Canet J, Gallart L, Gomar C, et al. Prediction of postoperative pulmonary complications in a population-based surgical cohort. Anesthesiology 2010;113:1338; with permission.

PERIOPERATIVE STRATEGIES TO DECREASE POSTOPERATIVE PULMONARY COMPLICATIONS

After identifying patients at high risk for PPC, one should use strategies to minimize risks and prevent complications. Some risk factors are not modifiable before surgery, whereas others may provide a target for risk reduction. Interventions that have proven to reduce PPC rates in high risk patients include the following:

- Preoperative:
  1. Smoking cessation (≥8 weeks is optimal);
  2. Optimizing airflow limitation in patients with COPD and asthma;
  3. Treat lower respiratory tract infections when present; and
  4. Lung expansion techniques – incentive spirometry and chest physical therapy.
- Intraoperative:
  1. Consider intraoperative analgesia with spinal, epidural, or regional technique when indicated;
  2. Avoid use of long-acting neuromuscular blockers;
  3. Intraoperative recruitment maneuvers to prevent atelectasis;
  4. Laparoscopic versus open surgery – consider less invasive surgery; and
  5. Fluid management – fluid optimization with goal-directed therapy.[54]

- Postoperative:
  1. Selective nasogastric tube decompression after abdominal surgery;
  2. Nutritional support;
  3. Lung expansion maneuvers; and
  4. Epidural analgesia.

With a comprehensive knowledge of the perioperative pulmonary assessment of patients undergoing surgery, it is possible to prevent perioperative pulmonary complications and improve outcomes.

SUMMARY

1. Almost 25% of postoperative deaths that occur during the first postoperative week are associated with PPCs.
2. The most significant predictors of the PPCs are ASA physical status, advanced age, dependent functional status, surgical site, and duration of surgery.
3. COPD, dyspnea, and smoking seem to confer only a moderate risk when compared with other patient-related factors and surgical site.
4. The overall risk of PPCs can be predicted using scores that incorporate readily available clinical data.
5. Do not routinely perform pulmonary function tests before high-risk noncardiothoracic surgery.

REFERENCES

1. Chun KY, Annabelle T, David YL, et al. Pulmonary complications after major abdominal surgery: National Surgical Quality Improvement Program analysis. J Surg Res 2015;198(2):441–9.
2. Sabate S, Mazo V, Canet J. Predicting postoperative complications: implications for outcomes and costs. Curr Opin Anesthesiol 2014;27:201.
3. Fergusson MK. Preoperative assessment of pulmonary risk. Chest 1999;115:585.
4. Hull NF. Trends in healthcare and the role of the anesthesiologist in the perioperative surgical home- the US perspective. Curr Opin Anesthesiol 2014;27:371.
5. Meyers JR, Lembeck L, O'Kane H, et al. Changes in functional residual capacity of the lung after operation. Arch Surg 1975;110:576.
6. Djokovic JL, Hedley-Whyte J. Prediction of outcomes of surgery and anesthesia in patients over 80. JAMA 1979;242:2301.
7. Sughimachi K, Ueo H, Natsusa Y, et al. Cough dynamics in esophageal cancer: prevention of postoperative pulmonary complications. Br J Surg 1982;69:734.
8. Hulzebos EH, Van Meteren NL, De Bie RA, et al. Prediction of postoperative pulmonary complications on the basis of preoperative risk factors in patients who have undergone coronary artery bypass graft surgery. Phys Ther 2003;83:8–16.
9. O'Donohue WJ Jr. Postoperative pulmonary complications. When are preventive and therapeutic measures necessary? Postgrad Med 1992;91:167.
10. Hall JC, Tarala RA, Hall JL, et al. A multivariate analysis of the risk of pulmonary complications after laparotomy. Chest 1991;99:923.
11. Gracey DR, Divertie MB, Didier EP. Preoperative pulmonary preparation of patients with chronic obstructive pulmonary disease: a prospective study. Chest 1979;76:123.
12. Dindo D, Demartines N, Clavien PA. Classification of surgical complications: a new proposal with evaluation in a cohort of 6336 patients and results of a survey. Ann Surg 2004;240:205.

13. Gronkjaer M, Eliasen M, Skov-Ettrup LS, et al. Preoperative smoking status and postoperative complications: a systemic review and meta-analysis. Ann Surg 2014;259:52.

14. Gupta H, Ramanan B, Gupta PK, et al. Impact of COPD on postoperative outcomes: results from the national database. Chest 2013;143:1599.

15. National Asthma Education and Prevention Program (NAEPP) Coordinating Committee. Expert panel report 3: guidelines for the diagnosis and management of asthma. Bethesda (MD): National Heart, Lung, and Blood Institute; 2007.

16. Kumar P, Goldstraw P, Yamada K, et al. Pulmonary fibrosis and lung cancer: risk and benefit analysis of pulmonary resection. J Thorac Cardiovasc Surg 2003;125: 1321.

17. Choi SM, Lee J, Park YS, et al. Postoperative pulmonary complications after surgery in patients with interstitial lung disease. Respiration 2014;87:287.

18. Tait AR, Malviya S. Anesthesia for the child with an upper respiratory tract infection: still a dilemma? Anesth Analg 2005;100:59.

19. Smetana GW, Lawrence VA, Cornell JE. American College of Physicians. Preoperative pulmonary risk stratification for noncardiothoracic surgery: systematic review for the American College of Physicians. Ann Intern Med 2006;144:581.

20. Phung DT, Wang Z, Rutherford S, et al. Body mass index and risk of pneumonia: a systematic review and meta-analysis. Obes Rev 2013;14:839.

21. Kaw R, Chung F, Pasupuleti V, et al. Meta-analysis of the association between obstructive sleep apnea and postoperative outcome. Br J Anaesth 2012; 109(6):897–906.

22. American Society of Anesthesiologists Task Force on Perioperative Management of Patients with Obstructive Sleep Apnea. Practical guidelines for the perioperative management of patients with obstructive sleep apnea: an updated report by the American Society of Anesthesiologists Task Force on perioperative management of patients with obstructive sleep apnea. Anesthesiology 2014;120:268.

23. Ramakrishna G, Sprung GW, Ravi BS, et al. Impact of pulmonary hypertension on the outcomes of non-cardiac surgery; predictors of perioperative morbidity and mortality. J Am Coll Cardiol 2005;45:1691.

24. Ji Q, Mei Y, Wang X, et al. Risk factors for pulmonary complications following cardiac surgery with cardiopulmonary bypass. Int J Med Sci 2013;10:1578.

25. Arozullah AM, Daley J, Henderson WG, et al. Multifactorial risk index for predicting postoperative respiratory failure in men after major non cardiac surgery. The National Veterans Administration Surgical Quality Improvement Program. Ann Surg 2000;232:242.

26. Arozullah AM, Khuri SF, Henderson WG, et al. Development and validation of a multifactorial risk index for predicting postoperative pneumonia after major non-cardiac surgery. Ann Intern Med 2001;135:847.

27. McCullock TM, Jensen NF, Girod DA, et al. Risk factors for pulmonary complications in the postoperative head and neck surgery patients. Head Neck 1997;19:372.

28. Nikolic I, Plavec D, Maloca I, et al. Stair climbing test with pulse oximetry as predictor of early postoperative complications in functionally impaired patients with lung cancer and elective lung surgery: prospective trail of consecutive series of patients. Croat Med J 2008;49:50.

29. Arozullah AM, Conde MV, Lawrence VA. Preoperative evaluation for postoperative pulmonary complications. Med Clin North Am 2003;112:219.

30. Ganai S, Lee KF, Merrill A, et al. Adverse outcomes of geriatric patients undergoing abdominal surgery who are at high risk for delirium. Arch Surg 2007;142: 1072.

31. Berdah SV, Picaud R, Jammes Y. Surface diaphragmatic electromyogram changes after laparotomy. Clin Physiol Funct Imaging 2002;22:69.
32. Ferreyra G, Long Y, Ranieri VM. Respiratory complications after major surgery. Curr Opin Crit Care 2009;15:342.
33. Brooks-Brunn JA. Predictors of postoperative pulmonary complications following abdominal surgery. Chest 1997;111:564.
34. Qaseem A, Snow V, Fillerman N, et al. Risk assessment for and strategies to reduce perioperative complications for patients undergoing noncardiothoracic surgery: a guideline from the American College of Physicians. Ann Intern Med 2006;144:575.
35. Rodgers A, Walker N, Schug S, et al. Reduction of postoperative mortality and morbidity with epidural or spinal anaesthesia: results from overview of random-ized trials. BMJ 2000;321:1493.
36. Yeager MP, Glass DD, Neff RK, et al. Epidural anesthesia and analgesia in high risk surgical patients. Anesthesiology 1987;66:729.
37. Major CP Jr, Greer MS, Russell WL, et al. Postoperative pulmonary complications and morbidity after abdominal aneurysmectomy: a comparison of postoperative epidural versus parenteral opioid analgesia. Am Surg 1996;62:45.
38. Cammu G, De Witte J, De Veylder J, et al. Postoperative residual paralysis in out-patients vs inpatients. Anesth Analg 2006;102:426.
39. Berg H, Roed J, Viby-Mogensen J, et al. Residual neuromuscular block is a risk factor for postoperative pulmonary complications. A prospective, randomized, and blinded study of postoperative pulmonary complications after atracurium, vecuronium and pancuronium. Acta Anaesthesiol Scand 1997;41:1095.
40. Abraham NS, Young JM, Solomon MJ. Meta-analysis of short-term outcomes after laparoscopic resection for colorectal cancer. Br J Surg 2004;91:1111.
41. Guller V, Jain N, Hervey S, et al. Laparoscopic vs open colectomy: outcomes comparison based on large nationwide database. Arch Surg 2003;138:1179.
42. Zacks SL, Sanders RS, Rutledge R, et al. A population based cohort study comparing laparoscopic cholecystectomy and open cholecystectomy. Am J Gaotroenterol 2002;97:334.
43. Lawrence VA, Page CP, Harris GD. Preoperative spirometry before abdominal procedures. A critical appraisal of its predictive value. Arch Intern Med 1989; 149:280.
44. Sun LY, Gershon AS, Ko DT, et al. Trends in pulmonary function testing before non-cardiothoracic surgery. JAMA Intern Med 2015;175(8):1410–2.
45. McAlister FA, Khan NA, Straus SE, et al. Accuracy of the preoperative assess-ment in predicting pulmonary risk after non-thoracic surgery. Am J Respir Crit Care Med 2003;167:741.
46. Archer C, Levy AR, McGregor M. Value of routine preoperative chest x-rays: a meta-analysis. Can J Anaesth 1993;40:1022.
47. Tisi GM. Preoperative evaluation of pulmonary function: validity, indications, and benefits. Am Rev Respir Dis 1979;119:293.
48. Fan ST, Lau WY, Yip WC, et al. Prediction of postoperative pulmonary complica-tions in esophagogastric cancer surgery. Br J Surg 1987;74:408.
49. Smith TB, Stonell C, Purkayastha S, et al. Cardiopulmonary exercise testing as a risk assessment method in non-cardiopulmonary surgery: a systematic review. Anaesthesia 2009;64:883.
50. Cataneo DC, Kobayasi S, Paccanaro RC, et al. Accuracy of six minute walk test, stair test and spirometry using maximal oxygen uptake as a gold standard. Acta Cir Bras 2010;25:194.

51. Canet J, Gallart L, Gomar C, et al. Prediction of postoperative pulmonary complications in a population based cohort. Anesthesiology 2010;113:1338.
52. Gupta H, Gupta PK, Fang X, et al. Development and validation of a risk calculator predicting respiratory failure. Chest 2011;140:1207.
53. Gupta H, Gupta PK, Schuller D, et al. Development and validation of a risk calculator for predicting postoperative pneumonia. Mayo Clin Proc 2013;88: 1241.
54. Cocoran T, Clarke S, Myles PS, et al. Perioperative fluid management strategies in major surgery: a stratified meta-analysis. Anesth Analg 2012;114:640.

Stratification and Risk Reduction of Perioperative Acute Kidney Injury

 CrossMark

Selma Ishag, MBBS, MD[a],*, Charuhas V. Thakar, MD[b,c]

KEYWORDS

- Acute kidney injury • Chronic kidney disease • Preoperative evaluation
- Renal protection strategies

KEY POINTS

- Acute kidney injury (AKI) is a frequently encountered complication in surgical patients and can lead to significant morbidity in the immediate and distant postoperative periods.
- Preoperative risk stratification is critical for informed consent and perioperative planning. Potential preoperative interventions, such as hematocrit and blood glucose optimization, and continuation of angiotensin-receptor blockers and statins may have a protective role.
- Perioperative renal protection strategies, including goal-directed fluid therapy, avoidance of hyperchloremic crystalloid solutions, and maintenance of hemodynamics within the renal autoregulation curve, are potentially invaluable in the prevention of AKI. Current advances in the development of biomarkers may offer the opportunity for early diagnosis and the implementation of therapeutic strategies.
- Increased awareness and concerted efforts by all perioperative physicians are needed to provide an improved outcome for surgical patients.

DEFINITION

Acute kidney injury (AKI) is a frequently encountered complication in surgical patients and can lead to significant morbidity in the immediate and distant postoperative periods. The most recent consensus for its diagnosis and staging by the Kidney Disease: Improving Global Outcomes (KDIGO) Work Group[1] defines AKI as a decrease in kidney function resulting in either an absolute increase in serum creatinine (sCr) of 0.3 mg/dL or more within 48 hours, an increase in sCr of 1.5 times from baseline that has occurred

a Division of General Anesthesiology, Barnes-Jewish Hospital, Washington University, South Campus, Campus Box 8054, 660 South Euclid Avenue, St Louis, MO 63110-1093, USA; b Division of Nephrology, Kidney CARE Program, University of Cincinnati, 231 Albert Sabin Way, Cincinnati, OH 45267, USA; c Renal Section, Cincinnati VA Medical Center, 231 Albert Sabin Way, Cincinnati, OH 45267, USA
* Corresponding author.
E-mail address: ishags@anest.wustl.edu

Anesthesiology Clin 34 (2016) 89–99
http://dx.doi.org/10.1016/j.anclin.2015.10.009   anesthesiology.theclinics.com
1932-2275/16/$ – see front matter © 2016 Elsevier Inc. All rights reserved.

within the prior 7 days, or a urine volume of 0.5 mL/kg/h or less for more than 6 hours.[1] Three stages of AKI have been classified according to these criteria (**Table 1**).

EPIDEMIOLOGY

The incidence of AKI varies within the range of 5.0% to 7.5% in all acute care hospitalizations and is approximately 20% in intensive care unit (ICU) admissions. Nearly 40% of AKI in hospitalized patients occurs in the perioperative period.[2] The incidence of AKI varies depending on the surgical setting (**Fig. 1**). Most of the authors' knowledge regarding AKI is from the cardiovascular surgery literature. This information is reviewed as well as emerging data from other surgical settings.

RISK STRATIFICATION BASED ON SURGICAL SETTING

Kheterpal and colleagues[3] developed a preoperative renal-risk index in *major noncardiovascular surgical procedures* that identified the following as independent risk factors for postoperative AKI: age greater than 59 years, body mass index (BMI) greater than 32, high-risk surgery (anticipated hospital stay of 2 or more days, emergency surgery, peripheral vascular disease, liver disease, and chronic obstructive pulmonary disease [COPD]). Based on the number of risk factors in patients with a normal baseline glomerular filtration rate (GFR), the incidence of postoperative renal failure, as defined by an absolute GFR of less than 50 mL/min, ranged between 0.3% and 4.3% (**Table 2**).

In bariatric patients undergoing *gastric bypass surgery*, the incidence of postoperative AKI as defined by an increase in sCr of 50% or dialysis requirement was 8.5%.[4] The higher BMI of gastric bypass patients is combined with other risk factors, namely, hyperlipidemia and preoperative use of angiotensin-converting enzyme inhibitors (ACEIs) or angiotensin receptor blockers (ARBs).

A study by Kim and colleagues[5] used a less sensitive definition for AKI of an increase in sCr of greater than 2 mg/dL above the baseline and/or dialysis in *intra-abdominal surgical procedures* and found an overall incidence of AKI of 1.1%, ranging from 0.2% in appendectomies and 0.3% for gastric bypass surgery to 3.5% in exploratory laparotomy patients.

In patients undergoing *orthopedic surgery*, a recent study by Kimmel and colleagues[6] describes an AKI incidence of 15% following elective total joint arthroplasty (TJA) in a population that was older and more obese and included patients with

Table 1		
Stages of severity of AKI according to AKIN criteria		
Stage	**Change in sCr**	**Urine Output**
I	Increased Cr 0.3 mg/dL or 1.5–2.0 fold of baseline	UOP <0.5 mL/kg/h for >6 h
II	Cr increase of >2–3 fold of baseline	UOP <0.5 mL/kg/h for >12 h
III	Cr increase >3 fold of baseline (or Cr >4 mg/dL with 0.5 mg/dL acute increase); AKI requiring dialysis	UOP <0.3 mL/kg/h for 24 h or anuria for 12 h

Abbreviations: AKIN, Acute Kidney Injury Network; Cr, creatinine; UOP, urine output.

Adapted from Kellum JA, Lameire N, Aspelin P, et al. Kidney Disease: Improving Global Outcomes (KDIGO) acute kidney injury work group. KDIGO clinical practice guideline for acute kidney injury. Kidney Int Suppl 2012;2:1–138; with permission.

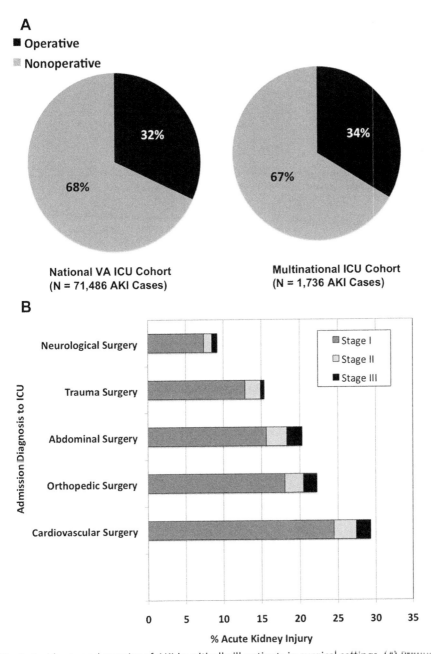

Fig. 1. Incidence and severity of AKI in critically ill patients in surgical settings. (*A*) Proportion of AKI cases attributable to surgical settings. (*B*) Incidence of AKI in major surgical settings in ICU. VA, veteran's administration. (*From* Thakar CV. Perioperative acute kidney injury. Adv Chronic Kidney Dis 2013;20(1):67–75; with permission.)

Table 2		
Incidence and risk factors of AKI after noncardiovascular surgery		
Risk Factors	Risk Category	AKI Frequency (%)
Age >59 y	Class I (0 risk factors)	0.3
BMI >32	Class II (1 risk factor)	0.5
Emergency surgery	Class III (2 risk factors)	1.3
High-risk surgery	Class IV (≥3 risk factors)	4.3
Peripheral vascular disease COPD Liver disease	—	—

From Thakar CV. Perioperative acute kidney injury. Adv Chronic Kidney Dis 2013;20(1):67–75; with permission.

preexisting renal dysfunction in comparison with the relatively younger, healthier patients studied by Weingarten and colleagues[7] who exhibited an incidence of less than 2% in elective TJAs. In a recent report based on a national inpatient survey, Nadkarni and colleagues[8] indicated that over a 10-year period, the incidence of AKI has increased 4-fold ($P<.0001$). Preoperative chronic kidney disease, which is prevalent in such patient populations, was among the most important risk factor for AKI. Additionally, postoperative events, including myocardial infarction, need for cardiac catheterization, sepsis, and need for transfusions, were most commonly associated with AKI. Most importantly, patients with perioperative AKI were at a significantly high risk of hospital mortality (odds ratio, 11.32, $P<.0001$); those who survived had a 2-times greater risk of an adverse discharge (defined as nursing home or long-term acute care). Thus, in an era when we are expected to see more than doubling of hip and knee surgeries, even a modest frequency of postoperative AKI can have significant impact on both patients and the health care system.

Transplant recipients are a particularly vulnerable group of patients to develop postoperative renal dysfunction for multiple reasons, including preexisting renal impairment, infections, and the use of nephrotoxic drugs and calcineurin inhibitors.[9] Postoperatively, one-third of *liver transplant* recipients develop AKI, with up to 17% of patients requiring dialysis.[10–13] Multiple factors contribute to this high incidence of AKI. In the immediate postoperative period, acute tubular necrosis and prerenal azotemia are the main causes, whereas sepsis and calcineurin inhibitor toxicity were implicated in this complication in postoperative weeks 2 to 4.[10] Risk factors associated with AKI in liver transplant recipients included serum albumin less than 3.2 g/dL, baseline impaired renal function, dopamine use, and graft dysfunction as well as bacterial infection/sepsis being associated with late AKI (2–4 weeks postoperatively).

Recently, Grimm and colleagues[14] found an incidence of postoperative renal failure necessitating dialysis in *lung transplant* patients to be 5.5%, which is consistent with previous studies. They described a Risk Stratification Score that includes race, diagnosis, BMI, preexisting renal function, diabetes, and so forth, and predicts a rate of renal failure of 3.1% in the lowest risk group, increasing up to 15.6% in the highest risk category.

Cardiac transplantation imposes its specific risks for AKI. Insulin requiring diabetes mellitus, preoperative renal dysfunction, and prolonged cold-ischemia time were associated with a higher incidence of AKI, whereas a higher preoperative albumin level was associated with a lower risk of dialysis-requiring renal dysfunction.[15–17]

In *kidney transplant* recipients, the diagnosis of AKI is complicated by repeated and rapid changes in graft function, in part secondary to different ischemia-reperfusion recovery courses, titration of immunosuppression dosages, and postoperative fluid shifts. Kidney transplant AKI is associated with poor long-term graft prognosis and may be represented by delayed graft function (DGF) as defined by the need for dialysis within the first posttransplant week. Postprocurement efforts to reduce DGF include machine perfusion, cold storage techniques, and reductions in cold ischemia time. Preorgan retrieval management goals, including mean arterial pressure, central venous pressure, vasopressor use, and so forth, instituted early before organ recovery was associated with significantly less DGF.[18]

The incidence of dialysis requiring AKI following *cardiac surgery* is less than 5%, with milder degrees of AKI occurring in up to 20% of patients. Multiple risk stratification systems have been validated, including the Cleveland Clinic Foundation, the Society of Thoracic Surgeons, and the Simplified Renal Index scores. Preoperative risk factors include female sex and older age as well as some consistently associated comorbidities, such as preexisting renal dysfunction, insulin-requiring diabetes mellitus, peripheral vascular disease, congestive heart failure, and COPD. Intraoperative risk factors are variable, probably indicating immeasurable events occurring during surgery and include use of intra-aortic balloon pump, hypothermic circulatory arrest, low output syndrome, vasopressor use, and number of blood transfusions. An association between exposure to and duration of cardiopulmonary bypass (CPB) has been consistently elucidated and may be a reflection of impaired renal perfusion from the nonpulsatile flow or an ischemic tissue injury from the proinflammatory state occurring with exposure to the CPB circuit. Performing off-pump cardiac bypass surgery may be a potentially beneficial and modifiable AKI risk factor.[2]

Vascular surgery patients have multiple comorbidities, such as diabetes and hypertension, that may contribute to preexisting renal dysfunction. AKI in open and endovascular aortic procedures has been extensively studied. Recently, Harris and colleagues[19] evaluated the AKI risk in a broad group of patients undergoing aortic, carotid, endovascular, and peripheral vascular procedures. Using the RIFLE criteria (sCr increase from baseline: risk $\geq$1.5 $\times$, injury $\geq$2.0 $\times$, and failure $\geq$3.0 $\times$), 48% of patients admitted to the surgical ICU developed AKI regardless of the surgical procedure. Diabetes, increasing critical illness severity, and sepsis were independent risk factors for AKI. Intraoperative blood loss and hypotension were associated with subsequent renal dysfunction as well as intraoperative and overall blood product transfusions. Interestingly, inpatient treatment with ACEIs and ARBs conferred a protective effect in this patient population. Using the KDIGO criteria whereby an increase in sCr of 50% or 0.3 mg/dL above the baseline defines AKI, Huber and colleagues[20] studied patients having a wide range of vascular surgery procedures and described AKI as the most common postoperative complication with an incidence of 12.7% in patients having peripheral revascularization procedures and up to 76% in patients having emergency open repair of ruptured aortic aneurysms. They also noted that using the National Surgical Quality Improvement Program criteria for AKI (increase in sCr >2 mg/dL from preoperative value or acute postoperative dialysis requirement), only 17% of patients diagnosed per the KDIGO criteria were captured. Despite increasing awareness of AKI, this still seems to be a grossly underreported complication, with only 20% of patients who had AKI having it listed in their discharge summaries.

Contrast-induced nephropathy (CIN), more recently referred to as contrast-induced AKI (CI-AKI), is the third most common cause of acute renal failure in hospitalized patients, after surgery and hypotension. It is defined as an absolute increase in sCr of 0.5 mg/dL or greater or a relative increase of 25% or greater occurring 48 to 72 hours after exposure to contrast media (CM). The most important patient-related risk factors for CIN are preexisting renal dysfunction and diabetes. The volume of CM used and its osmolarity as well as intra-arterial administration versus IV injection are all important procedure-related risk factors.[21] The Mehran risk score quantifies the risk of CIN and reliably predicts 1-year mortality.[22] Among other causes, CIN has been suggested as a factor in the development of AKI in 18.8% of patients undergoing endovascular aortic aneurysm repair, whereby AKI was defined using the Acute Kidney Injury Network (AKIN) and KDIGO criteria.[23]

PROGNOSIS

AKI is a significant complication in the perioperative period and is associated with increased mortality, myocardial infarction, heart failure, progression to chronic kidney disease (CKD), and end-stage renal disease during and after hospitalization. In hospitalized patients with heart failure, the 30-day readmission rate for heart failure was 21% in patients with AKI compared with 14% in those without AKI. AKI was found to be associated with a 30-day readmission rate of 16% in all hospitalized patients compared with 9% in patients who did not have AKI. In critically ill patients, the readmission rate of those without AKI was 12% versus 19% to 21% (depending on the severity of AKI).[24–30]

EARLY DIAGNOSIS/NOVEL BIOMARKERS

Currently, the consensus definitions of AKI use sCr levels as indicators of renal function. Various factors affect sCr levels, including muscle mass, age, sex, hydration status, and medications used. The sCr level does not begin to increase until 50% of kidney function is lost and there is a valuable time window between the renal injury event and change in sCr level that is potentially a missed therapeutic opportunity. An ideal test would be one that detects tissue injury, not loss of function. It should be tissue specific and generated by the damaged cells at a concentration proportional to the degree of damage; it should be expressed early and quickly decreased to facilitate its use to monitor the effect of implemented therapeutic measures. It should also be easy and reliable to measure. Several such biomarkers are being evaluated, and a kidney biomarker level seems to be on the horizon for use in the clinical setting.[31]

RENAL PROTECTION STRATEGIES

The recent review by Prowle and colleagues[32] on *fluid volume* management for prevention and attenuation of AKI emphasizes the importance of careful fluid balance and highlights the importance of cardiac output resuscitation. They discuss the obvious detrimental effect of fluid under resuscitation as well as the emerging evidence of decreased renal blood flow and GFR associated with increased renal subcapsular pressure and the development of abdominal compartment syndrome from overzealous fluid administration. This is of significance, especially in renal transplant recipients who traditionally received large volumes of fluids to maintain a high central venous pressure perioperatively and who were found to have worse long-term outcomes than those receiving moderate amounts of fluids. Maintenance of systemic blood pressure and cardiac output can be achieved by the addition of judicious amounts of vasopressors.

Fluid choice itself may have a significant impact on perioperative renal function. Normal saline (NS) has supraphysiologic levels of chloride. The infusion of large volumes of NS may cause hyperchloremic acidosis, renal vasoconstriction, and decreased GFR. Multiple studies have demonstrated the nephrotoxicity of starch-based fluids, whereas 4% albumin was deemed to be safe but expensive.[32]

Renal blood flow autoregulation occurs at mean arterial pressure (MAP) range of 80 to 160 mm Hg, outside of which blood flow to the kidneys becomes pressure dependent. This autoregulation is disrupted in chronic hypertensive patients and those who are acutely ill. Prolonged periods of relative or absolute hypotension are associated with AKI. At MAPs of 75 to 90 mm Hg, renal oxygen extraction was lower and GFR was higher when compared with MAP of 60 mm Hg in patients with vasodilatory shock. The use of vasoconstrictors to maintain systemic and renal perfusion pressure seems to outweigh their negative effect on renal vascular resistance.[32–34]

Ho and Power[35] showed in a meta-analysis that *furosemide* used for prevention or treatment of AKI was unlikely to directly improve either mortality or renal function. AKI incidence may be increased in dehydrated patients receiving furosemide together with other nephrotoxic agents, such as nonsteroidal antiinflammatory drugs, vancomycin, and gentamycin. A recent systematic review and meta-analysis by Yang[36] concluded that use of mannitol was not beneficial in AKI prevention and may be detrimental in patients exposed to CM. *Mannitol's* beneficial effects in kidney transplant recipients was described in older studies before current significant advances and needs to be further evaluated.

Blood glucose management for prevention of AKI has been the subject of extensive studies. Even though intensive insulin therapy whereby blood glucose is maintained at 80 to 110 mg/dL was initially found to reduce the incidence and severity of AKI in the surgical ICU setting, later studies associated it with significant hypoglycemia and associated morbidity and questionable survival benefit. The KDIGO Work Group weighs the balance between the benefit of glycemic control and the risk of hypoglycemia, thereby recommending insulin therapy to target blood glucose of 110 to 150 mg/dL.[1]

Perioperatively, *red blood cells* (RBCs) and other blood products are frequently transfused to replace blood loss and improve organ perfusion. Multiple studies have found an association between RBCs transfusion and renal dysfunction in patients undergoing cardiac and vascular surgery. Stored RBCs within the acceptable 42 days window of storage undergo changes known as storage lesion: irreversible changes that make them less deformable and more adherent to vascular endothelium resulting in decreased microvascular flow.[37,38] The recently published International Society of Nephrology's 0by25 initiative for AKI (zero preventable deaths by 2025) does empha size, however, the association of low hematocrit with AKI.[39] This point draws attention to the need for future research in preoperative optimization of comorbid conditions and risk modification efforts.

The *3-hydroxy-3-methylglutaryl coenzyme A reductase inhibitors (statins)*, by virtue of their antiinflammatory, antioxidant, and stabilization of endothelial membrane functions, have been the subject of multiple studies examining their role in AKI risk reduction when given preoperatively. Molnar and colleagues[40,41] addressed this after cardiac and major elective surgery. They did find an association between statin use and lower incidence of AKI, acute dialysis, and 30-day mortality in major elective surgery and lower levels of kidney injury markers in cardiac surgical patients but no reduction in kidney injury when defined as a doubling of sCr or dialysis requirement. Further studies found conflicting evidence for the benefit of statin use preoperatively; a meta-analysis by Mao and Huang[42] concluded that there is no significant association between statin use and risk of AKI overall, but their use may decrease the risk of CI-AKI. A more recent meta-analysis determined that preoperative statin therapy might be a promising choice in the cardiac surgery setting.[43] Further evidence is needed to quantify any benefit of preoperative statins in different patient populations.

ACEIs/ARB agents are commonly prescribed for patients with hypertension, cardiac failure, or diabetic nephropathy. Studies evaluating AKI and the preoperative use of

ACEIs/ARBs have yielded conflicting results. A systematic review and meta-analysis evaluated the more recent studies addressing the risk of AKI in patients who received preoperative renin-angiotensin system (RAS) inhibitors and concluded that preoperative use of RAS inhibitors was associated with a lower incidence of AKI.[44] The latest guidelines of the American College of Cardiology/American Heart Association on cardiovascular evaluation and management of patients undergoing noncardiac surgery recommend perioperative continuation of ACEIs/ARBs (class IIa).[45]

Sodium bicarbonate infusion has been extensively studied for the prevention of CI-AKI. The KDIGO Work Group concludes that benefit from bicarbonate solutions is possible but inconsistent. They raise the concern for costs of and errors during the preparation of the mixture in the hospital pharmacy; thus, they only recommend IV volume expansion with isotonic sodium chloride or bicarbonate solutions for the prevention of CI-AKI. Volume expansion may be preventative because of intrarenal vasodilation and directly by dilution of the contrast medium and countering of its tubulo-toxic effects. Bicarbonate solutions are suggested to be beneficial by virtue of alkalinization of urine, thereby decreasing free radical generation and reactive oxygen species scavenging.[1]

N-acetylcysteine (NAC) has vasodilatory and antioxidant effects. It has been studied in the prevention of CI-AKI and was generally found to be beneficial, but its effects on all-cause mortality or dialysis requirements have not been studied as much. The KDIGO Work Group recommends using NAC in patients at increased risk of CI-AKI given its low cost and low-risk profile.[1]

Considering that the mechanism for AKI is postulated to be secondary to a decrease in renal perfusion and ischemia, with activation of platelets, thromboxane, and inflammatory mediators, Garg and colleagues[46] investigated the effect of preoperative administration of *aspirin* (ASA) and the centrally acting α-2 agonist *clonidine* on postoperative AKI. They hypothesized that the antiplatelet aggregating effect of aspirin and the centrally mediated decrease in sympathetic output of clonidine with its concomitant antiinflammatory action would result in decreased incidence of AKI. They studied nearly 7000 patients with different degrees of renal function, who underwent major surgery defined as surgery requiring a hospital stay of more than 1 day. They concluded that neither preoperative ASA nor clonidine reduced the risk of AKI. This finding could be related to the increased risk of bleeding with ASA and hypotension with clonidine.

Dexmedetomidine, a highly selective α-2 agonist, has also been shown to have a beneficial effect in preventing AKI in animal studies. A recent randomized, triple-blinded, placebo-controlled study in patients undergoing coronary artery bypass grafting determined that the level of neutrophil gelatinase-associated lipocalin was significantly reduced by dexmedetomidine infusion, in a dose-dependent manner.[47]

SUMMARY AND RECOMMENDATIONS

In conclusion, more than one out of 3 cases of AKI in the hospital occurs in surgical patients. Even a mild degree of AKI carries with it the risk of increased morbidity and mortality. Preoperative risk stratification is critical for informed consent and perioperative planning. Potential preoperative interventions, such as hematocrit and blood glucose optimization, and continuation of ARB and statins may have a protective role. Perioperative renal protection strategies, including goal-directed fluid therapy, avoidance of hyperchloremic crystalloid solutions, and maintenance of hemodynamics within the renal autoregulation curve, are potentially invaluable in the prevention of AKI. Current advances in the development of biomarkers may offer the opportunity for early diagnosis and the implementation of therapeutic strategies. Increased awareness and concerted efforts by all perioperative physicians are needed to provide an improved outcome for surgical patients.

REFERENCES

1. Kellum JA, Lameire N, Aspelin P, et al. Kidney Disease: Improving Global Outcomes (KDIGO) Acute Kidney Injury Work Group. KDIGO clinical practice guideline for acute kidney injury. Kidney Int Suppl 2012;2:1–138.
2. Thakar CV. Perioperative acute kidney injury. Adv Chronic Kidney Dis 2013;20(1): 67–75.
3. Kheterpal S, Tremper KK, Englesbe MJ, et al. Predictors of postoperative acute renal failure after noncardiac surgery in patients with previously normal renal function. Anesthesiology 2007;107:892–902.
4. Thakar CV, Kharat V, Blanck S, et al. Acute kidney injury after gastric bypass surgery. Clin J Am Soc Nephrol 2007;2:426–30.
5. Kim M, Brady JE, Li G. Variations in the risk of acute kidney injury across intra-abdominal surgery procedures. Anesth Analg 2014;119(5):1121–32.
6. Kimmel LA, Wilson S, Janardan J, et al. Incidence of acute kidney injury following total joint arthroplasty: a retrospective review by RIFLE criteria. Clin Kidney J 2014;7:546–51.
7. Weingarten TN, Gurrieri C, Jarett PD, et al. Acute kidney injury following total joint arthroplasty: retrospective analysis. Can J Anaesth 2012;59:1111–8.
8. Nadkarni G, Patel A, Ahuja Y, et al. Incidence, risk factors, and outcome trends of acute kidney injury in elective total hip and knee replacement. Am J Orthop 2015. [Epub ahead of print].
9. Bloom RD, Reese PP. Chronic kidney disease after norenal solid organ transplantation. J Am Soc Nephrol 2007;18(12):3031–41.
10. Cabezuelo JB, Ramirez P, Rios A, et al. Risk factors of acute renal failure after liver transplantation. Kidney Int 2006;69:1073–80.
11. Valavathy N, Edelstein CL, Teitelbaum I, Acute renal failure and chronic kidney disease following liver transplantation. Hemodial Int 2007;11(Suppl 3):S7–12.
12. McCauley J, Van Thiel DH, Starzl TE, et al. Acute and chronic renal failure in liver transplantation. Nephron 1990;55:121–8.
13. Ojo AO, Held PJ, Port FK, et al. Chronic renal failure after transplantation of a non-renal organ. N Engl J Med 2003;349:931–40.
14. Grimm JC, Lui C, Kilic A, et al. A risk score to predict acute renal failure in adult patients after lung transplantation. Ann Thorac Surg 2015;99:251–7.
15. Greenberg A. Renal failure in cardiac transplantation. Cardiovasc Clin 1990;20: 189–98.
16. Boyle JM, Moualla S, Arrigain S, et al. Risks and outcomes of acute kidney injury requiring dialysis after cardiac transplantation. Am J Kidney Dis 2006;48: 787–96.
17. Ishani A, Erturk S, Hertz MI, et al. Predictors of renal function following lung or heart-lung transplantation. Kidney Int 2002;61:2228–34.
18. Cooper JE, Wiseman AC. Acute kidney injury in kidney transplantation. Curr Opin Nephrol Hypertens 2013;22:698–703.
19. Harris DG, Koo G, McCrone MP, et al. Acute kidney injury in critically ill vascular surgery patients is common and associated with increased mortality. Front Surg 2015;2:8.

20. Huber M, Ozrazgat-Baslanti T, Thottakkara P, et al. Mortality and cost of acute and chronic kidney disease after vascular surgery. Ann Vasc Surg 2015. [Epub ahead of print].
21. Azzalini L, Spagnoli V, Ly H. Contrast-induced nephropathy: from pathophysiology to preventive strategies. Can J Cardiol 2015. [Epub ahead of print].
22. Mehran R, Nikolsky E, Lasic Z, et al. A simple risk score for prediction of contrast-induced nephropathy after percutaneous coronary intervention: development and initial validation. J Am Coll Cardiol 2004;44(7):1393–9.
23. Saratzis A, Melas N, Mahmood A, et al. Incidence of acute kidney injury after endovascular abdominal aortic aneurysm repair. Eur J Vasc Endovasc Surg 2015; 49:534–40.
24. Ricci Z, Cruz D, Ronco C. The RIFLE criteria and mortality in acute kidney injury: a systematic review. Kidney Int 2008;73:538–46.
25. Coca SG, Yusuf B, Shlipak MG, et al. Long term risk of mortality and other adverse outcomes after acute kidney injury: a systematic review and meta-analysis. Am J Kidney Dis 2009;53:961–73.
26. Hansen MK, Gammelager H, Mikkelsen MM, et al. Post-operative acute kidney injury and five-year risk of death, myocardial infarction and stroke among elective cardiac patients: a cohort study. Crit Care 2013;17:R292.
27. Horkan CM, Purtle SW, Mendu ML, et al. The association of acute kidney injury in the critically ill and postdischarge outcomes: a cohort study. Crit Care Med 2015; 43:354–64.
28. Zeng X, McMahon GM, Brunelli SM, et al. Incidence, outcomes and comparisons across definitions of AKI in hospitalized individuals. Clin J Am Soc Nephrol 2014; 9:12–20.
29. Thakar CV, Parikh PJ, Liu Y. Acute kidney injury (AKI) and risk of readmissions in patients with heart failure. Am J Cardiol 2012;109:1482–6.
30. Christiansen CF. Hospital readmissions after acute kidney injury-why? Crit Care Med 2015;43(2):490–1.
31. Martensson J, Martling C-R, Bell M. Novel biomarkers of acute kidney injury and failure: clinical applicability. Br J Anaesth 2012;109(6):843–50.
32. Prowle JR, Kirwan CJ, Bellomo R. Fluid management for the prevention and attenuation of acute kidney injury. Nat Rev Nephrol 2014;10(1):37–47.
33. Brienza N, Giglio MT, Marucci M, et al. Does perioperative hemodynamic optimization protect renal function in surgical patients? A meta-analytic study. Crit Care Med 2009;37:2079–90.
34. Zarbock A, Milles K. Novel therapy for renal protection. Curr Opin Anaesthesiol 2015;28(4):431–8.
35. Ho KM, Power BM. Benefits and risks of furosemide in acute kidney injury. Anaesthesia 2010;65:283–93.
36. Yang B. Intravascular administration of mannitol for acute kidney injury prevention: a systematic review and meta-analysis. PLoS One 2014;9(1):e85029.
37. Habib RH, Zacharias A, Schwann TA, et al. Role of hemodilutional anemia and transfusion during cardiopulmonary bypass in renal injury after coronary revascularization: Implications on operative outcome. Crit Care Med 2005;33:1749–56.
38. O'Keefe SD, Davenport DL, Minion DJ, et al. Blood transfusion is associated with increased morbidity and mortality after lower extremity revascularization. J Vasc Surg 2010;51:616–21.
39. Mehta RL, Cerda J, Burdmann EA, et al. International Society of Nephrology's 0by25 initiative for acute kidney injury (zero preventable deaths by 2025); a human rights case for nephrology. Lancet 2015;385:2616–34.

40. Molnar AO, Coca SG, Devereaux PJ, et al. Statin use associates with a lower incidence of acute kidney injury after major elective surgery. J Am Soc Nephrol 2011; 22:939–46.
41. Molnar AO, Parikh CR, Coca SG, et al. Association between preoperative statin use and acute kidney injury biomarkers in cardiac surgical procedures. Ann Thorac Surg 2014;97:2081–8.
42. Mao S, Huang S. Statins use and the risk of acute kidney injury: a meta-analysis. Ren Fail 2014;36(4):651–7.
43. Wang J, Gu C, Gao M, et al. Pre-operative statin therapy and renal outcomes after cardiac surgery: a meta-analysis and meta-regression of 59,771 patients. Can J Cardiol 2015;31:1051–60.
44. Cheungpasiporn W, Thongprayoon C, Srivali N, et al. Pre-operative renin-angiotensin system inhibitors use linked to reduced acute kidney injury: a systematic review and met-analysis. Nephrol Dial Transplant 2015;30:978–88.
45. Fleisher LA, Fleischmann KE, Auerbach AD, et al. 2014 ACC/AHA guidelines on preoperative cardiovascular evaluation and management of patients undergoing noncardiac surgery: a report of the American College of Cardiology/American Heart Association Task Force on practice guidelines. J Am Coll Cardiol 2014; 64:e77–137.
46. Garg AX, Kurz A, Sessler DI, et al. Perioperative aspirin and clonidine and risk of acute kidney injury. JAMA 2014;312(21):2254–64.
47. Balkanay OO, Goksedef D, Omeroglu SN, et al. The dose-related effects of dexmedetomidine on renal functions and serum neutrophil gelatinase-associated lipocalin values after coronary artery bypass grafting: a randomised, triple-blind, placebo-controlled study. Interact Cardiovasc Thorac Surg 2015;20:209–14.

Perioperative Approach to Anticoagulants and Hematologic Disorders

Jisu Kim, MD, MSc*, Richard Huh, MD, Amir K. Jaffer, MD, MBA

KEYWORDS

- Preoperative evaluation • Coagulopathy • Coagulation disorder • Hemophilia
- Von Willebrand disease • Thrombocytopenia • Immune thrombocytopenia
- Drug-induced thrombocytopenia

KEY POINTS

- History and physical examination should guide further evaluation of bleeding risk rather than routine blood testing.
- Use a risk prediction model, such as the Caprini risk assessment, to stratify preoperative patients for their risk of postoperative venous thromboembolism (VTE) and prescribe therapies based on this risk. Patients with increased risk of bleeding may warrant mechanical prophylaxis as opposed to pharmacologic prophylaxis.
- Warfarin should be stopped 5 days before most major surgeries except in those patients having minor procedures (eg, certain dermatolgic surgeries and cataract surgeries) that can be performed while on warfarin.
- Apply evidence-based American College of Chest Physicians (ACCP) guidelines for the perioperative management of antithrombotic therapy and tailor bridging therapy depending on the risks and benefits.
- Target-specific oral anticoagulants (TSOACs) are indicated for VTE prophylaxis after major joint replacement, after VTE treatment, and for stroke prevention in atrial fibrillation. Given the various indications, dosages, and pharmacokinetics, it is important to review these details prior to prescribing them for patients.

COAGULATION DISORDERS

Accurate history and physical examination precede any assessment. To assess the risk of perioperative bleeding, a preoperative history should include questions that identify[1]

Department of Internal Medicine, Rush University Medical Center, 1653 West Congress Parkway, 10 Kellogg, Chicago, IL 60612, USA
* Corresponding author.
E-mail address: Jisu_Kim@rush.edu

Anesthesiology Clin 34 (2016) 101–125
http://dx.doi.org/10.1016/j.anclin.2015.10.010   anesthesiology.theclinics.com

- Excessive bruising
- Excessive bleeding
  - For longer than 3 minutes after brushing teeth
  - Frequent nose bleeds
  - Prolonged bleeding after cuts
  - After dental extractions, surgery, or childbirth
- History of occult or frank gastrointestinal or genitourinary tract blood loss
- Family history of hemophilia or a coinherited hematologic disorder
- Personal history of liver disease, hypersplenism, renal dysfunction, or hematologic or collagen vascular disease
- Current or recent use of medications that interfere with hemostasis

Physical examination should focus on signs of excessive bleeding, such as petechiae, hematomas, and purpura. In addition, signs of cirrhosis, such as jaundice, scleral icterus, and spider angiomata, may alert a clinician to potential postoperative bleeding complications.[1]

Assessment of Perioperative Bleeding Risk

The history and physical examination should guide further evaluation, rather than routine blood testing.[1–3] Recent American Society of Anesthesiologists (ASA) guidelines[4] noted coagulation abnormalities

- In 0.06% to 21.2% of asymptomatic or unselected patients, which led to 0% to 4% of cancellations or changes in management perioperatively
- In 3.4% to 29.1% of selected or indicated patients, with no reported changes in clinical management

Therefore, ASA guidelines do not recommend routine coagulation testing preoperatively in asymptomatic or nonselected patients; for the at-risk patients (bleeding disorders, renal or liver dysfunction, and type and invasiveness of procedure) undergoing regional anesthesia, insufficient data were available for the ASA to provide a recommendation.

Commonly obtained tests to assess bleeding risk include prothrombin time (PT), activated partial thromboplastin time (aPTT), and platelet count. PT and aPTT are tests were developed to test the integrity of the coagulation pathway, not designed to predict perioperative bleeding.[1,2] Abnormal platelet count, whether thrombocytopenia (<150,000) or thrombocytosis (>440,000), has been associated with higher risk of perioperative bleeding.[1] Other available tests include bleeding time, platelet function monitoring, thrombin time (TT), reptilase time, fibrinogen, and D dimer.[2]

For patients with an indication, the following provides an approach to common abnormalities that may be encountered preoperatively.

Assessment of the Coagulation Pathway

Approach to prothrombin time abnormality

PT reflects the extrinsic and common coagulation pathways.[5] It reflects the time it takes platelet-poor plasma to form a clot in the presence of tissue thromboplastin and calcium. Although there are different methods to report PT, the most accepted measurement is the international normalized ratio, which standardizes the results across different thromboplastin test reagents; normal range is 0.9 to 1.2. If PT (or aPTT) is prolonged, it should first be confirmed with a repeat peripheral blood sample.[2,5] Once confirmed, a systematic approach should be used (**Fig. 1**).

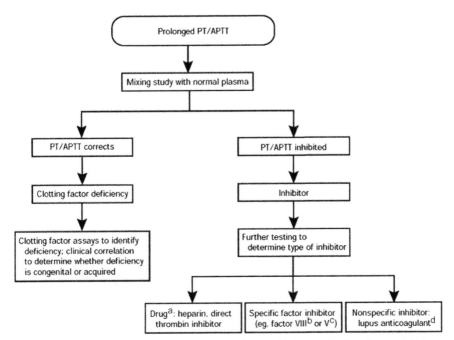

Fig. 1. Approach to a prolonged PT or APTT–distinguishing a clotting factor deficiency from a clotting factor inhibitor. [a] TT is prolonged and reptilase time is normal; [b] PT is normal; [c] PT is prolonged and inhibited; and [d] PT is typically normal but may be prolonged and inhibited when a mixing study is performed. (*From* Kamal AH, Tefferi A, Pruthi RK. How to interpret and pursue an abnormal prothrombin time, activated partial thromboplastin time, and bleeding time in adults. Mayo Clin Proc 2007;82(7):868; with permission.)

The first step in evaluating a prolonged clotting time (PT or aPTT) is a mixing study. This technique is performed by mixing a patient's plasma with normal donor plasma and, if correction of clotting time is noted, it is suggestive of factor deficiency.[2,5] If, however, the clotting time is not corrected, an inhibition is assumed in 1 or more of the coagulation pathways. This inhibitors can generally be classified into

- Medications: heparins and direct thrombin inhibitors
- Specific factor inhibitor(s)
- Nonspecific factor inhibitor(s): lupus anticoagulants (antibodies directed toward protein phospholipid complexes)

Practically, the mixing study may not be readily available on a daily basis in any particular institutional laboratory and, therefore, could lead to a delay in diagnosis. Therefore, it may be reasonable to combine and initiate multiple steps to evaluate the coagulopathy.

Key points

- Measure factors II, V, VII, and X and fibrinogen
  - Factors II, VII, IX, and X: vitamin K factors
    - Procoagulant proteins, which are depleted with decreased nutritional intake
    - Also decreased with warfarin use
    - Produced in liver, therefore also decreased in severe liver disease

- ○ Factor V: low in liver disease, thus helps distinguish between vitamin K deficiency state
- ○ Rare conditions
  - ▪ Congenital factor VII deficiency
  - ▪ Isolated congenital deficiencies of either factor X or V; distinguish from
- • Acquired isolated deficiency of factor X: amyloidosis
- • Acquired isolated deficiency of factor V: liver disease and myeloproliferative disease
- • Presence of an inhibitor: does not correct with mixing study
  - ○ PT inhibitors rarely present without also inhibiting the aPTT
    - ▪ Drugs: direct thrombin inhibitor, factor V inhibitor, and excess heparin in specimen
    - ▪ Lupus anticoagulant (LAC)

Approach to activated partial thromboplastin time abnormality

aPTT reflects the integrity of the intrinsic and common coagulation pathways.[5] Unlike PT, this is a nonstandardized time required for clot formation when a patient's plasma is mixed with phospholipid, calcium, and an activator; normal time is between 25 and 35 seconds.[2] aPTT becomes prolonged when the factor concentrations are reduced to approximately less than 30% of baseline. The test is most sensitive to factor VIII and IX deficiencies but does not reflect factor VII disorders. It is also sensitive to inhibition of thrombin. An evaluation for abnormal aPTT should start with a repeat, peripheral blood draw to ensure true abnormality, followed by a systematic approach starting with a mixing study (see **Fig. 1**).

Key points

- • Factor deficiencies: VIII, IX, XI, or XII. Also high-molecular-weight kininogen or prekallikrein
  - ○ Severe deficiencies of factor XII, high-molecular-weight kininogen, and prekallikrein result in aPTT prolongation but do not result in bleeding disorders.
  - ○ Congenital deficiencies of factors VIII (hemophilia A), IX (hemophilia B), and XI (hemophilia C) result in varying severity of bleeding. von Willebrand disease (vWD) is caused by a quantitative and qualitative deficiency in factor VIII and can be both congenital and acquired. These conditions are briefly discussed later.
  - ○ Warfarin use, liver disease, and consumptive coagulopathy (disseminated intravascular coagulation [DIC] and fibrinolysis) result in acquired factor deficiencies.
- • Presence of inhibitor
  - ○ Drugs: heparin, direct thrombin inhibitors (lepirudin, argatroban, alter both aPTT and PT); can be distinguished by measuring TT
  - ○ LAC: although aPTT prolonged, is a risk factor for thromboembolism. Further investigation includes testing for prolongation and inhibition of at least 1 of 2 phospholipid-based tests to prove phospholipid inhibition of the clotting time:
    - ▪ aPTT: shortening of the clotting time after addition of platelet phospholipid
    - ▪ Russell viper venom test: shortening of the clotting time after the addition of phospholipid
  - ○ Specific factor inhibitor: factor VIII inhibitor (acquired autoimmune hemophilia)
- • TT and reptilase time[2,5]: may help determine presence of heparin or direct thrombin inhibitor, because both drugs prolong TT, but not the reptilase time.

○ TT[2]: tests thrombin's ability to convert fibrinogen to fibrin in the final common pathway. Normal range is 15 to 19 seconds and is prolonged in conditions affecting either fibrinogen or thrombin (hypofibrinogenemia, abnormal fibrinogen, advanced liver disease, heparin, direct thrombin inhibitors, fibrinogen, and fibrinogen degradation products).

○ Reptilase time[2]: normal range is 14 to 21 seconds.

▪ TT prolonged, reptilase time normal: presence of heparin or direct thrombin inhibitor

▪ TT and reptilase time prolonged: low fibrinogen level or presence of fibrinogen degradation products

Approach to both prothrombin time and activated partial thromboplastin time abnormalities

If both coagulation tests are abnormal, this implies that the abnormality lies within any part (or multiple parts) of the coagulation pathway.[5]

Factor deficiencies can be due to deficiencies of vitamin K–dependent factors (supratherapeutic warfarin dose or anticoagulant rodenticide poisoning) and require confirmation of the factors. In addition, suspected overdose or poisoning cases can be confirmed with direct measurement of the plasma drug levels. Severe liver disease (due to acquired factor deficiencies) and consumptive coagulopathies, such as DIC, can also prolong both PT and aPTT.

Inhibition due to direct thrombin inhibitors, excess heparin in the sample, or potent LACs can also cause prolonged PT and aPTT. Lymphoproliferative disorders and monoclonal protein disorders can also be associated with nonspecific inhibitors of the PT and aPTT assay systems.

Bleeding time

The bleeding time test was originally developed to screen for bleeding disorders.[5] Because of lack of consistent results, however, due to both patient-dependent and operator-dependent factors, and no supporting data for its usefulness in predicting bleeding complications reliably, this test is no longer routinely performed preoperatively.

Hemophilia and Von Willebrand Disease

Hemophilia

Hemophilia is a congenital, X-linked bleeding disorder.[6] Although many other bleeding disorders have the hemophilia designation, this disorder classically refers to factor VIII (hemophilia A) and factor IX (hemophilia B) deficiencies. Hemophilia A is more common than hemophilia B and generally affects boys and men on the maternal side; the last estimate reported approximately 400,000 affected people in the world. Hemophilia should be suspected in patients with history of

• Early childhood easy bruising. Although history of bleeding is lifelong, some children may not have bleeding symptoms until they begin walking or running.

• Spontaneous bleeding without apparent known reason with particular focus on the joints, muscles, and soft tissues

• Excessive traumatic or surgical bleeding

• Family history of bleeding (approximately two-thirds of all patients)

In addition to these factors, special consideration should be made toward carriers of this disease. Because this is an X-linked disorder, obligate carriers are

- Daughters of hemophilia patient
- Mothers of 1 son with hemophilia who also has at least 1 other family member with hemophilia or a family member who is a known carrier of the hemophilia gene
- Mothers of 2 or more sons with hemophilia

Most carriers are asymptomatic; however, some may have decreased clotting factors near levels in the hemophilia range, particularly during trauma and surgery. Therefore, carriers with decreased clotting factors near the level of hemophilia should be categorized and managed as such. It is recommended that immediate female relatives of a person with hemophilia should have their clotting factor level assessed prior to any invasive intervention or childbirth or if they are symptomatic.

The severity of bleeding is correlated with the clotting factor level and the perioperative evaluation, monitoring, and treatment are complex and should be performed with the assistance of a hematologist. In general,[6,7]

- Comprehensive hemophilia treatment center or a similar plan is needed.
- Preoperative assessment of inhibitor screening and inhibitor assay should be completed within 1 week of surgery
- No procedure is too minor for adequate hemostasis planning (ie, dental procedure, endoscopy with biopsy, arterial blood gas, or arterial lines).
- Elective procedures should be scheduled early in the day and early in the week to ensure adequate laboratory support and availability of factor concentrates (or plasma).
- Anesthesiologists should have experience treating such bleeding disorders.
- Adequate laboratory support is needed to have reliable clotting factor level and inhibitor monitoring.

Treatment with viral inactivated plasma-derived or recombinant concentrates is preferred over cryoprecipitate or fresh frozen plasma (FFP). Cryoprecipitate, in turn, is preferred over FFP for hemophilia A, because it is generally difficult to achieve high enough factor VIII levels with FFP alone; FFP can be used for treatment of hemophilia B. Other options include desmopressin, tranexamic acid, and epsilon aminocaproic acid.

Desmopressin is a synthetic analogue of vasopressin that boosts plasma levels of factor VIII and vWF. Desmopressin can be used for mild or moderate hemophilia A (particularly carriers) and some platelet disorders; however, it is of no value to hemophilia B, because it does not affect factor IX. Individual response to Desmopressin is varied and difficult to predict.

Tranexamic acid competitively inhibits plasminogen activation to plasmin to promote clot stability. It is an antifibrinolytic agent that is renally excreted, so doses must be adjusted in patients with chronic kidney disease (CKD). It is an adjunctive therapy and could be useful for skin and mucosal surface bleeding, such as oral bleeding, epistaxis, or menorrhagia. Therefore, consideration can be made to use this agent in dental surgery. Due to its mechanism, there is a thromboembolic concern for this agent and it should not be given to patients with factor IX deficiency receiving prothrombin complex concentrates. If such dual therapy is needed, the prothrombin complex concentrate and tranexamic acid should be administered at least 12 hours apart. Tranexamic acid is contraindicated in hematuria, because it can cause obstructive uropathy by preventing clot dissolution in the ureters and lead to potentially permanent loss renal function.

Epsilon aminocaproic acid is similar to tranexamic acid but has shorter plasma half-life, lower potency, and higher toxicity and, therefore, is not preferred.[6]

No specific postoperative pharmacologic antithrombotic therapy is recommended at this time. In a small prospective study of hemophilia A and hemophilia B patients undergoing total knee or hip arthroplasty, the overall deep vein thrombosis (DVT) rate was much lower than in the normal healthy population. Due to the high rate of bleeding complications, however, the investigators recommended no pharmacologic DVT prophylaxis in hemophilia patients without a previous history of venous thromboembolic disorder.[8]

Hemophilia C (factor XI deficiency or Rosenthal syndrome)

Factor XI deficiency, an autosomal recessive disorder that affects both genders, is sufficiently prevalent in persons of Ashkenazi (European) Jewish descent and nearly all patients have prolonged aPTTs.[4,7] Approximately 3% of this population have sufficiently low factor XI levels associated with abnormal hemostasis and approximately 1% have excessive postoperative bleeding. In addition, this condition can be pretreated with FFP before surgery. Therefore, it may be reasonable to screen for factor XI deficiency in Ashkenazi Jewish patients preoperatively by using PTT. The authors recommend repeating an abnormal PTT level prior to proceeding with direct factor XI level measurement.

Von Willebrand disease

vWD is a bleeding disorder attributed to reduced levels of vWF activity and has multiple subtypes (**Table 1**).[7,9] Often it is due to congenital/genetic defect in the vWF gene; however, acquired von Willebrand syndrome (AVWS) is possible. AVWS has similar laboratory findings (decreased vWF antigen, vWF ristocetin cofactor activity, or factor VIII) and is usually caused by 3 possible mechanisms:

- Autoimmune clearance or inhibition of vWF – lymphoproliferative diseases, monoclonal gammopathies, systemic lupus erythematosus, other autoimmune disorders, and some cancers

Table 1
Types of von Willebrand disease

Type	Characteristics	Treatment
1	80% Of cases; quantitative defect	Desmopressin
2A	Abnormal multimer pattern; quantitative and qualitative defect	Desmopressin
2B	Rare; abnormal multimer pattern; quantitative and qualitative defect, autosomal dominant	Desmopressin may produce thrombocytopenia
2M	Qualitative defect; normal multimer pattern	Desmopressin
2N	Qualitative defect; vWF levels are normal; only factor VIII is reduced	Desmopressin effect may be too short-lived
3	Rare; low to nondetectable levels of vWF	Desmopressin usually not effective

With type 2B or when desmopressin acetate is not effective, vWF-containing factor VIII concentrates or cryoprecipitate may be used instead.

Data from Mensah PK, Gooding R. Surgery in patients with inherited bleeding disorders. Anesthesia 2015;70(Suppl 1):112–20; and Chair of group. The diagnosis, evaluation and management of von Willebrand disease. Bethesda (MD): National Heart, Lung, and Blood Institute, National Institutes of Health; 2007. (GPO #08-5832).

- Increased proteolysis of vWF – due to increased shear stress from ventricular septal defect, aortic stenosis, or primary pulmonary hypertension
- Increased binding of vWF to platelets or other cell surfaces. This large plasma glycoprotein (GP) mediates the adhesion of platelets at sites of vascular injury and binds and stabilizes factor VIII.

Some nonimmune mechanisms of AVWS have been described in hypothyroidism and in certain medications (valproic acid, ciprofloxacin, griseofulvin, and hydroxyethyl starch).

Preoperative testing in patients previously undiagnosed with VWD is difficult and requires careful preoperative history about previous hemostatic or any unexpected excessive bleeding issues. If vWD is diagnosed, however, a treatment plan should be made according to the severity of disease and the type of surgery:

- Major surgery: achieve 100% vWF preoperatively and maintain trough levels of 50% until adequate wound healing.
- Minor surgery: achieve 60% vWF level preoperatively and trough daily levels of 30% until wound healing.
- Dental extractions: achieve 60% vWF level preoperatively.
- Delivery and puerperium: 80% to 100% vWF level predelivery and trough levels of 30% for 3 to 4 days.

Other keypoints

- In type 1 vWD with vWF level greater than 10 IU/dL, desmopressin is the treatment of choice, because it produces a complete or partial response in more than 90% of the patients. Can be give within 40 to 60 minutes of surgery. Desmopressin increases endothelial cell release of factor VIII, vWF, and plasminogen activator. Goal vWF should be 80 IU/dL to 100 IU/dL and to raise factor VIII. Dosing consideration for tachyphylaxis should be made, due to depletion of endothelial stores.
- Type 2 and type 3 require vWF concentrate administration.
- Tranexamic acid is also an important adjunctive therapy as either intravenous or oral therapy.
- Cryoprecipitate can be used; however, ristocetin cofactor activity level should not exceed more than 50% and should be monitored while bleeding is controlled.
- If properly corrected, pharmacologic antithrombotic prophylaxis should be considered postoperatively.

Assessment of Platelet Count and Dysfunction

The platelet plug is the primary hemostatic mechanism, which initiates the rest of the coagulation cascade.[2] Normal platelet levels range between 150,000 per mm^3 and 440,000 per mm^3; typically, spontaneous bleeding is unlikely with counts greater than 10,000 per mm^3 to 20,000 per mm^3. In a healthy patient, pseudothrombocytopenia from platelet agglutination should always be excluded. Etiology can be categorized into decreased production, sequestration, or increased destruction of platelets (**Box 1**).

Acceptable preoperative platelet count depends on the surgical procedure. For adult patients, recent AABB (formerly, the American Association of Blood Banks) clinical practice platelet transfusion guidelines suggest prophylactic platelet transfusion to keep the level above certain levels, depending on the type of procedure[10]:

- Minor invasive procedures
  - Elective central venous catheter placement: greater than 20,000 per mm^3
  - Elective diagnostic lumbar puncture: greater than 50,000 per mm^3

Box 1
Causes of thrombocytopenia

Decreased production

Congenital
   Bernard-Soulier syndrome (loss of GPIb)
   Alport syndrome
   May-Hegglin anomaly
   Wiskott-Aldrich syndrome

Acquired
   Bone marrow infiltration
      Metastatic cancers
      Myelofibrosis
   Ineffective thrombopoiesis
      Folate, vitamin B_{12}, or iron deficiency
      Myelodysplastic syndrome

Increased destruction

Idiopathic

Drugs
   Immune mechanism (eg, penicillin, digitalis derivatives, sulfa compounds, quinine, quinidine
   phenytoin, heparin, and ampicillin)
   Nonimmune mechanism (eg, ticlopidine, mitomycin, cisplatin, and cyclosporine)

Drugs that alter platelet function (eg, nonsteroidal anti-inflammatory agents, β-lactam
antibiotics, heparin, isoniazid, penicillin, and aminoglycosides)

Autoimmune
   Chronic lymphocytic leukemia
   Systemic lupus erythematosus
   Thyroid disease
   Hypogammaglobulinemia
   Antiphospholipid syndrome
   Post-transfusion purpura
   Sepsis

Nonimmune
   Preeclampsia
   Hemolytic-uremic syndrome
   Thrombotic thrombocytopenic purpura
   Cardiopulmonary bypass
   DIC

- Major elective nonneuraxial surgery: greater than 50,000 per mm^3
- Cardiac surgery with cardiopulmonary bypass
  - Suggest platelet transfusion if exhibit perioperative bleeding with thrombocy-topenia and/or with evidence of platelet dysfunction
  - Against routine prophylactic platelet transfusion if not thrombocytopenic

Other procedural considerations[11]

- Neurosurgery, central nervous system trauma, ocular surgery: greater than 100,000 per mm^3
- Epidural catheter insertion or removal: greater than 50,000 to 80,000 per mm^3
- Vaginal delivery: greater than 50,000 per mm^3
- Miscellaneous minor procedures: greater than 50,000 per mm^3
  - Gastroscopy and biopsy

- ○ Transbronchial biopsy
- ○ Liver biopsy
- Bone marrow biopsy: no recommended threshold

Considerations prior to platelet transfusion

- Cause of thrombocytopenia must be established. This is especially important, because platelet transfusions are contraindicated in certain conditions, such as heparin-induced thrombocytopenia (HIT) and thrombocytopenic purpura/hemolytic uremic syndrome.
- Platelet count does not account for any underlying platelet dysfunction or other coagulopathies.
- Consider the risks of platelet transfusion:
  - ○ Fever = 1/14 per transfusion
  - ○ Allergic reaction = 1/50
  - ○ Bacterial sepsis = 1/75,000
  - ○ Transfusion-related acute lung injury = 1/138,000
  - ○ Hepatitis B infection = 1/2,652,580
  - ○ Hepatitis C infection = 1/3,315,729
  - ○ HIV infection = near 0 (95% CI, 0–1/1,461,888)

Thrombocytopenia

Preoperative finding of confirmed thrombocytopenia needs further investigation, especially for elective procedures, due to increased complications.[12] Evaluation requires a careful history (personal and family history as well as thorough medication history) and physical examination, in the context of the clinical setting. Peripheral smear is vital and all cell lines should be evaluated. Other testing includes liver and renal function tests, coagulation screen with D dimer, and lactate dehydrogenase (http://asheducationbook.hematologylibrary.org/content/2012/1/191.full). Pending these test results, further investigation may be required. Beyond initial evaluation and management, a hematology consultation may be appropriate.

Routine platelet testing in asymptomatic, otherwise healthy patients has been discouraged, mainly because the level often did not lead to changes in management.[1–4] An ASA task force guideline recommends considering clinical factors prior to preanesthesia coagulation studies, such as bleeding disorders, renal or liver dysfunction, medication use, and type and invasiveness of the procedure.[4]

More recent evidence, however, may suggest that preoperative platelet measurement and evaluation may have more utility than previously considered. Glance and colleagues[13] retrospectively reviewed patients having noncardiac surgery between 2008 and 2009 who had a preoperative platelet level done without an obvious indication (routine), using the National Surgical Quality Improvement Program database. The Current Procedural Terminology codes noted that the patients underwent general, vascular, or orthopedic surgery under general, spinal, or epidural anesthesia. They hypothesized that thrombocytopenic patients are more likely to receive erythrocyte transfusions and, secondarily, are more likely to have higher risk of mortality (ROM) and major complications. When compared with patients with normal platelet count

- Moderate to severe thrombocytopenia (<100,000 per mm^3) = 75% higher risk of receiving transfusion and 90% higher 30-day ROM (adjusted for preoperative risk and surgical complexity)

- Mild thrombocytopenia (101,000–150,000 per mm³) = 29% increased risk of transfusion and 31% higher ROM
- Thrombocytosis (≥450,000 per mm³) = 44% increased risk of transfusion but no increase in ROM
- One in 14 patients who had routine preoperative platelet testing had thrombocytopenia or thrombocytosis.

Given the high prevalence of platelet abnormalities noted in routine preoperative testing and its association with higher risk of blood transfusion, major complications, and death, the investigators questioned whether the recommendations discouraging preoperative testing are too restrictive. Therefore, unless the planned surgery is truly at low risk of bleeding, an argument can be made for routine preoperative platelet level evaluation.

For the scope of this review, the isolated thrombocytopenias are discussed: primary immune thrombocytopenia (ITP), drug-induced thrombocytopenia (DITP), heparin-induced thrombocytopenia (HIT), and DIC.

Primary immune thrombocytopenia

ITP is the most common isolated thrombocytopenia and is a diagnosis of exclusion.[12] The platelet antibody assays are not sensitive, although approximately 90% specific, and have some use in differentiating ITP from DITP. Liver disease and hypersplenism should be excluded with appropriate blood and imaging modalities (eg, ultrasound of the abdomen). Likewise, a chest radiograph can be helpful in identifying subclinical lymphadenopathy and infections, such as tuberculosis. Other laboratory tests recommended include complete blood and reticulocyte count, blood group, direct antiglobulin test, HIV and hepatitis C virus testing, and *Helicobacter pylori* testing.

In patients more than 60 years old, bone marrow biopsy can help diagnose myelodysplastic syndrome, because isolated thrombocytopenia may be an early presenting sign. In an otherwise healthy patient with a normal evaluation without any other obvious findings, however, a bone marrow biopsy is controversial.

Treatment of ITP is supportive and directed toward the spleen by inactivation of the antiplatelet antibody production and the subsequent destruction. The mainstay of treatment is corticosteroids, which prevent sequestration of antibody coated platelets. Gamma globulin or platelet transfusions can be used in urgent situations.[14]

Drug-induced thrombocytopenia

Development of drug-dependent antibody production against platelet GPs is the main cause of DITP.[12,15] If a patient is naïve to the drug, the decrease in platelet count can decrease over 1 to 3 weeks. With previous exposure to the drug, however, the decrease may become apparent within 2 to 3 days, sometimes hours. Although laboratory diagnosis methods are available (such as drug-dependent antiplatelet antibiody testing), the diagnosis of DITP is empirical and further supported when the platelet count returns to normal within 5 to 10 days after discontinuation of the suspected drug. This diagnosis can be easily confused with ITP, especially without a complete medication and other intake history, because the list of inciting medications, foods, and beverages is extremely long.

Treatment starts with discontinuation of the suspected drug, followed by supportive therapy, including corticosteroids, immunoglobulin therapy, plasma exchange, and platelet transfusions, depending on the severity of the condition.[15]

Heparin-induced thrombocytopenia

HIT should be suspected in any patient on heparin or LMWH therapy who develops a decrease of greater than 50% in platelet count from baseline or total platelet count of less than 100,000 per mm^3 with normal baseline counts.[12,16] It occurs in 0.5% to 5% of heparin-treated patients, typically after 5 to 10 days, but in patients with previous heparin exposure, HIT can have earlier onset (even within hours). Complications of HIT include venous or arterial thrombosis and necrotic skin lesions at heparin injection sites. Due to potentially emergent complications and delayed confirmatory testing, presumptive diagnosis must be made clinically. One tool is the 4 Ts pretest probability score[12,16]: thrombocytopenia, timing of platelet count decrease, thrombosis or other sequelae, other causes for thrombocytopenia (**Table 2**). In patients with high suspicion for HIT, heparin should be stopped immediately with an alternative anticoagulant administration even prior to the confirmatory test. Many tests are available, with individual pros and cons (**Table 3**); however, the current accepted gold standard test is the ^{14}C-serotonin release assay.

Disseminated intravascular coagulation

DIC is characterized by intravascular coagulation activation with microvascular thrombi formation.[12] This, in turn, causes thrombocytopenia and clotting factors depletion, leading to bleeding and end-organ complications.

Acute DIC manifests as a complication of several disease processes, notably sepsis, postoperative state, obstetric complication, blood transfusion reactions, and certain malignancies (acute promyelocytic leukemia). Clinically, a patient may have bleeding from various sites, including mucocutaneous and wound sites. In addition to thrombocytopenia, PT and aPTT are also abnormal.

Table 2
The 4 Ts for diagnosing heparin-induced thrombocytopenia

	Points (0, 1, or 2 for Each of 4 Categories: Maximum Possible Score = 8)		
	2	1	0
Thrombocytopenia	>50% Platelet fall to nadir ≥20 d	30%–50% Platelet fall or nadir 10–19	<30% Platelet fall or nadir <10
Timing[a] of onset of platelet fall (or other sequelae of HIT)	5–10 or ≤ day 1 with recent heparin (past 30 d)	>Day 10 or timing unclear; or <day 1 with recent heparin (past 31–100 d)	<Day 4 (no recent heparin)
Thrombosis or other sequelae	Proved new thrombosis; skin necrosis; or acute systemic reaction after intravenous unfractionated heparin bolus	Progressive or recurrent thrombosis; erythematous skin lesions; suspected thrombosis (proven)	None
Other cause(s) of platelet fall	None evident	Possible	Definite

Pretest probability score: 6 to 8 indicates high, 4 to 5 intermediate, and 0 to 3 low.
   [a] First day of immunizing heparin exposure considered day 0.
From Warkentin TE. Heparin-induced thrombocytopenia: diagnosis and management. Circulation 2004;110:e455; with permission.

Table 3
Comparison of heparin-induced antibody detection tests

Assay	Advantages	Disadvantages
Commercial PF4/polyanion–enzyme immunoassay[a]	Widely available; high sensitivity	Detects many nonpathogenic anti-PF4/polyanion IgA, IgM, and IgG antibodies (moderate specificity)
PF4/heparin–enzyme immunoassay that only detects IgG	Detecting only IgG improves specificity	Limited availability (research laboratories)
Platelet aggregation test (citrated platelet-rich plasma)	Many laboratories have conventional platelet aggregometers	Poor sensitivity and specificity; limited number of tests can be done; platelet donors required
Washed platelet activation assay (eg, serotonin release assay)	Highest sensitivity-specificity trade-off[b]	Technically demanding; limited availability (research laboratories); platelet donors required

In general, the greater the magnitude of a positive test result, the greater the likelihood that the patient has HIT; for example, most patients with HIT have serotonin release greater than 80% and optical density greater than 1.0 absorbance unit, that is, values well above the cutoffs defining a positive test.
   [a] Assay from GTI (Brookfield, Wisconsin) uses PF4/polyvinyl sulfonate, whereas assay from Stago (Asnières, France) uses PF4/heparin.
   [b] High sensitivity for clinical HIT (similar to enzyme immunoassays) but with greater diagnostic specificity than the enzyme immunoassays.
   From Warkentin TE. Heparin-induced thrombocytopenia: diagnosis and management. Circulation 2004;110:e456; with permission.

Chronic DIC has less obvious clinical or laboratory presentation and is seen in solid tumors and in large aortic aneurysms. Platelet count, in this situation, may only be moderately low or normal with modest elevation in D-dimer levels.
   Treatment of DIC should be directed at the underlying disease process.

Platelet Dysfunction

The qualitative aspect of platelet function and its evaluation can be challenging. On occasion, patients may present with history of bleeding issues (perioperative, menorrhagia, or easy bruising); may have disease processes, such as CKD; or may have medication history (aspirin or nonsteroidal anti-inflammatory drugs), which can guide the evaluation. For inherited platelet function disorders, however, there must be a high index of suspicion, because patients often lack any obvious clues.

Platelet Function Testing

The current gold standard is light transmission aggregometry. In this test, platelet-rich plasma is exposed to various agonists. The resulting agglutination/aggregation reactions are recorded and analyzed.
   Viscoelastic measure of coagulation, such as thromboelastograph and rotation thromboelastography, measure the whole spectrum of clot formation in real time on whole blood. This allows for an in vivo interaction measurement and has shown some utility in cardiac surgery, trauma, hepatobiliary surgery, and obstetrics.[2]
   Platelet function monitoring has also garnered some attention recently. Point-of-care tests (POCTs) have been developed and these tests are being studied for their utility in

assessing the effects of antiplatelet medications.[2,17] Rosengart and colleagues[18] retrospectively showed benefit of improved management of coronary artery bypass graft surgery after clopidogrel cessation by using POCTs instead of arbitrary time intervals. A recent Society of Thoracic Surgeons guideline update[19] recommended preoperative POCTs to identify patients with high residual platelet reactivity after usual doses of antiplatelet drugs and to monitor platelet function, which may help limit blood transfusion.

Inherited Platelet Function Disorders

If a patient is identified as having an inherited platelet function disorder, the patient should be prepared for surgery according to the risk of the procedure.[7] For minor procedures, tranexamic acid may be the only intervention, whereas for major procedures or severe platelet dysfunction, patients may require desmopressin or platelet transfusions. These patients may develop platelet or human leukocyte antigens–related antibodies with multiple transfusions, which may decrease any future platelet transfusion's effectiveness.

Glanzmann thrombasthenia

The autosomal recessive condition, Glanzmann thrombasthenia, causes reduction in the number and quality of the GPIIb/IIIa (fibrinogen) receptors on platelets and leads to decreased aggregation. Patients may have excessive bruising in early life, prolonged mucosal bleeding, and soft tissue or intracranial hemorrhage.

Recombinant factor VIIa could provide some hemostatic effect, if these patients are undergoing a minor procedure.

Bernard-Soulier syndrome

The autosomal recessive condition, Bernard-Soulier syndrome, reduces the number/function of GPIb/V/IX receptor on platelets. This results in decreased effectiveness of vWF binding and platelet adhesion. In addition, patients often have some thrombocytopenia with large platelets and may clinically present with bleeding diathesis.

Chronic Kidney Disease

CKD, independently of surgery, is associated with increased risk of bleeding.[20] This is likely multifactorial and has been attributed to platelet–vessel wall dysfunction. A recent meta-analysis of close to 700,000 patients undergoing cardiac surgery showed that approximately half of patients with normal kidney function required a red blood cell transfusion versus 75% of patients with CKD. In addition, CKD patients had 2-fold to 4-fold higher unadjusted relative risk of severe bleeding in cardiac and noncardiac settings (defined as >4 units of red blood cell transfusion). CKD was also associated with increased risk of reoperation due to bleeding. The investigators suggested improved preparation of CKD patients preoperatively:

- Preparation for rare blood type, specifically being mindful of potential antibody development if the patient is a future transplantation candidate
- Planning surgical technique
- Planning for duration of postoperative monitoring

Special Hematologic Considerations

Sickle cell anemia

Sickle cell diseases are a heterogeneous group of hemoglobin disorders that are usually in a chronic, compensated state.[21,22] Stressful situations, such as surgery, lead to multiple pathways, which can lead to vaso-occlusive pain crisis but also organ dysfunction. Pathophysiology is multifaceted but may include mechanisms driven by hypoxia and hypoperfusion as well as primary vascular endothelial damage, leading to ischemia.[22]

The preoperative testing should be based on clinical history and assessment of family origin. Patients from high-prevalence areas should be screened if not already aware of their status (**Box 2**), because heterozygosity may be diagnosed.[21]

For routine operations, complete blood cell count and high-performance liquid chromatography (or a suitable alternative) may be used. In emergency situations, complete blood cell count and sickle solubility test can be performed, which should be followed by a definitive testing.

Preoperative preparation of hemoglobin SS, hemoglobin S-C, and hemoglobin S/β-thalassemia patients includes[22]

- Adequate hydration, oxygenation monitoring, maintenance of normothermia, and pain/anxiety control
- Minor, nongeneral anesthetic surgeries may not require preoperative transfusion in a stable patient.
- For younger, stable patients undergoing low-risk to intermediate-risk procedures, preoperative transfusion can be considered. The practice of diluting sickle hemoglobin, however, is mostly based on case studies and needs to be balanced with the risk of iatrogenic complications of the transfusion itself.
- For patients with pulmonary disease or undergoing high-risk procedures, consideration should be made to decrease the hemoglobin S level to less than 30%, although some have suggested levels as high as 50% to 60% could be equally as effective.[23]

Glucose-6-phosphate dehydrogenase deficiency

Glucose-6-phosphate dehydrogenase (G6PD) deficiency is an X-linked disorder, which affects more men than women.[24] Certain drugs and foods as well as infection and metabolic stressors (such as surgery) can cause hemolysis. In general, hemolysis, if it occurs, is seen 1 to 3 days after contact with triggering factors. Although acute hemolysis is self-limited, in rare instances it may warrant treatment.

If G6PD deficiency is diagnosed preoperatively, careful planning is required to avoid any inciting triggers; this is the mainstay of the perioperative management. If hemolysis is suspected postoperatively, it should be evaluated with laboratory confirmation in addition to supportive therapy:

- Anemia
- Increased reticulocyte count by day 4 to 7
- Peripheral smear with Heinz bodies, schistocytes, reticulocytes
- Decreased haptoglobin
- Elevated bilirubin
- Urinalysis: brown color, hemosiderin, urobilinogen

Box 2

High-prevalence ethnic groups for hemoglobin S

North Africans, African Caribbeans, African Americans, Black British, Central and South Americans of partly African ethnicity, Greeks, Southern Italians (including Turks, Sicilians, Arabs, and Indians).

Adapted from Ryan K, Bain BJ, Worthington D, et al. Significant haemoglobinopathies: guidelines for screening and diagnosis. Br J Haematology 2010;149:37.

- Positive Coombs test
- Elevated lactate dehydrogenase

Thrombocytosis

Thrombocytosis, defined as platelet counts greater than 450,000 per mm^3, may be an incidental finding during a preoperative evaluation.[25] Thrombocytosis can be classified as primary (clonal), secondary (reactive), or familial. Primary thrombocytosis mostly affects adults and includes clonal disorders, such as essential thrombocythemia (ET), polycythemia vera, chronic myelogenous leukemia, and myelofibrosis.

ET is associated with giant platelets and dysplastic megakaryocytes. Due to abnormal platelet function, the patients have increased risk of bleeding as well as arterial thromboembolism (ATE) and VTE. Perioperatively, due to the prothrombotic state, there is an increase in ATE and VTE (incidence 5.3% and 1.1%, respectively). Bleeding risk also increases (incidence 10.5%). ET patients are treated if they have symptomatic disease, extreme thrombocytosis, and high-risk factors (age >60 years old, platelet count >1.5 million per mm^3, prior thrombosis or hemorrhage, and cardiovascular risk factors). Drug therapies include aspirin, hydroxyurea, anagrelide, interferon alfa, busulfan, and pipobroman. Given the high risk

- Elective surgery should be deferred and patients should be treated to decrease the platelet level to less than 400,000 per mm^3.
- In emergent situations when preoperative thrombocytosis cannot be lowered
  - Adequately hydrate to decrease the hyperviscosity
  - Encourage early postoperative ambulation and utilize mechanical thromboprophylaxis
  - Be judicious with pharmacologic thromboprophylaxis, due to the risk of bleeding.
  - May consider intraoperative and postoperative gabexate mesilate, as it has been reported to prevent thrombotic complications.
  - Consider platelet pheresis, when appropriate.

Secondary thrombocytosis has normal platelet structure and function and normal bone marrow. Treatment is geared toward the underlying cause, such as iron deficiency anemia, which is the most common noninfectious cause. Thrombotic complications are uncommon unless other prothrombotic risk factors are present.

VENOUS THROMBOEMBOLISM RISK STRATIFICATION AND PREVENTION

It is well known that VTE is a major cause of preventable death in hospitalized patients. It is approximated that 150,000 to 200,000 deaths per year occur in the United States; one-third of these deaths happen after surgery.[26] Despite knowledge of the risks of VTE, past analysis of hospital data showed that VTE prophylaxis was not as prevalent as hoped. The 2007 ENDORSE (Epidemiologic International Day for the Evaluation of Patients at Risk for Venous Thromboembolism in the Acute Hospital Care Setting) study, which analyzed 358 hospitals in multiple countries, found that only 58.5% of surgical patients deemed at risk for VTE (by ACCP guidelines) actually received guideline-recommended prophylaxis.[27] Since then, a variety of initiatives have brought attention to this matter, including a Call to Action by the Surgeon General in 2008[28] and another by the Joint Commission on Accreditation of Healthcare Organizations.[29] Furthermore, the Center for Medicare and Medicaid Services began to deny reimbursement for DVT or pulmonary embolism that occurred after hip or knee joint replacement surgery.

Methods for Venous Thromboembolism Prevention

Nonpharmacologic strategies for VTE prevention include early ambulation after surgery or devices like intermittent pneumatic compression devices (IPCs). Graduated compression stockings act by preventing venous distension in the lower extremities. A 2000 Cochrane review[30] examined trials that compared graduated compression stockings versus no prophylaxis in medical/surgical patients. The rate of DVT was 27% in the no prophylaxis group versus 13% in the graduated compression stocking group. In trials that added compression stockings to another method of prophylaxis, the DVT rate decreased from 15% to 2%.[30] There are also data regarding the effectiveness of IPCs for DVT prevention. IPCs work to improve venous circulation by periodic inflation and deflation of air-filled sleeves that encircle the lower legs. A meta-analysis by Vanek[31] found that IPCs reduced the rate of DVT by 18% (29% to 11%) compared with placebo and, when used in conjunction with compression stockings and foot pumps, reduced DVT rates from 15% to 8%.

Common pharmacologic treatments of VTE prevention include the use of aspirin, unfractionated heparin, LMWH, warfarin, and novel oral anticoagulants, which are now often referred to as TSOACs.

The effectiveness of aspirin in postoperative VTE prevention is unclear. A 2013 trial compared aspirin to LMWH for VTE prevention in 778 patients undergoing hip replacement. The patients in the aspirin group were found to have lower rates of VTE, but the rate did not achieve statistical significance for superiority.[32] The latest ACCP guidelines include aspirin on its list of agents to be considered for VTE prevention in joint replacement surgery, but evidence is not strong for its use over other chemical agents.

Key Points

Identifying surgical patients at risk for VTE

- The risk of VTE is dependent on several factors, notably a patient's individual risk factors for thrombosis and the type of surgery involved. Surgery itself can be associated with a prothrombotic state; the increase in plasminogen activator inhibitor-1 in the perioperative setting may increase the risk of VTE up to 100-fold.[33,34]
- The Caprini risk assessment model is a validated tool used to calculate the risk of VTE in surgical patients. A score is calculated by assigning points for various risk factors and then categorizing patients into 1 of 4 categories: very low risk, low risk, moderate risk, and high risk (**Table 4**).

The recommendations for VTE prophylaxis are as follows:

- Very low risk = Caprini score of 0 (incidence of VTE 0.5%)
  - Recommendations for prophylaxis include early ambulation (no chemical/mechanical prophylaxis).
- Low risk = Caprini score of 1 to 2 (incidence of VTE approximately 1.5%)
  - Mechanical prophylaxis recommended (preferably IPCs)
- Moderate risk = Caprini score of 3 to 4 (incidence of VTE approximately 3%)
  - LMWH/low-dose unfractionated heparin recommended (or IPCs in patients at high risk of bleeding)
- High risk = Caprini score of 5 or greater (incidence of VTE approximately 6%)
  - LMWH/low-dose unfractionated heparin recommended, with addition of graduated compression stockings or IPCs. If LMWH or low-dose unfractionated heparin is contraindicated, then fondaparinux or aspirin can be used.

Table 4
Caprini risk index

1 Point	2 Points	3 Points	5 Points
Age 41–60 y	Age 61–74	Age >75	Stroke less than
Minor surgery	Arthroscopic surgery	History of VTE	1 mo ago
Body mass index	Major open surgery	Family history of VTE	Elective
>25 kg/m^2	(>45 min)	Factor V Leiden	arthroplasty
Varicose veins	Laparoscopic surgery	Prothrombin 20210 A	Hip, pelvis,
Pregnancy/	(>45 min)	Lupus anticoagulant/	leg fracture
postpartum state	Malignancy	antiphospholipid	Acute spinal
Abnormal pulmonary	Confined to bed	antibody	cord injury
function test	(>72 h)	HIT	(less than
Acute congestive	Immobilizing	Thrombophilia	1 mo ago)
heart failure (in the	plastercast		
past month)	Central venous		
Bed rest	access		
Acute myocardial			
infarction			
History of unexplained			
or recurrent			
spontaneous			
abortion			
Inflammatory bowel			
disease			
Oral contraceptives/			
hormone replacement			
Sepsis (in the previous			
month)			
Serious lung disease/			
pneumonia (in the			
last month)			
Acute heart failure			

Venous Thromboembolism Prevention in Patients Undergoing Hip or Knee Replacement Surgery

Patients who undergo hip or knee replacement surgery are at increased risk of developing postoperative VTE. Thus, the current ACCP guidelines recommend extended VTE prophylaxis after surgery. IPCs are recommended during the inpatient stay. In addition to mechanical prophylaxis, pharmacologic prophylaxis for at least 10 to 14 days is recommended (IB recommendation). Prophylaxis may be extended for up to 35 days postoperatively (IIB recommendation).

PERIOPERATIVE MANAGEMENT OF THE PATIENT ON CHRONIC ANTICOAGULANT THERAPY

Management of antithrombotic therapy in the perioperative setting can be confusing for physicians. When should anticoagulation be held prior to surgery? Is bridging anticoagulation indicated postoperatively? If so, does bridging entail prophylactic dosing of subcutaneous heparin, LMWH, or full-dose anticoagulation (intravenous unfractionated heparin or therapeutic dosing of LWMH)? The latest ACCP guidelines is the recommended source for perioperative anticoagulation management.[35]

Key Points

Continuing warfarin during the surgical period

- Not all surgical procedures require temporary discontinuation of warfarin. Those procedures that can be safely performed without holding warfarin include
  - Dental procedures: restorations, uncomplicated extractions, endodontic surgery, prosthetic surgery, periodontal therapy, and dental hygiene
  - Gastrointestinal procedures: endoscopy (esophagogastroduodenoscopy, flexible sigmoidoscopy/colonoscopy without biopsy, diagnostic ERCP, push enteroscopy, and endoscopic ultrasound without biopsy)
  - Electroconvulsive therapy
  - Ophthalmologic procedures: cataract surgery, and trabeculectomy
  - Dermatologic procedures: Mohs surgery and simple excision/repair
  - Orthopedic procedures: joint aspiration, soft tissue injections, and minor foot procedure

Determination on whether or not to bridge

- Several factors need to be weighed when answering this question. The first consideration is weighing the risk of thromboembolism against the risk of bleeding. The risk of thromboembolism depends not only on the reason for chronic anticoagulation (atrial fibrillation, mechanical valve, or history of DVT/PE) but also on a patient's individual risk factor(s) (examples include advanced age, genetic hypercoagulable condition, and cancer). Patients can be risk stratified into low-risk, moderate-risk, or high-risk categories for perioperative thromboembolism. Atrial fibrillation and heart valves are discussed later.
- Low risk for VTE: VTE greater than 12 months ago and no other risk factors for thrombosis
- Moderate risk for VTE: VTE within the past 3 to 12 months, active cancer, nonsevere thrombophilia (like heterozygous factor V Leiden), and recurrent VTE
- High risk for VTE: VTE within the past 3 months, severe thrombophilia (protein C or S deficiency, antiphospholipid antibodies)
- Bridging is usually not recommended for patients falling into the low-risk VTE category. Therapeutic bridging is recommended for patients thought at high risk for postoperative VTE. Moderate-risk patients can be assessed on a case-by-case basis. In some patients, prophylactic bridging may be reasonable in the postoperative setting, whereas therapeutic bridging can be considered in other cases. The bleeding risk (based on the type of surgery/procedure) and provider/patient preferences may influence the decision on the type of bridging the patient receives. Although the distinction between low risk, moderate risk, and high risk outlined by the ACCP is based on observational data and not prospectively validated, it is a useful initial tool to help guide a clinician in the decision-making process.

Bridging in atrial fibrillation

- The goal in bridging anticoagulation for patients with atrial fibrillation is to minimize the risk of ATE, such as stroke or systemic embolism. Low-dose, or prophylactic-dose, bridging with LWMH has not been established in preventing ATE nor is thought biologically plausible to achieve this purpose. Therefore, when bridging patients in the perioperative setting, therapeutic dosing of LWMH or unfractionated heparin is to be used.
- Given the increased risk of bleeding in the postoperative period, careful consideration should be given as to which patients to bridge. Current ACCP guidelines

suggest using the $CHADS_2$ scoring system as a stratification tool. Although the CHA_2DS_2-VASc scoring system is now the clinical standard for assessing stroke risk in atrial fibrillation, its use has not been validated in the surgical population. As in the risk stratification for VTE, patients are grouped into low-risk, moderate-risk, and high-risk categories.

- ○ Low risk for ATE: $CHADS_2$ score of 0 to 2
- ○ Moderate risk for ATE: $CHADS_2$ score of 3 to 4
- ○ High risk for ATE: $CHADS_2$ score of 5 to 6 or $CHADS_2$ score of 3 to 4 but history of transient ischemic attack/stroke or intracardiac thrombus

- Bridging is not recommended for patients who fall in the low-risk category. Bridging in moderate-risk patients should be assessed on a case-by-case basis. Patient-specific factors and the bleeding risk associated with the procedure can help a clinician decide whether or not bridging is necessary. At this time, patients in the high-risk category are recommended to have bridging therapy.
- The recent BRIDGE trial supports the ACCP recommendation regarding non-bridging for low-risk patients but may raise questions regarding the overall safety of bridging for higher-risk patients with atrial fibrillation. In the study, patients with atrial fibrillation who underwent surgery were randomized to either a bridging strategy with therapeutic dosing of dalteparin (preoperatively and postoperatively) or to receive no bridging. The mean $CHADS_2$ score of the study group was 2.3. The nonbridging strategy was found noninferior in prevention of ATE. Furthermore, the bridging group was associated with an incidence of 3.2% for major bleeding versus 1.3% In the nonbridging group. These findings support no bridging up to a $CHADS_2$ score of 4 and reinforce the need to carefully consider which patients require perioperative bridging, because there is an increased risk of bleeding.[36]

Bridging for heart valves

- ACCP guidelines risk-stratify patients into low-risk, moderate-risk, and high-risk categories for ATE. Bridging involves the use of therapeutic dosing of LMWH or unfractionated heparin for patients at the highest risk for thromboembolism.
- Low risk for ATE: bileaflet aortic valve without atrial fibrillation and no other risk factors for stroke
- Moderate risk for ATE: bileaflet aortic valve and 1 of the following: atrial fibrillation, history of stroke/transient ischemic attack, hypertension, diabetes mellitus, congestive heart failure, and age greater than 75
- High risk for ATE: any mechanical mitral valve, older aortic valve, recent (<6 months) stroke, or transient ischemic attack

Target-specific Oral Anticoagulants

TSOACs have been approved by the Food and Drug Administration (FDA) and provide clinicians with alternative choices to vitamin K antagonists and aspirin (**Table 5**). Such medications have been used in practice for prevention of thromboembolism in the perioperative setting. Unlike warfarin, TSOACs do not require blood monitoring. Other potential advantages of these drugs over warfarin include that the drugs have an immediate anticoagulant effect (no need for bridging therapy when restarting medication in the perioperative setting), have less dietary restrictions, and have fewer drug-to-drug interactions. Disadvantages of TSOACs over warfarin include cost, short half-life of the medication, and lack of an effective reversal antidote. Also, TSOACs are not currently indicated for use in patients with prosthetic heart valves.

Table 5
Target-specific oral anticoagulants: mechanism of action, half-lives, and Food and Drug Administration–approved indications

Drug	Mechanism of Action	Time to Peak Plasma Concentration	Half-Life	Dosing Schedule	Food and Drug Administration Approved for Atrial Fibrillation	Food and Drug Administration Approved for Acute Venous Thromboembolism Treatment	Food and Drug Administration Approved for Venous Thromboembolism Prophylaxis After Hip and Knee Arthroplasty
Dabigatran	Thrombin inhibitor	1.5–2 h	15–17 h	Twice daily	Yes	Yes (bridging required)	No
Rivaroxaban	Factor Xa inhibitor	3–4 h	9–10 h	Once daily	Yes	Yes	Yes
Apixaban	Factor Xa inhibitor	3–4 h	8–15 h	Twice daily	Yes	Yes	Yes
Edoxaban	Factor Xa inhibitor	1–2 h	6–10 h	Once daily	Yes	Yes (bridging required)	No

TSOAC medications include the following: dabigatran (Pradaxa) is a direct thrombin (IIa) inhibitor, like argatroban. It is FDA approved for stroke prevention in nonvalvular atrial fibrillation (noninferior to warfarin in trials) as well as treatment of acute VTE (although it needs a parenteral bridge with heparin/LWMH at first). Dosing is twice a day; dose is reduced in patients with reduced creatinine clearance. Its main side effect centers on the gastrointestinal tract. Another potential disadvantage of dabigatran is its need to be stored in a separate bottle (away from other medications). Dabigatran is approved in multiple countries for VTE prevention in patients undergoing hip or knee joint replacement. The REMODEL and RENOVATE trials demonstrated that dabigatran was noninferior to enoxaparin in prevention of total VTE and all-cause mortality but not in the REMOBILIZE trial, which compared dabigatran to twice-daily dosing with enoxaparin.[37–39] Currently, dabigatran is not FDA approved in the United States for VTE prevention for joint replacement surgery. Rivaroxaban (Xarelto) is a factor Xa inhibitor, like heparin. It is the only TSOAC that is dosed daily (it lasts 8–12 hours, but factor Xa levels do not return to normal for 24 hours after dosing). Like other TSOACs, it is FDA approved for stroke prevention in patients with nonvalvular atrial fibrillation.

Rivaroxaban is also FDA approved for VTE prophylaxis in patients undergoing hip or knee joint replacement surgery. The RECORD trials compared the use of rivaroxoban versus enoxaparin in patients undergoing hip or knee replacement surgery. Compared with LWMH, rivaroxoban was associated with decreased rates of VTE and improved mortality rates. Incidence of major/clinically relevant bleeding was 2.8% in the rivaroxoban group versus 2.5% for enoxaparin.[40]

Apixiban (Eliquis) is a factor Xa inhibitor. Like the other oral Xa inhibitors, it is FDA approved for stroke prevention in atrial fibrillation (was found superior to warfarin in the AVERROES trial).[41] Apixiban is also approved for VTE prevention after hip or knee joint replacement surgery. Various trials have examined the efficacy of apixiban in VTE prevention in hip or knee replacement patients. The ADVANCE trial compared the use of apixiban 2.5 mg orally, twice a day, versus enoxaparin at 40 mg subcutaneously daily. The apixiban group was found to have a lower rate of VTE and a similar risk of bleeding compared with enoxaparin.[42,43] Apixiban is currently FDA approved in the United States for VTE prevention after hip and knee joint replacement surgery.

Edoxaban (Savaysa) is a factor Xa inhibitor that has been recently approved by the FDA for stroke prevention in patients with nonvalvular atrial fibrillation. It is also approved for the treatment of acute DVT or pulmonary embolism (after at least 5 days of parenteral drug treatment). Studies are ongoing to gauge its efficacy in postoperative VTE prevention for joint replacement (2 trials from Japan suggested a lower incidence of VTE when compared with enoxaparin).[44,45]

Other Key Points

When to hold anticoagulants prior to major surgery:

- LWMH: should be discontinued 24 hours prior to surgery
- Unfractionated heparin: should be discontinued 4 to 6 hours prior to surgery
- Warfarin: stop 5 days prior to surgery
- Fondaparinux: should be discontinued 72 to 96 hours prior to surgery
- TSOACs: the recommended time for discontinuation depends on several factors. The half-life of drug elimination, the risk of bleeding associated with the surgery in question, and whether a patient receives spinal or epidural anesthesia influences when a novel oral anticoagulant is stopped prior to a procedure.
  - Dabigatran: for patients with normal renal function, stop dabigatran 1 day prior to surgery in low-risk bleeding cases. For major surgery with a high

corresponding bleeding risk, dabigatran should be held for 2 to 3 days before surgery, which is approximately 4 to 5 half-lives of the drug. In patients with decreased renal function (creatinine clearance between 30 and 50 mL/min), dabigatran may need to be held for 5 days or more, because the drug is mostly excreted renally.
  o Rivaroxoban: for patients undergoing low-risk bleeding procedures, hold rivaroxoban 1 day before surgery. For major surgery, hold rivaroxoban 2 days prior to surgery (4–5 half-lives of the drug).
  o Apixiban: for patients undergoing low-risk bleeding procedures, stop apixiban 1 day before surgery. For major surgery, hold apixiban for 2 days prior to surgery (4–5 half-lives of the drug).

REFERENCES

1. Eckman MH, Erban JK, Singh SK, et al. Screening for the risk for bleeding or thrombosis. Ann Intern Med 2003;138(3):W15–24.
2. Thiruvenkatarajan V, Pruett A, Adhikary SD. Coagulation testing in the perioperative period. Indian J Anaesth 2014;58(5):565–72.
3. Seicean A, Schiltz NK, Seicean S, et al. Use and utility of preoperative hemostatic screening and patient history in adult neurosurgical patients. J Neurosurg 2012; 116:1097–105.
4. Committee on Standards and Practice Parameters, Apfelbaum JL, Connis RT, et al. Practice advisory for preanesthesia evaluation: an updated report by the American Society of Anesthesiologists Task Force on Preanesthesia Evaluation. Anesthesiology 2012;116(3):522–38.
5. Kamal AH, Tefferi A, Pruthi RK. How to Interpret and Pursue an Abnormal Prothrombin Time, Activated Partial Thromboplastin Time, and Bleeding Time in Adults. Mayo Clin Proc 2007;82(7):864–73.
6. Srivastava A, et al. Guidelines for the management of hemophilia. 2nd edition. Montreal (Quebec): World Federation of Hemophilia; 2012. p. 74.
7. Monagh DK, Gooding D. Surgery in patients with inherited bleeding disorders. Anaesthesia 2015;70(Suppl 1):112–20.
8. Buckner TW, Andrew L, Ragni MV, et al. Postoperative deep vein thrombosis (DVT) in patients with hemophilia undergoing major orthopedic surgery. Blood 2013;122(21):207.
9. Chair of group. The diagnosis, evaluation and management of von Willebrand disease. Bethesda (MD): National Heart, Lung, and Blood Institute; National Institutes of Health; 2007. GPO #08–5832.
10. Kaufman RM, Djulbegovic B, Gernsheimer TG, et al. Platelet Transfusion: A Clinical Practice Guideline from the AABB. Ann Intern Med 2015;162(3): 205–13.
11. Lin Y, Foltz LM. Proposed guidelines for platelet transfusion. B C Med J 2005; 47(5):245–8.
12. Stasi R. How to approach thrombocytopenia. Hematology 2012;2012:191–7.
13. Glance LG, Blumberg N, Eaton MP, et al. Preoperative thrombocytopenia and postoperative outcomes after noncardiac surgery. Anesthesiology 2014;120(1): 62–75.
14. Cines DB, Blanchette VS. Immune thrombocytopenic purpura. N Engl J Med 2002;346(13):995–1008.
15. Aster RH, Bougie DW. Drug-induced immune thrombocytopenia. N Engl J Med 2007;357(6):580–7.

16. Warkentin TE. Heparin-induced thrombocytopenia: diagnosis and management. Circulation 2004;110:e454–8.

17. Lippi G, Favaloro EJ, Salvagno GL, et al. Laboratory assessment and perioperative management of patients on antiplatelet therapy: From the bench to the bedside. Clin Chim Acta 2009;405:8–16.

18. Rosengart TK, Romeiser JL, White LJ, et al. Platelet activity measured by a rapid turnaround assay identifies coronary artery bypass frafting patients at increased risk for bleeding and transfusion complications after clopidogrel administration. J Thorac Cardiovasc Surg 2013;146(5):1259–66.

19. Ferraris VA, Saha SP, Oestreich JH, et al. 2012 update to the society of thoracic surgeons guideline on use of antiplatelet drugs in patients having cardiac and noncardiac operations. Ann Thorac Surg 2012;94:1761–81.

20. Acedillo RR, Shah M, Devereaux PJ, et al. The risk of perioperative bleeding in patients with chronic kidney disease: a systemic review and meta-analysis. Ann Surg 2013;258(6):201–13.

21. Ryan K, Bain BJ, Worthington D, et al. Significant haemoglobinopathies: guidelines for screening and diagnosis. Br J Haematol 2010;149:35–49.

22. Firth PG. Anaesthesia for peculiar cells-a century of sickle cell disease. Br J Anaesth 2005;95:287–99.

23. Vichinsky EP, Haberkern CM, Neumayr L, et al. A comparison of conservative and aggressive transfusion regimens in the perioperative management of sickle cell disease. The Preoperative Transfusion in Sickle Cell Disease Study Group. N Engl J Med 1995;333(4):206–13.

24. Elyassi AR, Rowshan HH. Perioperative management of the glucose-6-phosphate dehydrogenase deficient patient: a review of literature. Anesth Prog 2009;56: 86–91.

25. Harrison CN, Bareford D, Butt N, et al. Guideline for investigation and management of adults and children presenting with a thrombocytosis. Br J Haematol 2010;149:352–75.

26. Horlander KT, Mannino DM, Leeper KV. Pulmonary embolism mortality in the United States, 1979-1998: an analysis using multiple-cause mortality data. Arch Intern Med 2003;163(14):1711–7.

27. Cohen AT, Tapson VF, Bergmann JF, et al. Venous thromboembolism risk and prophylaxis in the acute hospital care setting (ENDORSE study): a multinational cross-sectional study. Lancet 2008;371(9610):387–94.

28. US Department of Health and Human Services. Surgeon general's call to action to prevent deep vein thrombosis and pulmonary embolism. 2008. Available at: http://www.surgeongeneral.gov/topics/deepvein. Accessed August 5, 2015.

29. U.S. Department of Health and Human Services and Joint Commission on Accreditation of Health Care Organizations. Available at: http://www.hhs.gov/; http://www.jointcommission.org/. Accessed August 5, 2015.

30. Amaragiri SV, Lees TA. Elastic compression stockings for prevention of deep venous thrombosis. Cochrane Database Syst Rev 2000;(3):CD001484.

31. Vanek VW. Meta-analysis of effectiveness of intermittent pneumatic compression devices with a comparison of thigh-high to knee-high sleeves. Am Surg 1998;64: 1050–8.

32. Anderson DR, Dunbar MJ, Bohm ER, et al. Aspirin versus low-molecular-weight heparin for extended venous thromboembolism prophylaxis after total hip arthroplasty: a randomized trial. Ann Intern Med 2013;158(11):800–6.

33. Jaffer AK. Perioperative management of warfarin and antiplatelet therapy. Cleve Clin J Med 2009;76(4):S37–44.

34. Gould MK, Garcia DA, Wren SM, et al. Prevention of VTE in nonorthopedic surgical patients. Chest 2012;141(Suppl 2):e227S–77S.
35. Douketis JD, Spyropoulos AC, Spencer FA, et al. Perioperative management of antithrombotic therapy: antithrombotic therapy and prevention of thrombosis, 9th ed: American College of Chest Physicians evidence-based clinical practice guidelines. Chest 2012;141(2 Suppl):e326S–50S.
36. Douketis JD, Spyropoulos AC, Kaatz S, et al. Perioperative bridging anticoagulaton in patients with atrial fibrillation. N Engl J Med 2015;373(9): 823–33.
37. Eriksson BI, Dahl OE, Rosencher N, et al. Oral dabigatran etexilate vs. subcutaneous enoxaparin for the prevention of venous thromboembolism after total knee replacement: the RE-MODEL randomized trial. J Thromb Haemost 2007; 5(11):2178–85.
38. Eriksson B, Dahl OE, Huo MH, et al, RE-NOVATE II Study Group. Oral thrombin inhibitor dabigatran versus enoxaparin for thromboprophylaxis after primary total hip arthroplasty (RE-NOVATE II). A randomized, double-blind, non-inferiority trial. Thromb Haemost 2011;105(4):721–9.
39. RE-MOBILIZE Writing Committee, Ginsberg JS, Davidson BL, et al. Oral thrombin inhibitor dabigatran etexilate vs North American enoxaparin regimen for prevention of venous thromboembolism after knee arthroplasty surgery. J Arthroplasty 2009;24(1):1–9.
40. Turpie AG, Lassen MR, Eriksson BI, et al. Rivaroxoban for the prevention of venous thromboembolism after hip or knee arthroplasty. Pooled analysis of four studies. Thromb Haemost 2011;105(3):444–53.
41. Connolly SJ, Eikelboom J, Joyner C, et al. Apixaban in patients with atrial fibrillation. N Engl J Med 2011;364:806–17.
42. Lassen MR, Raskob GE, Gallus A, et al, ADVANCE-2 Investigators. Apixiban versus Enoxaparin for thromboprophylaxis after knee replacement (ADVANCE-2): a randomized double-blind trial. Lancet 2010;375(9717):807–15.
43. Lassen MR, Gallus A, Raskob GE, et al, for the ADVANCE-3 Investigators. Apixiban versus enoxaparin for thromboprophylaxis after hip replacement. N Engl J Med 2010;363:2487–98.
44. Raskob G, Cohen AT, Eriksson BI, et al. Oral direct factor Xa inhibition with edoxaban for thromboprophylaxis after elective total hip replacement: a randomised double-blind dose-response study. J Thromb Haemost 2010;104(3):642–9.
45. Fuji T, Wang CJ, Fujita S, et al. Safety and efficacy of edoxaban, an oral factor Xa inhibitor, versus enoxaparain for thromboprophylaxis after total knee arthroplasty: the stars e-3 trial. Thromb Res 2014;134(6):1198–204.

Innovative Treatment/
Preparation Programs

Preoperative Anemia
Evaluation and Treatment

Ankit J. Kansagra, MD[a],*, Mihaela S. Stefan, MD[b]

KEYWORDS

- Preoperative period • Transfusion • Surgery • Optimization
- Patient blood management

KEY POINTS

- Preoperative anemia is the most frequent hematological condition identified before surgery.
- Preoperative anemia is associated with an increased likelihood of red blood cell (RBC) transfusion, which in turn has been associated with increased morbidity, mortality, and length of stay.
- Preoperative optimization of patients undergoing elective surgical procedures associated with significant blood loss, along with strategies to minimize intraoperative blood loss, shows promise for reducing postoperative transfusions and improving outcomes.
- Patients should be evaluated as early as possible in the preoperative pathway to coordinate optimization of patient hemoglobin and iron stores.
- Further research should evaluate if correcting preoperative anemia improves postoperative outcomes.

INTRODUCTION
Definition

Anemia is defined as a condition in which the body has a decreased amount of circulating erythrocytes, or RBCs, (and consequently their oxygen carrying capacity) compared with age-matched controls.[1] The World Health Organization (WHO) defines anemia as hemoglobin less than 13 g/dL in adult men (15 years of age and above) and less than 12 g/dL in adult nonpregnant women (15 years of age and above).[2,3] The WHO acknowledges, however, that these values were chosen somewhat arbitrarily; most laboratories define anemia as the lowest 2.5% of the distribution of hemoglobin values from a normal, healthy population.[2]

[a] Department of Hematology/Oncology, Baystate Medical Center, Tufts University, 376 Birnie Avenue, Springfield, MA 01199, USA; [b] Division of Hospital Medicine, Department of General Medicine, Tufts University, 759 Chestnut Street, S2660, Springfield, MA 01199, USA
* Corresponding author.
E-mail address: ankit.kansagramd@baystatehealth.org

Anesthesiology Clin 34 (2016) 127–141
http://dx.doi.org/10.1016/j.anclin.2015.10.011
anesthesiology.theclinics.com
1932-2275/16/$ – see front matter © 2016 Elsevier Inc. All rights reserved.

Epidemiology

Prevalence in general population

In the United States, prevalence estimates of anemia are approximately 5% in the general population, with preschool, pregnant, and elderly populations affected most significantly. In those older than 65, the prevalence of anemia climbs to 11%[4] and increases to more than 30% in those older than 85 years.[5]

Prevalence in surgical population

The reported prevalence of anemia in surgical patients varies largely due to the criteria for definition of anemia, population studied, and type of surgery. In studies published after 2000, preoperative anemia was found in 34% of all veterans undergoing noncardiac surgeries, in 46% of colorectal surgeries, in 25% to 45% of hip and knee surgeries, in 46% of elderly patients undergoing hip fracture surgery, and in 75% of patients with advanced colon cancer undergoing colectomy.[5,6]

Bleeding and blood loss are expected in major surgical procedures (especially cardiac, orthopedic, gynecologic, and cancer) despite the use of techniques to reduce blood loss; for example, a patient undergoing a major orthopedic surgery can lose as much as 1 litre of blood perioperatively.

Elderly patients and those with comorbidities, such as renal disease, cancer, heart failure, and diabetes mellitus, have an increased risk of being anemic.[5] Female patients are also at an increased risk of being anemic compared with men, likely because female patients have lower circulating blood volume and if the amount of blood loss is the same it may result in a higher probability of postoperative anemia.[7]

In 2011, the availability of allogenic whole blood/RBCs in the United States was approximately 14.5 million units, and 13.7 million units were transfused.[8] It is estimated that yearly 60% to 70% of all RBC units are transfused to surgical patients.[9,10] In the United States, the whole blood/RBC transfusion rate in 2011 was 44.0 allogenic units per 1000 overall population; although this rate is lower than in 2008, it is still substantially higher than the rates reported in Canada and in European countries.[11] It is postulated that the decline in transfusion is an indicator of better blood management practices, including a reduction in transfusion rates in surgical patients.

PREOPERATIVE OPTIMIZATION OF PATIENTS AND ANEMIA EVALUATION
Should Evaluation for Anemia Be Part of the Preoperative Risk Assessment and Optimization?

The preoperative evaluation can be considered to serve 2 broad purposes: (1) to risk stratify patients in order that providers and patients and their families are well informed on the risks in undergoing the surgical procedure and (2) to proactively identify and optimize preoperatively modifiable factors and thus improve a patient's chance for a successful outcome.

Although several studies suggest that anemia is associated with an increase in postoperative transfusions, morbidity, and mortality, patients with anemia frequent proceed with surgery without optimization and often the hemoglobin is measured only a few days before surgery when there is little to be done for work-up and treatment.[12,13] One of the reasons may be the belief that anemia is readily correctable by means of transfusion, giving clinicians a sense that it is not a problem that necessarily needs to be addressed before surgery. Preoperative assessment provides an opportunity for proactive recognition and management of the anemia and may avoid postoperative anemia and blood transfusions.

Which Surgeries Require Measurement of Hemoglobin Preoperatively and When Should the Test be Scheduled?

Anemia screening should be individualized based on a patient's symptoms, age, and comorbidities; type of surgery; and anticipated blood loss.

As a general rule a complete blood cell count is indicated in

- Surgery with potential for large (>15% estimated blood volume) blood loss
- Surgery with potential for moderate (>10% estimated blood volume) blood loss and
  - Known or suspected anemia, or
  - An established coagulation abnormality, or
  - Known or suspected RBC antibodies, or
  - Symptomatic anemia

A hemoglobin measurement is not indicated for low-risk surgeries or healthy, young patients undergoing surgeries with anticipated minimal blood loss.

The preoperative office visit represents an opportunity for timely detection and management of perioperative anemia before elective surgery. The decision to complete a work-up for diagnostic evaluation of anemia depends on the severity of anemia and the urgency of the surgery, and each case must be evaluated separately. To be able to appropriately manage a patient found to be anemic, however, the hemoglobin has to be determined at least 3 to 4 weeks prior to the surgery.

What Should Be the Target Hemoglobin Preoperatively?

Generally speaking, there is no reason to think that a patient undergoing an elective surgery should have a different target from a normal range; however, the decision to postpone surgery to achieve this target has to be individualized to the patient and type of procedure.

Only a few good-quality studies have evaluated the effect of preoperative hemoglobin on postoperative outcomes. One study, which assessed a cohort of patients who refused blood transfusions for religious reasons, found that there was an increase in mortality in patients with a hemoblogin level less than 7 g/dL preoperatively.[14] When deciding the threshold for hemoglobin, other factors to consider include patient age and presence of comorbidities. In a large retrospective study of 310,311 veterans aged 65 years and older who underwent major noncardiac surgery, Wu and colleagues[15] showed a 1.6% increase in postoperative mortality with every percentage point decrease in hematocrit value (Hct) from normal range.

An approximate estimate of calculating the hemoglobin/Hct after surgery can be obtained by modifying a calculator of allowed blood loss in surgery by replacing the allowed blood loss value with the actual estimated blood loss and lowest acceptable Hct with postoperative Hct. It should also be taken into account that in addition to the blood loss with the surgery, postoperative anemia is worsened by hemodilution, inflammatory cytokine release after surgery, decrease in gastrointestinal uptake, and decreased erythropoietin production.[16–19]

A calculator for the amount of allowed blood loss is provided at: https://www.openanesthesia.org/maximum_abl_calculation/.

Allowed blood loss = Estimated blood volume × (Initial Hct – Lowest acceptable Hct)/Initial Hct; average blood volume = 75 mL/kg for adult men and 65 mL/kg for adult women

When Should the Surgery Be Postponed for Anemia Work-up and Treatment?

Several recent consensus guidelines recommend routine preoperative anemia management for elective surgery.[20,21] Elective surgery offers the potential for preoperative work-up and optimization of hemoglobin before surgery and, when possible, patients with unexpected preoperative anemia should be rescheduled until evaluation and treatment are finalized.

In 2011, the Network for Advancement of Transfusion Alternatives, which included a multidisciplinary panel of physicians from 13 countries, including the United States, published practice guidelines for detection, evaluation, and management of anemia in elective orthopedic surgeries; it may be reasonable to consider these recommendations for any surgery with potential significant blood loss.[20]

The group has the following recommendations:

1. Patients should have a hemoglobin level measured 28 days before the scheduled surgery.
2. Target hemoglobin before the surgery should be in the normal range.
3. If anemia is identified, further testing should be performed to evaluate for nutritional deficiencies, chronic renal insufficiency, and/or chronic inflammatory disease.
4. Nutritional deficiencies should be treated and erythropoietin-stimulating agents (ESAs) may be used in patients in whom nutritional deficiencies have been ruled out or corrected.

An example of a pathway for evaluation of anemia prior to an elective procedure is given in **Fig. 1**.

PREOPERATIVE ANEMIA, PERIOPERATIVE BLOOD TRANSFUSIONS, AND POSTOPERATIVE OUTCOMES

Preoperative anemia contributes to postoperative anemia and increases the chance of RBC transfusion,[22–24] which in itself is associated with adverse outcomes.[25] In a large study of more than 6000 noncardiac surgical patients, the subgroup with preexisting anemia required 5 times more blood than nonanemic patients.[26]

Several retrospective observational studies suggest that transfusions are associated with increased rates of infection, ischemic complications, and death[12,13] and that preoperative anemia is associated with an increase in postoperative complications, length of hospital stay, and mortality.[15,26–29] Preoperative anemia, postoperative anemia, and blood transfusion are interlinked, however, and sick patients are more likely to be transfused and develop complications. Identifying the independent effect of each is challenging and anemia is often a sign of an underlying disease that could have an impact on surgical outcomes.

Randomized controlled trials did not find any difference in mortality of patients assigned to restrictive transfusion (hemoglobin <8 g/dL) compared with those assigned to liberal transfusion strategy (hemoglobin ≥10 g/dL),[30,31] but these studies did not address specifically the impact of perioperative anemia on the outcomes.

Mortality

Preoperative anemia was found an independent risk factor for in-hospital, 30-day, and 90-day mortality after several types of surgery. A large retrospective study using a

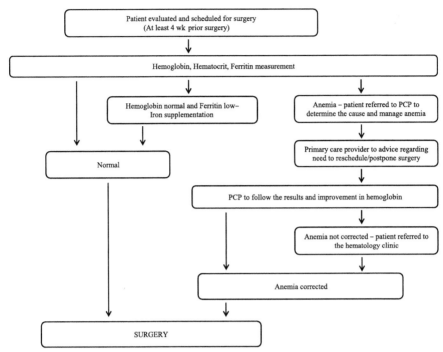

Fig. 1. Preoperative anemia pathway for a patient scheduled for an elective surgery. For hospitals with a preoperative clinic for risk assessment and optimization, anemia assessment and management can be performed in the clinic.

National Surgical Quality Improvement Program database found that patients with preexisting anemia has an increased risk for mortality, especially if they also had preexisting cardiovascular disease and an increased risk in a composite outcome of myocardial infarction, stroke, renal insufficiency, or death within 30 days of surgery.[6]

Postoperative Complications

The vast majority of evidence suggest that preoperative anemia has a deleterious impact on the medical postoperative outcomes and complications in both elective and emergent surgical populations. In patients with hip fracture, anemia on admission had been associated with an increase length of hospital stay and readmission rate and with worse postoperative function.[32–34] In elective cardiac and noncardiac surgeries, preexisting anemia is associated with increased risk of infective complications, respiratory failure, renal failure, delirium in the elderly, and perioperative cardiac events.[28,35–37] The relationship with functional outcomes after elective orthopedic surgeries is not clear, with some more recent studies finding that postoperative anemia is not related to quality-of-life and functional outcome.[38,39]

EVALUATION FOR ANEMIA

Preoperative evaluation for patients at risk of being anemic or who are anemic include the following:

1. Detailed medical and surgical history
2. Review of prior medical records

3. Physical examination
4. Review of existing laboratory results
5. Ordering laboratory tests if indicated

The 3 main causes of anemia are:

- Blood loss
- Underproduction of RBCs
- Increased destruction of RBCs

History

History should inquire about symptoms of bleeding; chronic diseases, which may be associated with anemia; past history of anemia; medications; and symptoms related to anemia.

Various history-taking clues that can aid in the evaluation of anemia are described briefly (**Box 1**).[3,40]

Answering the following questions helps define a framework for further work-up:

1. Is the patient bleeding (now or in the past)?
2. Is the patient iron deficient? If so, why?
3. Is the patient folate or vitamin B_{12} deficient? If so, why?
4. Is the patient's bone marrow suppressed? If so, why?
5. Is there any evidence of increased RBC destruction?

Box 1
Etiology of anemia

Blood loss (acute or chronic)

- Gastrointestinal tract (ie, hematemesis or hematochezia)
- Genitourinary tract (ie, hematuria)
- Respiratory tract (ie, hemoptysis or nose bleeds)
- Menstrual history
- Recent surgeries (direct loss or secondary bleeding [eg, retroperitoneal hemorrhage after cardiac catheterization])

Chronic medical problems

- Renal disease
- Inflammatory disease (eg, rheumatoid arthritis or inflammatory bowel disease)
- Congestive heart failure
- Prosthetic valves
- Malignancy
- Infections (eg, HIV)
- Liver disease
- Intestinal malabsorption, celiac disease

Past history of anemia and prior treatment

- History of transfusions
- Splenectomy
- Blood donation

Medications

- Nonsteroidal anti-inflammatory drugs
- Antibiotics (eg, cephalosporin and sulfa drugs)
- Chemotherapeutic agents
- Dapsone
- Anticonvulsants (eg, phenytoin and carbamazepine)
- Herbal and over-the-counter medications

Family history

- Sickle cell anemia
- Thalassemia
- Hereditary spherocytosis

Social history

- Nutritional status especially in older adults (eg, tea and toast diet)
- Alcohol usage

Signs, Symptoms, and Physical Examination

Symptoms related to anemia can result from 2 factors: decreased oxygen delivery to tissues and, in patients with acute bleeding, the added effect of hypovolemia. Many patients, however, are asymptomatic/minimally symptomatic although they have anemia, and the diagnosis of anemia is found on routine preoperative laboratory work.

Patients can complain of symptoms, such as fatigue, weakness, lightheadedness or dizziness, chest pain, and decreased exercise tolerance. Patients with chronic anemia or congenital forms of anemia (eg, sickle cell disease [SCD] and hereditary spherocytosis) may not report symptoms until hemoglobin decreases to less than 5 g/dL.

Physical examination findings of pallor, jaundice, or scleral icterus may suggest a hemolytic anemia. Other signs of underlying disease may include cardiac murmurs, hepatosplenomegaly, lymphadenopathy, petechial rash, or blood on digital rectal examination.[3]

Laboratory Evaluation

Initial laboratory evaluation of anemia includes complete blood cell count, peripheral blood smear, and a reticulocyte count. **Fig. 2** describes a practical approach to the work-up of anemia.

Two important RBC indices that help determine the cause of anemia include mean corpuscular value (MCV) (ie, size of an RBC) and reticulocyte production index (RPI) (measurement of reticulocyte response with correction for the degree of anemia and reticulocyte maturation time). Most laboratory reports calculate RPI; however, if that is not available, it can be calculated as RPI = reticulocytes (percent) $\times$ (Hct $\div$ 45) $\times$ (1 $\div$ RMT) [Reticulocyte maturation time (RMT) is used to correct for the longer life span of prematurely released reticulocytes in blood – a phenomenon of increased red blood cell production. To find out reticulocyte maturation time, use the following guidelines. For the Hct value for the patient use the given maturation time in provided equation,

- HCT 36-45, the maturation time = 1.0
- HCT 26-35, the maturation time = 1.5

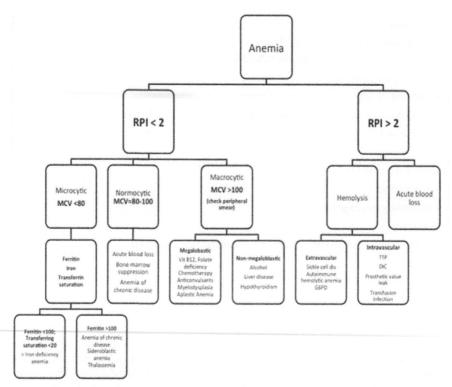

Fig. 2. Differential diagnosis of anemia flow diagram. This list of causes is not meant to be exhaustive; only the most common are included. DIC, disseminated intravascular coagulation; G6PD, Glucose-6-Phosphate Dehydrogenase deficiency; MCV, mean corpuscular volume; RPI, reticulocyte production induction; TTP, thrombotic thrombocytopenia. Items listed in bold indicate laboratory investigation. (*Adapted from* Vieth JT, Lane DR. Anemia. Emerg Med Clin North Am 2014;32(3):613–28; with permission; and *Data from* Patel MS, Carson JL. Anemia in the preoperative patient. Anesthesiol Clin 2009;27(4):751–60.)

- HCT of 16-25, the maturation time = 2
- HCT 15 and below, the maturation time = 2.5].
- An RPI greater than 2 indicates an appropriate bone marrow response and differential diagnosis includes blood loss or hemolysis.
- Next steps include
  ○ Assessing for sources of blood loss: careful history, stool guaiac, and endoscopy/colonoscopy if indicated
  ○ Assessing for hemolysis: lactate dehydrogenase, haptoglobin, and peripheral smear. An elevated direct bilirubin and lactate dehydrogenase and a low haptoglobin level along with a positive direct and indirect Coombs test point toward hemolysis.
  ○ Peripheral smear should be reviewed for clues to underlying process and hemoglobin electrophoresis may be helpful. Various peripheral smear findings are described in **Table 1**.
- An RPI less than 2 indicates hypoproliferative anemia or an inappropriate/attenuated bone marrow response to anemia.
- The next step includes checking the MCV and further characterizing the anemia as microcytic, normocytic, or macrocytic and a peripheral blood smear. **Fig. 2** also

Table 1
Common peripheral smear findings and their associated disease

Abnormal Peripheral Blood Smear Findings	Associated Disease State
Schistocytes	Microangiopathic hemolytic anemia Hemolysis
Spherocytes	Hereditary spherocytosis Autoimmune hemolytic anemia
Sickle cells	SCD
Burr cells	Chronic renal failure
Target cells	Hemoglobinopathies IDA
Teardrop cells	Leukoerythroblastic syndrome – for example, myelofibrosis and myelodysplasia
Nucleated RBCs	Severe hemolysis Myelophthisic condition – for example, myelofibrosis
Rouleaux formation	Multiple myeloma
Blasts	Leukemia Lymphoma Myelodysplasia
Smudge cells	Chronic lymphocytic luekemia

Adapted from Vieth JT, Lane DR. Anemia. Emerg Med Clin North Am 2014;32(3):613–28; with permission; and *Data from* Bain BJ. Diagnosis from the blood smear. N Engl J Med 2005;353(5):498–507.

describes the most common causes of anemia based on MCV. **Table 2** describes the laboratory parameters that help differentiate between most common causes of anemia (iron deficiency anemia [IDA] and anemia of chronic disease).

A hematology consultation prior to surgery in patients with newly diagnosed anemia is recommended in the following situations:

1. Abnormal cells in circulation (eg, nucleated RBCs and blasts)
2. Increase/decrease in absolute counts for granulocyte, lymphocyte, monocyte, or platelets, which likely suggests a complex hematological problem (eg, leukemia, aplastic anemia, myelodysplasia, or myeloproliferative neoplasm)
3. Lack of improvement of anemia after 3 to 4 weeks of adequate treatment

Table 2
Differential diagnosis of microcytic anemia

Causes of Hypochromic Anemia	Serum Iron (Fe)	Ferritin	Total Iron Binding Capacity	Percentage Saturation
Iron deficiency	Decreased	Low (<100)	Increased	Decreased (<16%)
Anemia of chronic disease	Decreased	Normal	Decreased	Decreased
Thalassemia	Normal/increased	Normal	Normal	Normal/increased

Adapted from Vieth JT, Lane DR, Anemia. Emerg Med Clin North Am 2014;32(3):613–28; with permission; and *Data from* Goodnough LT, Maniatis A, Earnshaw P, et al. Detection, evaluation, and management of preoperative anaemia in the elective orthopaedic surgical patient: NATA guidelines. Br J Anaesth 2011;106(1):13–22.

TREATMENT OF ANEMIA

Management of perioperative anemia is driven by the cause of the anemia and urgency of the surgery.

Nutritional Deficiency

Iron deficiency anemia

Once a diagnosis of IDA is made, it is important to identify the underlying cause, such as blood loss, and treat it. Ferrous sulfate is an inexpensive and easy way of correcting iron deficiency. An appropriate daily dose for treating IDA in adults is in the range of 150 to 200 mg/d of elemental iron. Various iron preparations are available, including ferrous sulfate, 325 mg (65 mg elemental iron), or ferrous gluconate, 325 mg (36 mg elemental iron), given 2 or 3 times a day. There is no evidence of one more effective than another. Oral iron is more readily absorbed in an acidic gastric environment and, therefore, often given with ascorbic acid. Clinical response with feeling of well-being is noted within first few days, with laboratory improvement of hemoglobin by approximately 2 g/dL over 3 weeks. Occasionally patients may not respond to oral iron and need intravenous iron and further evaluation of underlying causes. Common clinical conditions include nonadherence, concomitant uses of antacids, *Helicobacter pylori* infection, malabsorption (eg, celiac disease), and ongoing blood losses.[40,41]

Vitamin B$_{12}$ or folate deficiency

Patients with gastric surgeries (subtotal gastrectomy or bariatric surgery), pure vegetarians, and pregnant women on Mediterranean diets are at a risk of vitamin B$_{12}$ deficiency. Intramuscular vitamin B$_{12}$ is given at a dose of 1000 μg every day for 7 days, followed by 1000 μg weekly for 4 weeks. Hemoglobin concentration begins to rise within 10 days and normalizes within 8 weeks. Folate deficiency, very uncommon in the United States, is treated with folic acid, 1 mg/d orally, for 1 to 4 months.[42]

Stimulation of Erythropoiesis

Several randomized controlled trials have evaluated the role of ESAs in correcting preoperative anemia and avoiding or reducing postoperative blood transfusion in various surgical settings (orthopedic, cardiovascular, and oncological). The American Society of Anesthesiologists (ASA) Task Force on Preoperative Blood Management recommends ESAs with or without iron in select patient populations (eg, renal insufficiency, anemia of chronic disease, and refusal of transfusion).[43]

The current recommendation for perioperative use of epoetin alfa (Procrit) as it appears on the package insert is[44]

- 300 Units/kg per day subcutaneously for 15 days total: administered daily for 10 days before surgery, 1 dose on the day of surgery and then for 4 days after surgery, or
- 600 Units/kg subcutaneously in 4 doses administered 21, 14, and 7 days before surgery and on the day of surgery.

The package insert also recommends deep venous thrombosis prophylaxis during epoetin alfa therapy. Suggested precautions and contraindications for the use of ESAs in-patient with preoperative anemia are listed[44,45]:

- Uncontrolled hypertension (systolic blood pressure >160 mm Hg and diastolic blood pressure >90 mm Hg)
- Pure RBC aplasia that begins after treatment with erythropoietin protein drugs

- Previous history of thrombotic vascular events (myocardial infarction/cerebro-vascular accident/transient ischemic attack/deep vein thrombosis/pulmonary embolism). Using ESAs to target a hemoglobin level of greater than 11 g/dL increased the risk of serious adverse cardiovascular reactions.
- Previous history of seizures
- Risk factors predisposing to preoperative deep vein thrombosis (eg, immobility and fracture joint)
- Hypercoagulable disease states (eg, positive lupus anticoagulant)
- Cancer diagnosis/treatment (in past 3 years); not an absolute exclusion, consider each patient individually; if proceeding, close monitoring and Hb not to exceed 13.5 g/dL

Red Cell Transfusion

Allogeneic transfusion

In 2006 the ASA launched a task force to establish new guidelines for perioperative blood management. In an updated report in February 2015, the ASA task force strongly recommends a restrictive strategy for blood transfusion and administration of RBCs with hemoglobin level less than 6 g/dL. To determine who would benefit from blood transfusion when hemoglobin level falls between 6 g/dL and 10 g/dL is based on factors like potential or actual ongoing bleeding (rate and magnitude), intravascular volume status, signs of organ ischemia, and adequacy of cardiopulmonary reserve.[43]

The task force also recommends administration of unit-by-unit transfusion with interval re-evaluation. In the published updates in 2015, the task force endorses use of transfusion algorithms, especially those based on thromboelastographic testing, and blood ordering schedules. The ASA has selected restrictive transfusion strategy in the perioperative period as 1 of the top 5 Choosing Wisely initiatives.

Autologous transfusion

Over the past several years, there has been a steady decline in the use of preoperative autologous blood donations (PADs). Compared with 2008, 59.4% fewer units of autologous blood were transfused in 2011. Approximately half of all autologous donations were not used in 2011.[11] This decline can be explained by a combination of several factors, including a decreasing real and perceived risk of disease transmission through allogeneic transfusion, the adoption of better patient blood management (PBM) practices, and the increasing logistical and cost constraints of PAD programs. Various national societies recommend that PADs be considered exclusively for patients refusing necessary allo-transfusion (eg, religious belief), those with RBC alloantibodies necessitating rare blood unavailable in volumes likely to be required, and, possibly, selected healthy individuals planning procedures with at least a 50% risk of requiring 3 or more units of transfusion.[46]

PREOPERATIVE ANEMIA MANAGEMENT IN PATIENTS WITH SICKLE CELL DISEASE

Surgical procedures in patients with SCD are associated with significant risk of perioperative complications. Surgical stress and trauma can increase the rate of anemia and sickle cell formation, and RBC transfusions are often used to preserve oxygen carrying capacity and to dilute the sickle cells. The Transfusion Alternatives Preoperatively in Sickle Cell Disease study is a multicenter randomized control trial that demonstrated a lowered risk of postoperative complications in patients with SCD undergoing medium-risk surgery when preoperative hemoglobin level was increased to 10 g/dL. Based on these results, an expert panel reviewing recommendations in management of SCD recommends RBC transfusion to bring preoperative hemoglobin level to 10 g/dL prior to any surgical procedures involving general anesthesia.[47,48]

Hematology consultation should be considered in patients with SCD receiving hydroxyurea therapy, planning to undergo high-risk surgery (eg, neurosurgery, prolonged anesthesia, or cardiac bypass), or those with hemoglobin SC or hemoglobin SB plus thalassemia.

PATIENT BLOOD MANAGEMENT

PBM, a term has that emerged in the past few years, is a patient-centered evidence-based multidisciplinary approach to improve the care of patients who may need transfusion.[7,49–51]

PBM has 3 main pillars:

1. Optimization of blood volume and RBC mass preoperative, which includes anemia screening, assessment, and management
2. Minimization of blood loss and blood conservation modalities
3. Making patient-centered decisions for transfusions

Many transfusions may be avoided if, for example, patients' iron deficiency is treated and patients have enough time to generate their own RBCs. Still there is a significant challenge to making sure that anemia is diagnosed and treated in a timely manner. Implementation of a PBM program represents a great opportunity to address the perioperative anemia and reduce the need for transfusions. This requires, however, a collaborative strategy to include primary care providers, surgeons, transfusion specialists, anesthesiologists, and the hospitals and, most importantly, a change in the culture of health care providers.

SUMMARY

Preoperative anemia is the most frequent hematological condition identified before surgery and the most common cause is iron deficiency. Preoperative anemia is associated with an increased likelihood of RBC transfusion, which in turn has been associated with increased morbidity, mortality, and length of stay. Anemia is often overlooked in the preoperative evaluation based on the misconception that it is easily corrected with blood transfusions. Patients should be evaluated as early as possible in the preoperative pathway to coordinate optimization of the patient hemoglobin and, when possible, patients with unexpected preoperative anemia should be rescheduled until evaluation and treatment are finalized.

REFERENCES

1. Skjelbakken T, Langbakk B, Dahl IM, et al. Haemoglobin and anaemia in a gender perspective: the Tromso Study. Eur J Haematol 2005;74(5):381–8.
2. Bryan LJ, Zakai NA. Why is my patient anemic? Hematol Oncol Clin North Am 2012;26(2):205–30, vii.
3. Vieth JT, Lane DR. Anemia. Emerg Med Clin North Am 2014;32(3):613–28.
4. Dubois RW, Goodnough LT, Ershler WB, et al. Identification, diagnosis, and management of anemia in adult ambulatory patients treated by primary care physicians: evidence-based and consensus recommendations. Curr Med Res Opin 2006;22(2):385–95.
5. Shander A, Knight K, Thurer R, et al. Prevalence and outcomes of anemia in surgery: a systematic review of the literature. Am J Med 2004;116(Suppl 7A): 58S–69S.

6. Leichtle SW, Mouawad NJ, Lampman R, et al. Does preoperative anemia adversely affect colon and rectal surgery outcomes? J Am Coll Surg 2011; 212(2):187–94.

7. Munoz M, Gómez-Ramírez S, Kozek-Langeneker S, et al. 'Fit to fly': overcoming barriers to preoperative haemoglobin optimization in surgical patientsdagger. Br J Anaesth 2015;115(1):15–24.

8. McLean E, Cogswell M, Egli I, et al. Worldwide prevalence of anaemia, WHO Vitamin and Mineral Nutrition Information System, 1993-2005. Public Health Nutr 2009;12(4):444–54.

9. Wells AW, Mounter PJ, Chapman CE, et al. Where does blood go? Prospective observational study of red cell transfusion in north England. BMJ 2002; 325(7368):803.

10. Patel MS, Carson JL. Anemia in the preoperative patient. Anesthesiol Clin 2009; 27(4):751–60.

11. Whitaker BI. The 2011 National Blood collection and utilization survery report. 2011. Available at: http://www.aabb.org/research/hemovigilance/bloodsurvey/Documents/11-nbcus-report.pdf. Accessed July 27, 2015.

12. Shokoohi A, Stanworth S, Mistry D, et al. The risks of red cell transfusion for hip fracture surgery in the elderly. Vox Sang 2012;103(3):223–30.

13. Weber WP, Zwahlen M, Reck S, et al. The association of preoperative anemia and perioperative allogeneic blood transfusion with the risk of surgical site infection. Transfusion 2009;49(9):1964–70.

14. Carson JL, Noveck H, Berlin JA, et al. Mortality and morbidity in patients with very low postoperative Hb levels who decline blood transfusion. Transfusion 2002; 42(7):812–8.

15. Wu WC, Schifftner TL, Henderson WG, et al. Preoperative hematocrit levels and postoperative outcomes in older patients undergoing noncardiac surgery. JAMA 2007;297(22):2481–8.

16. Weiss G, Goodnough LT. Anemia of chronic disease. N Engl J Med 2005;352(10): 1011–23.

17. Tilg H, Ulmer H, Kaser A, et al. Role of IL-10 for induction of anemia during inflammation. J Immunol 2002;169(4):2204–9.

18. Clemens J, Spivak JL. Serum immunoreactive erythropoietin during the perioperative period. Surgery 1994;115(4):510–5.

19. Garcia-Erce JA, Cuenca J, Muñoz M, et al. Perioperative stimulation of erythropoiesis with intravenous iron and erythropoietin reduces transfusion requirements in patients with hip fracture. A prospective observational study. Vox Sang 2005; 88(4):235–43.

20. Goodnough LT, Maniatis A, Earnshaw P, et al. Detection, evaluation, and management of preoperative anaemia in the elective orthopaedic surgical patient: NATA guidelines. Br J Anaesth 2011;106(1):13–22.

21. Leal-Noval SR, Muñoz M, Asuero M, et al. Spanish consensus statement on alternatives to allogeneic blood transfusion: the 2013 update of the "Seville Document". Blood Transfus 2013;11(4):585–610.

22. Melis M, McLoughlin JM, Dean EM, et al. Correlations between neoadjuvant treatment, anemia, and perioperative complications in patients undergoing esophagectomy for cancer. J Surg Res 2009;153(1):114–20.

23. Gombotz H, Rehak PH, Shander A, et al. Blood use in elective surgery: the Austrian benchmark study. Transfusion 2007;47(8):1468–80.

24. Spahn DR. Anemia and patient blood management in hip and knee surgery: a systematic review of the literature. Anesthesiology 2010;113(2):482–95.

25. Glance LG, Dick AW, Mukamel DB, et al. Association between intraoperative blood transfusion and mortality and morbidity in patients undergoing noncardiac surgery. Anesthesiology 2011;114(2):283–92.

26. Dunne JR, Malone D, Tracy JK, et al. Perioperative anemia: an independent risk factor for infection, mortality, and resource utilization in surgery. J Surg Res 2002; 102(2):237–44.

27. Hagino T, Ochiai S, Sato E, et al. The relationship between anemia at admission and outcome in patients older than 60 years with hip fracture. J Orthop Traumatol 2009;10(3):119–22.

28. Kulier A, Levin J, Moser R, et al. Impact of preoperative anemia on outcome in patients undergoing coronary artery bypass graft surgery. Circulation 2007; 116(5):471–9.

29. Beattie WS, Karkouti K, Wijeysundera DN, et al. Risk associated with preoperative anemia in noncardiac surgery: a single-center cohort study. Anesthesiology 2009;110(3):574–81.

30. Carson JL, Terrin ML, Noveck H, et al. Liberal or restrictive transfusion in high-risk patients after hip surgery. N Engl J Med 2011;365(26):2453–62.

31. Foss NB, Kristensen MT, Jensen PS, et al. The effects of liberal versus restrictive transfusion thresholds on ambulation after hip fracture surgery. Transfusion 2009; 49(2):227–34.

32. Gruson KI, Aharonoff GB, Egol KA, et al. The relationship between admission hemoglobin level and outcome after hip fracture. J Orthop Trauma 2002;16(1):39–44.

33. Halm EA, Wang JJ, Boockvar K, et al. The effect of perioperative anemia on clinical and functional outcomes in patients with hip fracture. J Orthop Trauma 2004;18(6):369–74.

34. Lawrence VA, Silverstein JH, Cornell JE, et al. Higher Hb level is associated with better early functional recovery after hip fracture repair. Transfusion 2003;43(12): 1717–22.

35. Carson JL, Duff A, Poses RM, et al. Effect of anaemia and cardiovascular disease on surgical mortality and morbidity. Lancet 1996;348(9034):1055–60.

36. Musallam KM, Tamim HM, Richards T, et al. Preoperative anaemia and postoperative outcomes in non-cardiac surgery: a retrospective cohort study. Lancet 2011;378(9800):1396–407.

37. Marcantonio ER, Goldman L, Orav EJ, et al. The association of intraoperative factors with the development of postoperative delirium. Am J Med 1998;105(5):380–4.

38. Vuille-Lessard E, Boudreault D, Girard F, et al. Postoperative anemia does not impede functional outcome and quality of life early after hip and knee arthroplasties. Transfusion 2012;52(2):261–70.

39. So-Osman C, Nelissen R, Brand R, et al. Postoperative anemia after joint replacement surgery is not related to quality of life during the first two weeks postoperatively. Transfusion 2011;51(1):71–81.

40. Hershko C, Camaschella C. How I treat unexplained refractory iron deficiency anemia. Blood 2014;123(3):326–33.

41. Tefferi A. Anemia in adults: a contemporary approach to diagnosis. Mayo Clin Proc 2003;78(10):1274–80.

42. Stabler SP. Clinical practice. Vitamin B12 deficiency. N Engl J Med 2013;368(2): 149–60.

43. American Society of Anesthesiologists Task Force on Perioperative Blood Management. Practice guidelines for perioperative blood management: an updated report by the American Society of Anesthesiologists Task Force on Perioperative Blood Management. Anesthesiology 2015;122(2):241–75.

44. Procrit [Package Insert]. Available at: http://assets.procrit.com/shared/product/procrit/procrit-prescribing-information.pdf. Accessed July 27, 2015.
45. Ralley FE. Erythropoietin and intravenous iron in PBM. Transfus Apher Sci 2014; 50(1):16–9.
46. Vassallo R, Goldman M, Germain M, et al. Preoperative autologous blood donation: waning indications in an era of improved blood safety. Transfus Med Rev 2015;29(4):268–75.
47. Howard J, Malfroy M, Llewelyn C, et al. The Transfusion Alternatives Preoperatively in Sickle Cell Disease (TAPS) study: a randomised, controlled, multicentre clinical trial. Lancet 2013;381(9870):930–8.
48. Yawn BP, Buchanan GR, Afenyi-Annan AN, et al. Management of sickle cell disease: summary of the 2014 evidence-based report by expert panel members. JAMA 2014;312(10):1033–48.
49. Building a Better Patient Blood Management Program. 2015. Available at: http://www.aabb.org/pbm/Documents/AABB-PBM-Whitepaper.pdf. Accessed July 27, 2015.
50. Isbister JP. The three-pillar matrix of patient blood management–an overview. Best Pract Res Clin Anaesthesiol 2013;27(1):69–84.
51. What is Patient Blood Management. Available at: http://www.blood.gov.au/patient-blood-management-pbm-whatispbm. Accessed July 27, 2015.

Preoperative Nutrition and Prehabilitation

Ruchir Gupta, MD, Tong J. Gan, MD, MHS, FRCA*

KEYWORDS

- Nutrition • Prehabilitation • Preoperative optimization • Functional capacity
- Immunonutrition

KEY POINTS

- Identifying patients who are nutritionally deficient allows us to intervene preoperatively to optimize their nutritional status.
- The development of a carbohydrate beverage that is also clear liquid has allowed patients to be brought to the operating room in a fed state, thereby reducing insulin resistance postoperatively and postoperative hypoglycemia.
- Physical exercise training programs have demonstrated an improvement in both physical fitness and clinical outcomes in patients with major comorbidities (ie, cardiac failure, ischemic heart disease, and chronic obstructive pulmonary disease).
- The 6-minute walk test is a simple test that does not require expensive equipment and allows evaluation of exercise tolerance.
- The contribution of cardiopulmonary exercise testing to the evaluation of perioperative risk, the subsequent development of a training program, and the use of indices to both risk stratify as well as measure improvement after a training program allow a personalized preoperative program to be developed for each patient.

INTRODUCTION

Enhanced recovery after surgery (ERAS) is the natural evolution of what were previously referred to as *fast track* programs and seeks to implement a series of preoperative, intraoperative, and postoperative interventions to improve and enhance recovery from surgery and anesthesia after major surgical procedures. These goals are achieved by instituting measures that will minimize the effects of surgical stress and encourage early active patient mobilization and participation in the immediate postoperative period. Using evidence-based protocols, care is coordinated between

Department of Anesthesiology, Health Science Center, Stony Brook University School of Medicine, L4-060, Stony Brook, NY 11794, USA
* Corresponding author. Department of Anesthesiology, Stony Brook University, Stony Brook, NY 11794.
E-mail address: tong.gan@stonybrookmedicine.edu

Anesthesiology Clin 34 (2016) 143–153
http://dx.doi.org/10.1016/j.anclin.2015.10.012   anesthesiology.theclinics.com
1932-2275/16/$ – see front matter © 2016 Elsevier Inc. All rights reserved.

the various members of the health care team from the preoperative clinic to the intra-operative care and postoperative care team. This coordination of care combined with evidence-based clinical management interventions are the 2 main pillars of the enhanced recovery strategy. Two important aspects of the ERAS pathway are nutrition and prehabilitation.

PREOPERATIVE NUTRITION ASSESSMENT AND OPTIMIZATION

The prevalence of malnutrition in patients undergoing surgery varies by type of surgery as well as by patient population. Patients with advanced age, weight loss, and a lack of nutritional support are at greater risk of malnutrition.[1] The presence of malnutrition preoperatively in patients undergoing surgery has been associated with an increased risk of postoperative complications, prolonged length of hospital stay, delayed recovery of bowel function,[2,3] higher rates of readmission,[4] and an increased incidence of postoperative death. As a result, there has been an increased focus on perioperative nutrition; several consensus guidelines have been developed to address this issue by various societies.[5–8] Among these are the guidelines for elective colon surgery and rectal/pelvic surgery[9] from the Enhanced Recovery After Surgery Society.

One of the main goals in ERAS is the optimization of patients' preoperative nutritional status and instituting strategies to prevent perioperative starvation, which can lead to negative protein balance.[6] Through the utilization of supplemental nutritional drinks[10] and the avoidance of overnight fast, the risk of postoperative insulin resistance is also reduced.[11]

DETECTING MALNUTRITION BEFORE SURGERY

The early guidelines from the Enhanced Recovery After Surgery Society focused primarily on colorectal procedures. Malnutrition and weight loss in this population is common because of tumor-related cachexia and decreased oral food intake caused in part by gastrointestinal tract obstruction. Furthermore, malnutrition continues to be a prognostic indicator of poor outcome in terms of survival and response to surgical treatment.[6,12,13]

Although much effort has been devoted in developing tools for preoperative nutrition risk screening, it remains unclear which screening system best predicts the risk of developing nutrition-related complications. Traditional anthropometric nutritional assessment using body weight, serum nutritional factor levels (such as low serum albumin, pre-albumin, and transthyretin), skin fold thickness and functional measurements of muscle strength have fallen out of favor due to their limited value in determining actual nutritional risk before surgery. Thus, several diverse measurements have been combined into subjective scoring systems including the Subjective Global Assessment (SGA) questionnaire,[14] the nutritional risk screening (NRS) 2002,[15] Reilly's NRS[16] and the nutritional risk indicator (NRI) scoring systems (**Table 1**). A combination of objective and subjective nutritional assessment tools may be better than either alone.

Once a patient is identified as nutritionally at risk, oral nutritional supplementation should be initiated and a dietician should be involved in further nutritional care of the patient. Although there is a lack of consensus in the interval when nutritional supplementation should occur, 5 to 7 days seems to be the most commonly recommended time period.[5] If patients are deemed to be at severe nutritional risk (ie, weight loss >10%–15% per 6 months; body mass index <18.5 kg/m^2; SGA grade C [see **Table 1**]; serum albumin less than 30 g/L), it would be reasonable to consider delaying surgery until the nutritional deficit is corrected, if only partially.

Table 1
Tools for preoperative nutrition risk screening

Scoring System	Indices Tested	Categorizations
SGA[17]	Patients' medical history (*weight change, dietary intake change, gastrointestinal symptoms and changes in functional capacity*) and physical examination (*loss of subcutaneous fat, muscle wasting, ankle or sacral edema and ascites*) are evaluated.	SGA A: well nourished SGA B: moderately malnourished SGA C: severely malnourished
NRS[18]	Patients are characterized by scoring the components *undernutrition* and *severity of disease* in 4 categories (absent, mild, moderate, and severe). Patients can have a score of 0–3 for each component and a total score of 0–6; any patient with a total score ≥3 is considered to be at nutritional risk.	Score 1: Patients are admitted to the hospital because of complications associated with a chronic disease. Patients are weak but out of bed regularly. Protein requirement is increased but can be covered by oral diet or supplements in most cases. Score 2: Patients are confined to bed because of an illness, for example, following major abdominal surgery or a severe infection. Protein requirement is substantially increased but can be covered, although artificial feeding is required in many cases. Score 3: Patients are in intensive care with assisted ventilation, inotropic drugs, and so forth.
Reilly's NRS[16]	The following information is evaluated: weight loss (*amount and duration*); body mass index for adults (*weight in kg/height in m²*) and percentile charts for children; food intake (*appetite and ability to eat and retain food*); stress factors (*effect of medical condition on nutritional requirements*).	7–15 *High risk* 4–6 *Moderate risk* 0–3 *Low risk*
NRI[19]	Recent weight loss and serum albumin concentration are evaluated. NRI = (1.489 × serum albumin [g/L]) + (41.7 × current weight/ usual weight)	≥97.5 *Well nourished* 83.5%–97.5% *Moderately malnourished* <83.5% *Severely malnourished*

Data from Refs.[16–19]

ROLE OF TOTAL PARENTERAL NUTRITION

Although enteral nutrition stimulates hormone secretion, promotes the portal circulation, and maintains the barrier and immune function of the intestinal mucosa, it is not often possible because of preexisting gut dysfunction. Therefore, enteral support combined with parenteral nutrition support is often considered as an alternative to purely enteral feeding. Total parenteral nutrition (TPN) is a commonly used means for nutritional support to compensate for any such deficiency of enteral nutrition.

TPN solutions provide complete nutritional support because they contain fat emulsion, vitamins, and trace elements. However, there are risks associated with TPN use, which include pneumothorax, hemothorax, electrolyte imbalances, refeeding syndrome, and central vein catheter infection. It is suggested that preoperative TPN support be administered for 7 to 10 days.

Peripheral parenteral nutrition (PPN) has also been used because of its relative ease compared with TPN. Unfortunately, PPN solutions generally do not provide enough energy and nutrients for full nutritional support. Modified PPN solutions have been tried, whereby a 2-in-1 (dextrose + amino acids) formula or fat emulsion is used.[20] However, even with these formulations, multiple vitamins and trace elements are often omitted.

AVOIDING INSULIN RESISTANCE AND POSTOPERATIVE HYPERGLYCEMIA

Major surgical trauma results in a transient reduction in insulin sensitivity, leading to an increase in glucose production, decrease in tissue uptake of glucose, and glycogen synthesis, resulting in hyperglycemia.[21] Not only does hyperglycemia result in an increased risk of complications[22,23] but aggressive treatment of this hyperglycemia in the postoperative period can lead to hypoglycemia with its associated negative sequelae.

Because of its effect in reducing the postoperative development of insulin resistance, preoperative carbohydrate treatment is commonly advocated as part of multimodal fast-track surgery or ERAS pathways. Improved postoperative insulin sensitivity has been shown to result from preoperative ingestion of a carbohydrate drink, using minimally invasive surgical methods, administering epidural anesthesia, and avoiding preoperative malnutrition.[10] The traditional mantra of fasting from midnight to the day of surgery and nil per os has been abandoned in all recent fasting guidelines in light of ample evidence for improved insulin responsiveness in patients receiving oral intake of clear fluids up to 2 hours before induction of anesthesia.[24,25] Preoperative carbohydrate treatment is meant to replicate normal metabolic responses to eating breakfast,[24] thereby stimulating endogenous insulin release, which will switch off the overnight fasting metabolic state and decrease peripheral insulin resistance in response to the surgical stress response.

Several commercially available formulations of a preoperative carbohydrate drink have been developed, but only one, Clearfast, is available in the United States. Clearfast contains 21 g of monosaccharides, 38 g of polysaccharides, and 230 calories per 12 ounces. A less expensive alternative to Clearfast is Gatorade, which also provides monosaccharides (80 g/12 oz) and caloric replenishment (80 cal/oz) but lacks polysaccharides. Another formulation of Gatorade, Gatorade prime, provides a more robust nourishment per 12 oz (69 g of monosaccharides, 6 g of polysaccharides, and 300 calories) and may be a suitable alternative for the ERAS program in centers with budgetary constraints.

Interestingly, a Cochrane study by Smith and colleagues,[26] which included 27 trials and involved 1976 participants, found that preoperative carbohydrate treatment was associated with only a small and possibly clinically insignificant reduction in length of hospital stay when compared with placebo or fasting in adult patients undergoing elective surgery. Furthermore, they found that preoperative carbohydrate treatment did not increase or decrease postoperative complication rates when compared with placebo or fasting. However, the investigators cautioned about the lack of adequate blinding in many of the studies, which precludes a definitive conclusion.

IMMUNONUTRITION

Recent studies have shown that irrespective of a patient's baseline nutritional status, supplementation of preoperative oral nutritional formulations with specific immune-modulating substrates, such as glutamine, arginine, and omega-3 fatty acids, improves surgical outcomes.[27–29] The anabolic and immune modulatory properties of long-chain polyunsaturated fatty acid of the omega-3-fatty acid family have been demonstrated to be beneficial in the perioperative period.[30]

Glutamine plays a crucial role not just as a source of metabolic fuel but also as an aid for preservation of small bowel function.[31] Additionally, it aids in the preservation of T-lymphocyte responsiveness during major surgery.[32] Arginine is a nonessential amino acid that also stimulates T-cell function and improves microcirculation via the formation of nitric oxide.

Clinical studies have not confirmed the positive effects of immunonutrition that were seen in earlier animal models.[33] However, recent reviews and meta-analyses on the various formulas of immunonutrition concluded that perioperative immune nutrition improves surgical outcome.[34] It remains unclear, however, as to when administration (preoperative, intraoperative, or postoperative) should occur and what the optimum dosage should be.

PREHABILITATION: PHYSICAL ACTIVITY AND HEALTH OUTCOMES

Prehabilitation is defined as "the process of enhancing the functional capacity of the individual to enable him or her to withstand a stressful event".[35] Thus, a physical exercise training program preoperatively before elective surgery is an example of prehabilitation.

There is increasing evidence that good functional capacity has multiple benefits in almost every context of health and disease,[36] and poor functional capacity resulting from physical inactivity is one of the most important public health issues facing our generation.[37]

It has also been shown that patients who are fitter and more physically active have better outcomes as it relates to underlying conditions, such as coronary artery disease,[38] heart failure,[39] hypertension, diabetes, chronic obstructive pulmonary disease (COPD), depression, dementia, chronic kidney disease, cancer, and stroke.[40] Furthermore, the evidence supports that the incidence of chronic diseases, such as type 2 diabetes, osteoporosis, obesity, depression, and cancer of the breast, kidney, and colon, is also reduced with increasing physical activity. Despite the slight increase in the risk of complications, such as myocardial ischemia or even death during physical training, the overall benefit of enhanced physical status outweighs this short-lived period of elevated risk.[40]

PREHABILITATION: EXERCISE TRAINING BEFORE A PHYSIOLOGIC CHALLENGE

Preoperative exercise training is both feasible and safe in patients with a spectrum of severe cardiac and pulmonary disease. Indeed, physical exercise training programs have demonstrated an improvement in both physical fitness and clinical outcomes in patients with major comorbidities (ie, cardiac failure, ischemic heart disease, and COPD).[40]

Patients with malignancy often receive neoadjuvant chemotherapy and radiation therapy, which is administered weeks before a surgical procedure and usually require 6 to 12 weeks of recovery. This recovery period has opened up a window of opportunity to train patients before major cancer surgeries when previously the pressure of reducing the time between diagnosis and surgery prevented such an intervention. There are preliminary nonrandomized data from patients undergoing elective colorectal cancer surgery within an ERAS program that have shown the feasibility of providing a cardiopulmonary exercise testing (CPET)–guided structured responsive interval exercise training program.

Such a program is delivered 3 times a week for 6 weeks in a hospital setting after neoadjuvant chemoradiotherapy and before surgery.[41] The control population was made up of patients unable to engage with the exercise program for logistical reasons (eg, distance of residence from the hospital). A follow-on randomized study, in patients scheduled to undergo elective colorectal surgery within an ERAS program, is currently underway to evaluate the efficacy of a CPET-guided structured responsive training program in maintaining physical fitness after neoadjuvant chemoradiotherapy.[42]

In summary, the incremental exercise test can be used to measure the efficacy of prehabilitation exercise training programs. An effective training program would be expected to result in an increase in the anaerobic threshold (AT) and/or maximum oxygen consumption (VO_{2peak}). These variables can be reliably measured and can, therefore, be used to compare patient groups from different clinical centers and compare outcomes in clinical trials. The question that remains is whether a preoperative exercise training program can improve morbidity and mortality.

EXERCISE PROGRAMS

Is there evidence that a preoperative exercise program leads to better postoperative outcomes? Although exercise training programs have been shown to be beneficial in a variety of conditions, including COPD, stroke, heart failure, and intermittent claudication,[43] the overall long-term benefits of such interventions are less well evaluated.

Patients with increased risk may benefit from prehabilitation programs that include endurance and strength training, high-intensity training schedules, and the use of nutritional and pharmaceutical adjuncts. These programs often use CPET to determine their effectiveness.[44] CPET integrates expired gas analysis (oxygen and carbon dioxide concentrations) with the measurement of ventilatory flow, thereby enabling calculation of oxygen uptake (VO_2) and carbon dioxide production under conditions of varying physiologic stress imposed by a range of defined external workloads.[40]

The incremental exercise test to the limit of tolerance using cycle ergometry (incremental ramp test) has been used extensively in both clinical practice and clinical trials. It permits the accurate determination of exercise capacity and also allows the identification of the site of exercise limitation when this is abnormal.[45] The advantages of this exercise protocol are that it evaluates the exercise response across the entire range of functional capacity, allows assessment of the normalcy or otherwise of the exercise response, permits identification of the site of functional exercise limitation, and gives an appropriate frame of reference for training or rehabilitation targets. Additionally, the initial work rate is low, and there is a short duration of high-intensity exercise. The entire protocol consists of 8 to 12 minutes of exercise.

The typical test profile for this exercise includes 3 minutes of resting measurement, 3 minutes of unloaded cycling (cycling against no resistance), followed by a continuously increasing ramp until physical exhaustion. CPET determines perioperative aerobic capacity. This capacity is measured by the AT, which is the VO_2 at which anaerobic adenosine triphosphate (ATP) synthesis starts to supplement aerobic ATP synthesis. AT is also the point that CO_2 production increases more than VO_2 during gas exchange.

Consequently, it is thought that myocardial ischemia occurs at or above the AT such that patients with low AT are at risk for early ischemia. As a result, AT is useful in the risk stratification of patients (**Table 2**).[44]

To date 24 cohort studies (more than 4000 patients) have shown a remarkably consistent relationship between physical fitness (defined using CPET-derived variables) and postoperative outcome.[40]

These studies were conducted over a period of 21 years (1993–2014); the surgical procedures included were 5 major abdominal, 1 colon, 1 rectal, 1 cystectomy, 5 abdominal aortic aneurysm repairs, 1 major hepatobiliary, 1 hepatic resection, 1 Whipple, 3 liver transplants, 4 upper gastrointestinal, and 2 bariatric. The indices used in the studies were AT and VO_{2Peak} and their respective relationship with the risk threshold. The outcome of these studies varied as well, with morbidity being the primary outcome in 13 studies, mortality being the primary outcome in 11 studies, and morbidity and mortality being the primary outcome in 3. Among these studies, a significant relationship was found between the AT and risk threshold as well as the VO_{2Peak} and the risk threshold. In the 4 studies that only tested the AT and risk threshold, a significant association was found in all the studies. In the one study that tested VO_{2Peak} and AT, a significant association was found. Remarkably there was only one study that showed no association with AT or VO_{2Peak} and risk threshold.

6-minute Walk Test

The 6-minute walk test (6MWT) is a simple test that does not require expensive equipment but rather requires patients to walk the longest distance possible in a set interval of 6 minutes, through a walking course (corridor) preferably 30 m long. Patients have the option of stopping or slowing down at any time and then resume their walking, depending on their degree of fatigue. Even though other parameters can be monitored during the test, such as arterial pressure and/or heart rate, the number of times patients have to stop during the test, the speed of walking or even changes in respiratory gases (measured using a portable instrument) and oxygen saturation, the distance walked in 6 minutes is simple and most useful.[46]

Because the 6MWT lasts for a short duration and the actual walking is on a flat surface rather than an incline or on a rugged surface, the 6MWT has come to be considered a submaximal test under the pretense that walking 6 minutes on a flat surface would not allow patients to reach their maximal capacity.[46] However, in most studies, the longest distance walked during the 6MWT has shown a medium to high correlation with the actual VO_2 measured at the peak of the maximal exercise test. There is also a strong correlation with the VO_{2peak} and the VO_2 at the end of the 6MWT.[47] In fact, the

Table 2		
Using the AT for risk stratification of patients		
AT level (mL/min/kg)	**Recommendations**	
>11	Perioperative mortality of <1% and unlikely to need higher level of care	
≤11	Perioperative mortality of 18% and should be considered for intensive recovery, PACU, high dependency unit, or ICU	
<8	Perioperative mortality of 50% and should be considered and prepared for extended ICU stay	

Abbreviations: ICU, intensive care unit; PACU, postanesthesia care unit.

Data from Davies SJ, Wilson RJ. Preoperative optimization of the high-risk surgical patient. Br J Anaesth 2004;93(1):121–8.

Vo_2 at the end of the walking test was actually greater than the VO_{2peak}. Consequently, the 6MWT does not seem to have the features of a submaximal test.

Enright and Sherrill[48] have developed equations to calculate the distance walked by a healthy adult during 6MWT. These equations are as follows:

6MWT distance = (7.57 × height cm) − (5.02 × age) − (1.76 × weight kg) − 309 m for men

6MWT distance = (2.11 × height cm) − (2.29 × weight kg) − (5.78 × age) + 667 m for women

These data also show the relationship between anthropometric variables, sex, age, and the 6MWT distance.[49] The 6MWT distance is inversely correlated with age,[50] which is greater in men than women by an average of nearly 76 m.

SUMMARY

Taken together, these concepts support the notion of individualized medicine whereby the right treatment is administered to the right patient at the right time. Identifying patients who are nutritionally deficient allows us to intervene preoperatively to optimize their nutritional status. In some cases, TPN therapy may be needed, either as an adjunct or exclusively, to achieve this goal. Additionally, debunking the traditional mantra of fasting for 8 hours before surgery, the development of a carbohydrate beverage that is also clear liquid has allowed patients to be brought to the operating room in a fed state, thereby reducing insulin resistance postoperatively and postoperative hypoglycemia.

Finally, the contribution of CPET to the evaluation of perioperative risk, the subsequent development of a training program, and the use of indices to both risk stratify as well as measure improvement after a training program allow a personalized preoperative program to be developed for each patient. Based on the available literature it seems such a training program may need to be 6 weeks in duration, but more studies are needed to elucidate the optimal intervention duration.[42]

REFERENCES

1. Frances N, Kennedy RH, Ljungqvist L, et al. Manual of fast track recovery for colorectal surgery. London: Springer; 2012.
2. Lohsiriwat V, Chinswangwatanakul V, Lohsiriwat S, et al. Hypoalbuminemia is a predictor of delayed postoperative bowel function and poor surgical outcomes in right-sided colon cancer patients. Asia Pac J Clin Nutr 2007;16(2):213–7.
3. Lohsiriwat V, Lohsiriwat D, Boonnuch W, et al. Pre-operative hypoalbuminemia is a major risk factor for postoperative complications following rectal cancer surgery. World J Gastroenterol 2008;14(8):1248–51.
4. Zhang JQ, Curran T, McCallum JC, et al. Risk factors for readmission after lower extremity bypass in the American College of Surgeons National Surgery Quality Improvement Program. J Vasc Surg 2014;59(5):1331–9.
5. Weimann A, Braga M, Harsanyi L, et al. ESPEN guidelines on enteral nutrition: surgery including organ transplantation. Clin Nutr 2006;25(2):224–44.
6. Braga M, Ljungqvist O, Soeters P, et al. ESPEN guidelines on parenteral nutrition: surgery. Clin Nutr 2009;28(4):378–86.
7. Ukleja A, Freeman KL, Gilbert K, et al. Standards for nutrition support: adult hospitalized patients. Nutr Clin Pract 2010;25(4):403–14.

8. Chambrier C, Sztark F. French clinical guidelines on perioperative nutrition. Update of the 1994 consensus conference on perioperative artificial nutrition for elective surgery in adults. J Visc Surg 2012;149(5):e325–36.

9. Nygren J, Thacker J, Carli F, et al. Guidelines for perioperative care in elective rectal/pelvic surgery: Enhanced Recovery After Surgery (ERAS(R)) Society recommendations. Clin Nutr 2012;31(6):801–16.

10. Lassen K, Soop M, Nygren J, et al. Consensus review of optimal perioperative care in colorectal surgery enhanced recovery after surgery (ERAS) group recommendations. Arch Surg 2009;144(10):961–9.

11. Ljungqvist O. Modulating postoperative insulin resistance by preoperative carbohydrate loading. Best Pract Res Clin Anaesthesiol 2009;23(4):401–9.

12. Schiesser M, Kirchhoff P, Müller MK, et al. The correlation of nutrition risk index, nutrition risk score, and bioimpedance analysis with postoperative complications in patients undergoing gastrointestinal surgery. Surgery 2009;145(5):519–26.

13. Sungurtekin H, Sungurtekin U, Hanci V, et al. Comparison of two nutrition assessment techniques in hospitalized patients. Nutrition 2004;20(5):428–32.

14. Detsky AS, Baker JP, O'Rourke K, et al. Predicting nutrition-associated complications for patients undergoing gastrointestinal surgery. JPEN J Parenter Enteral Nutr 1987;11(5):440–6.

15. Kondrup J, Allison SP, Elia M, et al. ESPEN guidelines for nutrition screening 2002. Clin Nutr 2003;22(4):415–21.

16. Reilly HM, Martineau JK, Moran A, et al. Nutritional screening–evaluation and implementation of a simple nutrition risk score. Clin Nutr 1995;14(5):269–73.

17. Detsky AS, McLaughlin JR, Baker JP, et al. What is subjective global assessment of nutritional status? JPEN J Parenter Enteral Nutr 1987;11(1):8–13.

18. Kondrup J, Rasmussen HH, Hamberg O, et al. Nutritional risk screening (NRS 2002): a new method based on an analysis of controlled clinical trials. Clin Nutr 2003;22(3):321–36.

19. Buzby GP, Knox LS, Crosby LO, et al. Study protocol: a randomized clinical trial of total parenteral nutrition in malnourished surgical patients. Am J Clin Nutr 1988; 47(2 Suppl):366–81.

20. Liu MY, Tang HC, Hu SH, et al. Influence of preoperative peripheral parenteral nutrition with micronutrients after colorectal cancer patients. Biomed Res Int 2015;2015:535431.

21. Thorell A, Nygren J, Ljungqvist O. Insulin resistance: a marker of surgical stress. Curr Opin Clin Nutr Metab Care 1999;2(1):69–78.

22. Doenst T, Wijeysundera D, Karkouti K, et al. Hyperglycemia during cardiopulmonary bypass is an independent risk factor for mortality in patients undergoing cardiac surgery. J Thorac Cardiovasc Surg 2005;130(4):1144.

23. Gustafsson UO, Thorell A, Soop M, et al. Haemoglobin A1c as a predictor of postoperative hyperglycaemia and complications after major colorectal surgery. Br J Surg 2009;96(11):1358–64.

24. Ljungqvist O, Soreide E. Preoperative fasting. Br J Surg 2003;90(4):400–6.

25. Brady M, Kinn S, Stuart P. Preoperative fasting for adults to prevent perioperative complications. Cochrane Database Syst Rev 2003;(4):CD004423.

26. Smith MD, McCall J, Plank L, et al. Preoperative carbohydrate treatment for enhancing recovery after elective surgery. Cochrane Database Syst Rev 2014;(8):CD009161.

27. Braga M, Gianotti L, Nespoli L, et al. Nutritional approach in malnourished surgical patients: a prospective randomized study. Arch Surg 2002;137(2):174–80.

28. Braga M, Gianotti L, Vignali A, et al. Preoperative oral arginine and n-3 fatty acid supplementation improves the immunometabolic host response and outcome after colorectal resection for cancer. Surgery 2002;132(5):805–14.

29. Tepaske R, Velthuis H, Oudemans-van Straaten HM, et al. Effect of preoperative oral immune-enhancing nutritional supplement on patients at high risk of infection after cardiac surgery: a randomised placebo-controlled trial. Lancet 2001; 358(9283):696–701.

30. Ryan AM, Reynolds JV, Healy L, et al. Enteral nutrition enriched with eicosapentaenoic acid (EPA) preserves lean body mass following esophageal cancer surgery: results of a double-blinded randomized controlled trial. Ann Surg 2009; 249(3):355–63.

31. Zheng YM, Li F, Zhang MM, et al. Glutamine dipeptide for parenteral nutrition in abdominal surgery: a meta-analysis of randomized controlled trials. World J Gastroenterol 2006;12(46):7537–41.

32. O'Riordain MG, Fearon KC, Ross JA, et al. Glutamine-supplemented total parenteral nutrition enhances T-lymphocyte response in surgical patients undergoing colorectal resection. Ann Surg 1994;220(2):212–21.

33. Lobo DN, Williams RN, Welch NT, et al. Early postoperative jejunostomy feeding with an immune modulating diet in patients undergoing resectional surgery for upper gastrointestinal cancer: a prospective, randomized, controlled, double-blind study. Clin Nutr 2006;25(5):716–26.

34. Zhu X, Herrera G, Ochoa JB. Immunosuppression and infection after major surgery: a nutritional deficiency. Crit Care Clin 2010;26(3):491–500, ix.

35. Ditmyer MM, Topp R, Pifer M. Prehabilitation in preparation for orthopaedic surgery. Orthop Nurs 2002;21(5):43–51 [quiz: 52–4].

36. Fiuza-Luces C, Garatachea N, Berger NA, et al. Exercise is the real polypill. Physiology (Bethesda) 2013;28(5):330–58.

37. Kohl HW 3rd, Craig CL, Lambert EV, et al. The pandemic of physical inactivity: global action for public health. Lancet 2012;380(9838):294–305.

38. Thompson PD, Franklin BA, Balady GJ, et al. Exercise and acute cardiovascular events placing the risks into perspective: a scientific statement from the American Heart Association Council on Nutrition, Physical Activity, and Metabolism and the Council on Clinical Cardiology. Circulation 2007;115(17):2358–68.

39. Belardinelli R, Georgiou D, Cianci G, et al. Randomized, controlled trial of long-term moderate exercise training in chronic heart failure: effects on functional capacity, quality of life, and clinical outcome. Circulation 1999;99(9): 1173–82.

40. Levett DZ, Grocott MP. Cardiopulmonary exercise testing, prehabilitation, and enhanced recovery after surgery (ERAS). Can J Anaesth 2015;62(2):131–42.

41. West MA, Lythgoe D, Barben CP, et al. Cardiopulmonary exercise variables are associated with postoperative morbidity after major colonic surgery: a prospective blinded observational study. Br J Anaesth 2014;112(4):665–71.

42. US National Institutes of Health. The effect of chemotherapy and surgery for cancer on exercise capacity. Clinicaltrials.gov. Identifier: NCT01325883.

43. Lane R, Ellis B, Watson L, et al. Exercise for intermittent claudication. Cochrane Database Syst Rev 2014;(7):CD000990.

44. Davies SJ, Wilson RJ. Preoperative optimization of the high-risk surgical patient. Br J Anaesth 2004;93(1):121–8.

45. Whipp BJ, Davis JA, Torres F, et al. A test to determine parameters of aerobic function during exercise. J Appl Physiol Respir Environ Exerc Physiol 1981; 50(1):217–21.

46. Faggiano P, D'Aloia A, Gualeni A, et al. The 6 minute walking test in chronic heart failure: indications, interpretation and limitations from a review of the literature. Eur J Heart Fail 2004;6(6):687–91.
47. Riley M, McParland J, Stanford CF, et al. Oxygen consumption during corridor walk testing in chronic cardiac failure. Eur Heart J 1992;13(6):789–93.
48. Enright PL, Sherrill DL. Reference equations for the six-minute walk in healthy adults. Am J Respir Crit Care Med 1998;158(5 Pt 1):1384–7.
49. Hamilton DM, Haennel RG. Validity and reliability of the 6-minute walk test in a cardiac rehabilitation population. J Cardiopulm Rehabil 2000;20(3):156–64.
50. Gibbons WJ, Fruchter N, Sloan S, et al. Reference values for a multiple repetition 6-minute walk test in healthy adults older than 20 years. J Cardiopulm Rehabil 2001;21(2):87–93.

Special Considerations

Preoperative Evaluation of Patients with Diabetes Mellitus

Joshua D. Miller, MD, MPH[a],*, Deborah C. Richman, MBChB, FFA(SA)[b]

KEYWORDS

- Diabetes • Glycemic control • Hyperglycemia • Hemoglobin A1c • Insulin pump
- Preoperative evaluation

KEY POINTS

- Diabetes is a chronic secondary diagnosis affecting more than 9% of the population.
- Uncontrolled diabetes can result in poor short- and long-term surgical outcomes.
- Complications from the disease affect nearly every organ system and can greatly impact perioperative risk.
- Careful consideration should be given to patients with diabetes undergoing surgery in order to ensure best possible outcomes.

INTRODUCTION

There are more than 29 million people in the United States with diabetes; it is estimated that by 2050, one in 3 individuals will have the disease.[1,2] Of those with diabetes, 90% to 95% have type 2, with the remainder having type 1 or other secondary forms. Total costs from diabetes have been estimated at $245 billion with $176 billion in direct medical costs.[1] Interestingly, the annual number of newly diagnosed cases has leveled off in the last 5 years after a steady increase since 1980, which saw the number of new cases in the United States triple from 493,000 in 1980 to 1.4 million in 2013.[3] This is despite a persistent increase in obesity, to which the high prevalence of type 2 diabetes (T2DM) has been attributed. After circulatory diseases, diabetes is the second most common diagnosis at time of hospital discharge.[4]

At least 50% of patients with diabetes are expected to undergo surgery in their lifetime, and 28% of patients with diabetes will have coronary artery bypass graft (CABG)/ surgery.[5] Diabetes is associated with prolonged recovery following surgery as well as

[a] Department of Medicine, Stony Brook Medicine, Stony Brook, NY 11794-8154, USA;
[b] Department of Anesthesiology, Stony Brook Medicine, Stony Brook, NY 11794-8480, USA
* Corresponding author.
E-mail address: Joshua.Miller@stonybrookmedicine.edu

Anesthesiology Clin 34 (2016) 155–169
http://dx.doi.org/10.1016/j.anclin.2015.10.008   anesthesiology.theclinics.com

increases in hospital length of stay, morbidity, and mortality.[6,7] Complications from uncontrolled diabetes can impact multiple organ systems and affect perioperative risk. This review helps the clinician gain an understanding of principles in diabetes assessment and management in patients undergoing surgery.

PATIENT EVALUATION OVERVIEW

History and physical examination are key. Patients should be asked if they have ever been told that they have diabetes or high blood sugar. Patients should also be screened for risk factors for undiagnosed diabetes like obesity, metabolic syndrome, diabetogenic medications, and family history of diabetes. Preoperative evaluation should begin with a detailed history of disease type, chronicity, known complications, and understanding of glycemic control and self-management (**Box 1**). This evaluation in turn will inform perioperative management decisions regarding risk stratification and pharmacologic management.

Classification

Type 1 diabetes (T1DM) results from autoimmune pancreatic beta cell destruction with insulin deficiency (**Table 1**). Although the disease was previously thought to only affect pediatric patients, it is now also frequently diagnosed in adults. Coexisting autoimmune disease exists in as many as 8% of patients with T1DM (adrenal insufficiency, autoimmune thyroid disease, or myasthenia gravis).[8] Patients with T1DM are managed almost exclusively with exogenous insulin administered in a manner so as to mimic normal physiologic pancreatic insulin secretion (basal/bolus), either by subcutaneous injection (multiple daily insulin injections) or by continuous subcutaneous insulin infusion (insulin pump). Importantly, basal insulin should never be withheld in patients with T1DM as this can precipitate ketosis.

T2DM is multifactorial in cause, owing to the effects of obesity on insulin resistance, the inability of pancreatic insulin secretion to maintain euglycemia, inappropriate counter-regulatory glucagon production, and unchecked hepatic gluconeogenesis. Factors associated with development of T2DM occur along a continuum. Therefore, patients with prediabetes can also experience similar adverse perioperative outcomes.[9]

Box 1
Elements of preoperative diabetes risk assessment

1. Diabetes type

2. Disease duration/context of initial diagnosis

3. If type 1 diabetes: coexisting autoimmune diseases, history of DKA

4. Known complications

5. Associated comorbidities

6. Home diabetes regimen (oral agents, insulin type/frequency, last medication adjustment)

7. Frequency/severity of hypoglycemia

8. Hemoglobin A1c (if known)

9. Renal function

10. If insulin pump use, obtain settings from patient or primary endocrinologist

Abbreviation: DKA, diabetic ketoacidosis.

Table 1
Classification of diabetes

Type	Risk Factors	Cause	Treatment Principles
TIDM	• Other autoimmune disease	• Autoimmune pancreatic beta cell destruction	• Exogenous insulin replacement (MDII or CSII)
T2DM	• Obesity • Family history • Age >45 y • History of GDM	• Insulin resistance • Pancreatic insufficiency • Inappropriate glucagon response/hepatic gluconeogenesis	• Improve insulin sensitivity/pancreatic insulin secretion • Decrease hepatic gluconeogenesis • Slow gastric emptying/induce early satiety
Secondary forms	• Acute/chronic pancreatitis • CFRD • Pancreatectomy • Pancreatic cancer • Glucocorticoid use • Antirejection medication use	• Insulin resistance • Pancreatic insufficiency	• Depending on primary cause

Abbreviations: CFRD, cystic fibrosis-related diabetes; CSII, continuous subcutaneous insulin infusion (insulin pump); GDM, gestational diabetes mellitus; MDII, multiple daily insulin injections.

Diabetes can also develop secondary to medications (ie, glucocorticoids, antirejection agents) or from other pancreatic causes, such as pancreatitis, malignancy, or a postpancreatectomy state.

Diabetes-Related Complications: Impact on Perioperative Risk

Long-standing, uncontrolled diabetes can result in microvascular and macrovascular complications, the presence of which can greatly impact perioperative risk (**Table 2**). Complications from the disease can develop in as few as 6 years following diagnosis.[10,11] For these reasons, it is important for the clinician to ascertain the degree of preoperative glycemic control and any known complications in order to make preparations for surgery and the postoperative period.

Perioperative cardiac events are more common in patients with diabetes. Hollenberg and colleagues found diabetes to be one of 5 independent risk factors for postoperative myocardial ischemia. Insulin-requiring diabetes is one of the 5 clinical risk factors on the Revised Cardiac Risk Index. This index looked for major cardiac complications, including cardiac arrest, myocardial infarction, heart failure, and heart block.[12,13] Preoperative assessment of cardiac risk is done according to the American College of Cardiology/American Heart Association's guidelines.[14]

Surgical site infection is another concern in patients with diabetes. Neutrophil dysfunction associated with hyperglycemic states is one proposed cause.[15] Glycosylation of immunoglobulins is also a suggested mechanism of impaired immunity and subsequent infection risk.[16] Diabetes is recognized as a mediator of accelerated aging, accentuated with poor glycemic control. Thus, organ systems in patients with diabetes may be functionally older than chronologic age.

Autonomic Dysfunction

Patients should be assessed for autonomic instability; if present, perioperative management should be altered to mitigate the risks of this dysfunction (**Table 3**). Diabetic

Table 2
Diabetes complications and perioperative considerations

Complication	Perioperative Implication
Cardiovascular disease	
Myocardial ischemia/infarction Stroke Heart failure	Major cause of perioperative morbidity and mortality
Autonomic neuropathy	
Cardiovascular	Risk of arrhythmia, consider telemetry
Cystopathy	Urinary retention, increased risk of UTI
Gastroparesis	Delayed gastric emptying, risk of reflux
Hypoglycemia unawareness	More frequent glucose monitoring
Nephropathy	Avoid IV contrast/nephrotoxic agents Appropriate hydration Monitor renal function
Peripheral neuropathy	Risk of skin breakdown, ulceration
Retinopathy	Can acutely worsen with blood loss
Cheiroarthropathy	Difficult intubation, positioning and IV access
Impaired immunity/wound healing	Surgical site infection

Abbreviations: IV, intravenous; UTI, urinary tract infection.

autonomic neuropathy is found in greater than 25% of patients with T1DM and higher numbers of patients with T2DM, usually with earlier onset in the latter.[17] The pathophysiology is multifactorial but primarily due to hyperglycemia and its effects at the mitochondrial level, with the release of free radicals, intracellular signaling disturbances, and dysfunction of the sodium/potassium/adenosinetriphosphatase pump.[18]

Gastroparesis
A syndrome of delayed gastric emptying and gastric dilatation is a feature of autonomic neuropathy of diabetes. It is thought to be due to vagal neuropathy and is a risk factor for

Table 3
Common clinical presentations of autonomic dysfunction

Organ System	Symptoms	Comments
CAN	• Resting tachycardia • Loss of heart rate variability • Postural hypotension • Exercise intolerance • Dizziness • Silent ischemia • Abnormal baroreceptor responsiveness	Dominant sympathetic system Earliest manifestation of CAN Indicates inability to increase heart rate, blood pressure, and cardiac output
Genitourinary	• Impotence • Urinary retention	
Gastrointestinal	• Gastroparesis • Diarrhea	
Peripheral	• Abnormal sweating • Inability to perceive hypoglycemia	

Abbreviation: CAN, cardiovascular autonomic neuropathy.

aspiration and subsequent chemical pneumonitis with possible bacterial contamination and infection. Risks for significant pneumonitis are associated with one or more of the following characteristics of aspirated material: high acidity (pH <2.5), high-volume (>0.4 mL/kg) or particulate material. Recommendations to lower the risk of aspiration on induction of anesthesia include (1) promote gastric emptying with a prokinetic agent like metoclopramide,[19] (2) avoid solid food intake for at least 8 hours preoperatively, and (3) administer antacid preoperatively.

Cardiac autonomic neuropathy

The sympathetic and parasympathetic nervous systems work in conjunction to maintain normal cardiovascular function. Heart rate, blood pressure, contractility, cardiac electrical conduction, and vascular tone are all controlled by the autonomic nervous system. Cardiac autonomic neuropathy (CAN) is a feature of both T1DM and T2DM with associated increased mortality in those with greater autonomic dysfunction.[20–22] Some associate the mortality with early cardiac death, whereas others see the association as a marker for overall severity of disease.[23–25] In addition to mortality risk, patients with diabetes and CAN are at an increased risk of intraoperative instability with hypotension on induction and more frequent need of intraoperative vasopressor support.[5]

Other intraoperative effects include blunted hemodynamic response to intubation and increased risk of hypothermia.[26] Significant hypothermia is a risk factor for poor wound healing and surgical site infection. Hypothermia also impairs the metabolism of some anesthetic agents. Persistent drug levels can compound another possible risk of CAN: impaired response to hypoxia with decreased ventilatory drive.[27] The risk of cardiorespiratory arrest in patients with CAN is higher, both with the concomitant administration of anesthesia and sudden unrelated death.[21,28,29] Patients with CAN also suffer more ischemic strokes.[30] Silent ischemia as a result of CAN leads to delayed treatment of myocardial ischemia and infarction. With a lack of the classic anginal symptoms, fatigue, dizziness, dyspnea, sweating, palpitations, nausea, and vomiting may be the only signs of myocardial ischemia.

COMORBIDITIES ASSOCIATED WITH DIABETES MELLITUS

As mentioned, T1DM is seen in conjunction with other autoimmune diseases. These diseases need to be individually assessed for perioperative risk. Secondary diabetes arises from several comorbidities and their treatments, and each has different implications:

- Cystic fibrosis may be the underlying cause of diabetes.
- Chronic pancreatitis is usually associated with a chronic pain syndrome; patients are often on high-dose opiates and, thus, can have tolerance to opioids and anesthesia.
- Transplant antirejection medications and glucocorticoids can lead to hyperglycemia and overt diabetes; transplant history and current status need to be evaluated.

Diabetes is part of the constellation of disease states in metabolic syndrome (hypertension, hyperglycemia, increased abdominal circumference, and hyperlipidemia). Obesity has perioperative implications, including risk of obstructive sleep apnea, difficult intubation, positioning difficulties, and increased postoperative complications. In a recently published study examining obesity-related outcomes, it was found that patients undergoing bariatric surgery who had metabolic syndrome had a greater risk of pulmonary complications and increased mortality as compared with those without metabolic syndrome.[31]

MEDICATION CONSIDERATIONS

Table 4 outlines oral diabetes agents and insulins commonly encountered by the perioperative clinician. Familiarity with the mechanism of action and contraindications in the perioperative period are key.

Newer classes of diabetes medications are frequently being introduced. Although there has been more experience with older agents, such as metformin, insulin sensitizers, and secretogogues, there has not yet been consensus on the perioperative approach to patients taking newer agents, such sodium-glucose cotransporter-2 (SGLT2) inhibitors, glucagonlike peptide-1 analogues, or dipeptidyl peptidase-4 inhibitors.

Metformin, a biguanide, is renally cleared. There has been long-standing concern for the development of lactic acidosis in patients taking the medication.[32] Given the risk for renal impairment, hemodynamic instability, and potential need for imaging with radiocontrast dye, the American Association of Clinical Endocrinologists and the American Diabetes Association recommend against the use of metformin in hospitalized patients.[33] Although some guidelines do allow for continuation of metformin after receipt of intravenous (IV) contrast in patients with normal serum creatinine,[34] general practice is to withhold the medication 24 to 48 hours before elective surgical or radiological procedure. Owing to the potential for ketosis in patients receiving SGLT2 inhibitors, the medications are also held in the 24- to 48-hour preoperative period. Insulin secretogogues, such as sulfonylureas and meglitinides, carry a risk of hypoglycemia in patients with impaired renal function and decreased oral intake. They are generally withheld on the morning of and evening before surgery.

Holding diabetes medications can often result in hyperglycemia in the perioperative period. This effect is compounded by a relative hypoinsulinemia in the perioperative period due to an increase in circulating catecholamines. Use of institutional rapid-acting insulin correction protocols with frequent blood sugar monitoring in preanesthesia can improve preprocedure glycemic control and lessen the burden of hyperglycemia intraoperatively. Such protocols should also be used in postoperative patients and should account for prandial carbohydrate intake once regular diet is resumed. Ultimately, decision to resume patients' home diabetes medication regimen at time of discharge should be based on stable renal function, dietary intake, overall functional status, and type of surgical procedure. Communication with the patients' diabetes clinician should take place to ensure safe transition of care.

PHYSICAL EXAMINATION CONSIDERATIONS FOR THE ANESTHESIOLOGIST
Airway

Standard airway examination techniques are appropriate for patients with diabetes but may not identify all difficult intubations. Musculoskeletal effects of diabetes include glycosylation of joints and ligaments, most noticeably in the cervical spine and metacarpals. The stylohyoid ligament can also be involved. Cheiroarthropathy is the name given to this complication of diabetes, which is present in more than 50% of patients with the disease. It involves tightening of the skin and soft tissues and leads to limited joint mobility. Shoulder pain from adhesive capsulitis, carpal tunnel syndrome, Dupuytren contracture, and flexor tendinitis are common findings.

Treatment includes improved glycemic control, stretching exercises, and simple analgesics/antiinflammatories. The classic prayer sign (2 hands held together with palms facing each other with inability to approximate) has been frequently noted. Using this abnormality, Nadal and colleagues[35] found that the palm print (or lack thereof) was 100% sensitive in predicting difficult intubations in patients with diabetes. This same pathology may lead to difficulty with IV placement and patient positioning.

Cardiovascular

Standard preoperative cardiovascular examination with attention to signs of heart failure, cerebrovascular and peripheral vascular disease, and the presence of signs of diabetic foot and peripheral neuropathy should be performed.

Autonomic Dysfunction

Autonomic dysfunction can be assessed clinically at the bedside (**Table 5**). Abnormalities of the parasympathetic system usually present before those of the sympathetic system.

Surgical Site Infection Screening

Patients should be screened for skin infections and dental caries as possible niduses for wound infection, especially in high-risk patients (ie, joint replacement, CABG).

Preoperative Laboratory Testing

It is reasonable to measure glucose and renal function preoperatively. If a hemoglobin A1c (HbA1c) has not been done in the preceding 3 months or patients report poor control on home testing, an HbA1C level gives an indication of control in the preceding 2 to 3 months. Elevated HbA1c is associated with worse postoperative outcomes, and consideration should be given to delaying surgery in order to pursue medical optimization. Institution-specific practices exist regarding optimal HbA1c before procedure. The authors generally recommend considering postponement of elective surgery with HbA1c greater than 9%, depending on the surgical procedure.

Elevated HbA1c is associated with higher perioperative glucose levels, elevated C-reactive protein, and complications.[36,37] Preoperative hyperglycemia is an independent risk factor for increased cardiovascular mortality in patients undergoing noncardiac, nonvascular surgeries.[9]

The American Heart Association's guidelines are followed for ordering an electrocardiogram. In patients with suspected metabolic syndrome or undiagnosed diabetes, it is reasonable to check an HbA1C. If there are symptoms of dehydration, diabetic ketosis (DKA), or hyperosmolar hyperglycemic state (HHS), electrolytes and a venous blood gas should be checked. If DKA/HHS is discovered, established protocols should be followed for management.[38]

Preoperative Instructions

As with any surgery, patients should be advised on a healthy lifestyle and preoperative conditioning (appropriate diet, increasing exercise levels, and remaining compliant with medication instructions). Smoking cessation should be strongly recommended. Patients with sleep apnea should be encouraged to comply with continuous positive airway pressure instructions. The American Society of Anesthesiologists offers guidelines regarding oral intake in the immediate preoperative period.[39] If there is a concern about aspiration, it is reasonable to extend the fasting period.

Anesthesia Plan

Patients with diabetes should be preferentially scheduled as first cases, which allows for optimization of glycemic control preoperatively. In shorter ambulatory cases, patients may even be in recovery eating breakfast at their regular time with minimal effect on blood glucose. For patients undergoing longer procedures with higher metabolic impact, glucose levels can be monitored and corrected as needed.

Blood glucose should be checked on admission to the preoperative holding area. Hypoglycemia, if present, can be corrected with IV fluids, and surgery should proceed

Table 4
Oral diabetes agents and insulins

			Noninsulin Agents		
Class	Examples	Mechanism of Action	Metabolism	Perioperative Considerations
Alpha-glucosidase inhibitors	Acarbose	Delayed digestion of complex carbohydrates and lower postprandial glycemia	GI tract, excreted in urine	Cause flatus and diarrhea; limit use perioperatively
Biguanides	Metformin Metformin ER	Decreases hepatic gluconeogenesis/improves insulin sensitivity	Excreted in urine; not metabolized by the liver	Risk of lactic acidosis, which is increased in CHF, liver, or renal failure; hold for 24–48 h preoperatively
DPP-4 inhibitors	Alogliptin Linagliptin Saxagliptin Sitagliptin Vildagliptin	Inhibit the enzyme, DPP-4, resulting in increased levels of incretin hormones leading to increased insulin and decreased glucagon secretion	Minor, hepatic metabolism	Low risk of hypoglycemia; limit use if risk for pancreatitis
Incretin mimetics (GLP-1 agonists)	Albiglutide Dulaglutide Exenatide Liraglutide	Simulate pancreatic glucose-dependent; decrease satiety/weight loss	Minor systemic metabolism; excreted in urine	Can cause nausea and delayed gastric emptying; limit use if risk for pancreatitis; hold perioperatively
Meglitinides	Nateglinide Repaglinide	Increase pancreatic ATP-dependent insulin secretion	Hepatic metabolism; excreted in feces	Hypoglycemia risk significant; avoid in renal failure; hold perioperatively while NPO
SGLT2	Canagliflozin Dapagliflozin Empagliflozin	Cause increased renal excretion of glucose	Glucoronidation; excreted in urine	Increased risk of vulvocandidiasis and UTI; reports of DKA
Sulfonylureas	Glimepiride Glipizide Glyburide	Increase ATP-dependent insulin secretion by pancreatic beta cells	Hepatic metabolism; excreted in urine and feces	Hypoglycemia risk significant; avoid in renal failure; hold perioperatively while NPO
Thiazolidinediones	Pioglitazone Rosiglitazone	Insulin sensitizer by activation of PPARs	Hepatic metabolism; excreted in urine and feces	Use with extreme caution in CHF; hold perioperatively

Insulins

Example	Brand Name	Perioperative Considerations
Rapid acting (time to onset <15 min, duration 3 h)		
Aspart Lispro Glulisine	Novolog Humalog Apidra	Use for glucose correction perioperatively; greater effect in those with renal failure or who are insulin naïve
Short acting (time to onset 1 h, duration 5–6 h)		
Regular	Humulin-R Novolin-R	Use limited to intravenous insulin infusion perioperatively
Intermediate acting (time to onset 2–4 h, duration 10–15 h)		
NPH	Humulin-N Novolin-N	Useful for continuous enteral feeds and in pregnancy; (previously used more frequently for basal insulin)
Long acting (time to onset 0.5–2.0 h, duration 20–24 h)		
Detemir Glargine	Levemir Lantus	Allow at least 30–60 min when transitioning from insulin infusion to SC basal insulin
Mixed insulins (intermediate + rapid- or short-acting insulin)		
NPH/aspart NPH/lispro NPH/regular	Novolog 70/30 Humalog 70/30 Humalog 75/25 Humalog 50/50 Humulin 70/30 Novolin 70/30	Use limited to outpatient setting; convert to rapid-acting + long-acting insulin regimen during hospitalization; consult with endocrinologist for expert guidance
Concentrated insulins		
U-300 U-500	Toujeo Humulin-R U500	Highly specialized use; Consult with endocrinologist for expert guidance.

Abbreviations: CHF, congestive heart failure; DKA, diabetic ketoacidosis; DPP-4, dipeptidyl peptidase-4; ER, extended release; GI, gastrointestinal; GLP-1, glucagon-like peptide 1; NPH, neutral protamine Hagedorn; NPO, nil per os; PPAR, peroxisome proliferator-activated receptors; SC, subcutaneous; UTI, urinary tract infection.

Table 5
Assessment of autonomic dysfunction

Test		Response
Valsalva maneuver		Initial increase in heart rate and subsequent decrease after end of maneuver
Change in heart rate	On moving from supine to standing	Maximum rate by the 15th beat and decreasing maximally by the 30th beat
	Response to 6 deep breaths in 1 min (repeated 3 times)	Should be >15-beat variability between the highest and lowest heart rate (<5 beat/min difference implies severe dysfunction)
Change in blood pressure	Measurement supine and then 2 min after standing	Normal should not decrease >10 mm Hg (severe dysfunction implied if decrease >20 mm Hg)
	Increase in diastolic blood pressure with 5 min sustained	Normal should increase by >16 mm Hg

with regular blood glucose checks. Institutional policies exist regarding frequency of glycemic monitoring perioperatively. Hourly glucose checks while under anesthesia are common but may be more frequent in unstable patients. Preoperative hyperglycemia should also be corrected with rapid-acting insulin. Subcutaneous insulin injection is appropriate for most patients; however, IV insulin infusion can provide a more reliable response, especially in patients undergoing more invasive procedures. Although hyperglycemia should not be grounds for automatic case cancellation, it should be corrected before surgery starts. Hyperglycemic patients with T1DM should be assessed for DKA/HHS; if present, case cancellation should be strongly considered until the metabolic abnormality is corrected.

Intraoperative Glycemic Monitoring

Consensus regarding goal glycemic end points in hospitalized patients has been difficult to establish because of the inconsistency in trial data. Understanding that tight glycemic control may only be appropriate for specific populations of inpatients, the American Diabetes Association has outlined goal glycemic control for various hospitalized patients (**Box 2**).[40]

It is important for the perioperative clinician to be familiar with their institutional point-of-care (POC) glucose-monitoring device. Only certain POC devices are approved by regulatory agencies for use in hospital and critical care settings because of inconsistencies in test results in patients with poor peripheral perfusion, hypovolemia, shock, hypothermia, and/or acid/base disturbances. Thus, finger stick/capillary blood samples may not be appropriate for certain patients undergoing major surgery (eg, cardiothoracic, vascular or major colorectal procedures). Manufacturer recommendations should be followed closely, and arterial/venous blood samples may be more appropriate in these situations.

Postoperative Glycemic Considerations

As the sympathetic nervous system is stimulated by the stress of surgery, both increased glycogenolysis and increased release of free fatty acids is seen, leading to elevated blood glucose levels. There have been conflicting reports in the literature surrounding

> **Box 2**
> **American Diabetes Association's glycemic targets in hospitalized patients**
>
> *Critically ill patients*
>
> - Initiate insulin therapy for persistent hyperglycemia greater than 180 mg/dL to maintain a goal glucose of 140 to 180 mg/dL.
> - Consider tighter targets if clinically appropriate and safe to do so.
> - Consider use of institutional intravenous insulin drip protocol.
>
> *Noncritically ill patients*
>
> - Use preprandial goal glucose less than 140 mg/dL with random glucose less than 180 mg/dL.
> - Consider tighter targets if clinically appropriate and safe to do so.
>
> *Medication choice*
>
> - Use of oral diabetes agents in hospitalized patients is not recommended for most clinical settings.
> - Insulin protocols should account for carbohydrate intake; sole use of sliding-scale correction insulin is discouraged.
>
> *Modified from* American Diabetes Association. Diabetes care in the hospital, nursing home, and skilled nursing facility. Sec. 13. In standards of medical care in diabetes. Diabetes Care 2015;38(Suppl 1):S80–5.

appropriate glycemic control in the hospital.[40–43] Although the pendulum of inpatient glycemic end points continues to swing, there is persistent and significant evidence supporting the role of tighter glycemic control in certain postoperative populations. Specifically, following cardiac surgery, patients may benefit from tighter glucose control. Data from the 17-year prospective Portland Diabetes Project demonstrated the importance of a protocolized insulin infusion regimen in patients undergoing cardiothoracic surgery. Specifically, implementation of an IV insulin infusion resulted in reduction of postoperative deep sternal wound infections (DSWI) by nearly 66%, resulting in a total net savings to the hospital of $4638 per patient.[44] Rates of DSWI dramatically increased in patients with higher postoperative blood glucose as did mortality and length of stay.

Regulatory agencies and third-party payers have recognized the significance of perioperative glycemic control on clinical outcomes in the era of value-based purchasing. The Joint Commission's Surgical Care Improvement Project (SCIP), a subset of the National Quality Hospital Measures created by the Centers for Medicare and Medicaid Services called for tighter glycemic control (blood glucose ≤180 mg/dL) in the 18 to 24 hours following the anesthesia end time. In early 2015, the Joint Commission temporarily suspended the SCIP-INF-4 measure for postoperative glycemic control citing concern that the measure may adversely affect the way clinicians and hospitals provide care.[45] Some institutions reported increases in rates of hypoglycemia commensurate with tighter postoperative blood sugar goals. It is thought, however, that regulatory efforts aimed at raising awareness of perioperative glycemic control will likely be reimplemented in the future. Therefore, the authors recommend persistent attention to perioperative glycemic control and implementation of safe and effective insulin protocols based on recognized standards of care.[40]

Continuous Subcutaneous Insulin Infusion (Insulin Pumps)

Insulin pump technology has improved markedly in recent years. Although most patients using pumps have T1DM, there are growing numbers of people with T2DM using them; the perioperative clinician will undoubtedly encounter pumps during patient care. Insulin pumps are designed to provide a continuous basal supply of insulin in a manner mimicking the healthy pancreas as well as to meet prandial needs (bolus). Rapid-acting analogue insulin is infused through a small cannula (infusion set) placed under the skin by patients at 2- to 3-day intervals. An hourly basal rate is programmed to anticipate for trends in normal basal insulin secretion in the nondiabetic pancreas (ie, the dawn phenomenon accounting for early morning increases hepatic gluconeo-genesis and insulin resistance). Prandial insulin is administered based on a predeter-mined insulin-to-carbohydrate ratio (accounting for food intake) and correction factor (accounting for preprandial hyperglycemia). Mealtime boluses are entirely patient directed and depend highly on the ability to accurately assess mealtime carbohydrate intake (ie, carbohydrate counting). Although there has recently been improvement in and greater utilization of continuous glucose monitoring systems (CGMS), there does not currently exist a close-looped insulin pump delivery system. Some pump + CGMS combination systems have the ability to automatically suspend basal insulin in the event of hypoglycemia, and advancements in automated insulin delivery are undoubtedly forthcoming.

Intraoperative insulin pump use depends on multiple factors and involves multidis-ciplinary coordination to ensure patient safety. Consultation by the institution's endo-crinology service is imperative and will help guide the surgical team in appropriate management practices. Communication with patients' endocrinologists in advance of surgery is imperative. The type of surgery impacts the appropriateness of pump continuation during the procedure. Should the decision be made to continue insulin pump therapy intraoperatively, it is important that the surgical team inspects and ex-amines the insulin infusion site to determine if its location on the skin would impede the surgical approach. If so, the authors recommend discontinuation of the insulin pump and implementation of alternative insulin administration (subcutaneous or IV) preoper-atively. At most centers, pump patients undergoing high-risk cardiac, vascular, or open abdominal surgeries are transitioned to IV insulin infusion preoperatively. Lower-risk, shorter procedures may be appropriate for pump continuation with careful intraoperative monitoring of glycemic control.

SUMMARY/DISCUSSION

Diabetes is a chronic secondary diagnosis affecting more than 9% of the population. Uncontrolled diabetes can result in poor short- and long-term surgical outcomes. Complications from the disease affect nearly every organ system and can greatly impact perioperative risk. Modern treatment regimens mimicking natural pancreatic function, better monitoring, and evidence-based recommendations help improve long-term and perioperative outcomes. Careful consideration should be given to pa-tients with diabetes undergoing surgery in order to ensure the best possible results.

REFERENCES

1. American Diabetes Association. 2015 diabetes fact sheet. Available at: http://professional.diabetes.org/admin/UserFiles/0-Sean/Documents/Fast_Facts_3-2015.pdf. Accessed September 5, 2015.
2. Danaei G, Finucane MM, Lu Y, et al. National, regional, and global trends in fast-ing plasma glucose and diabetes prevalence since 1980: systematic analysis of health examination surveys and epidemiological studies with 370 country-years and 2.7 million participants. Lancet 2011;378(9785):31–40.

3. Geiss LS, Wang J, Cheng YJ, et al. Prevalence and incidence trends for diagnosed diabetes among adults aged 20 to 79 years, United States, 1980-2012. JAMA 2014;312(12):1218–26.

4. Centers for Disease Control and Prevention. Distribution of first-listed diagnoses among hospital discharges with diabetes as any-listed diagnosis, adults aged 18 years and older, United States, 2010. Available at: http://www.cdc.gov/diabetes/statistics/hosp/adulttable1.htm.

5. Burgos LG, Ebert TJ, Asiddao C, et al. Increased intraoperative cardiovascular morbidity in diabetics with autonomic neuropathy. Anesthesiology 1989;70(4):591–7.

6. Gandhi GY, Nuttall GA, Abel MD, et al. Intraoperative hyperglycemia and perioperative outcomes in cardiac surgery patients. Mayo Clin Proc 2005;80(7):862–6.

7. Lauruschkat AH, Arnrich B, Albert AA, et al. Prevalence and risks of undiagnosed diabetes mellitus in patients undergoing coronary artery bypass grafting. Circulation 2005;112(16):2397–402.

8. Kota SK, Meher LK, Jammula S, et al. Clinical profile of coexisting conditions in type 1 diabetes mellitus patients. Diabetes Metab Syndr 2012;6(2):70–6.

9. Noordzij PG, Boersma E, Schreiner F, et al. Increased preoperative glucose levels are associated with perioperative mortality in patients undergoing noncardiac, nonvascular surgery. Eur J Endocrinol 2007;156(1):137–42.

10. U.K. prospective diabetes study 16. Overview of 6 years' therapy of type II diabetes: a progressive disease. U.K. Prospective Diabetes Study Group. Diabetes 1995;44(11):1249–58.

11. Fonseca VA. Defining and characterizing the progression of type 2 diabetes. Diabetes Care 2009;32(Suppl 2):S151–s156.

12. Hollenberg M, Mangano DT, Browner WS, et al. Predictors of postoperative myocardial ischemia in patients undergoing noncardiac surgery. The Study of Perioperative Ischemia Research Group. JAMA 1992;268(2):205–9.

13. Lee TH, Marcantonio ER, Mangione CM, et al. Derivation and prospective validation of a simple index for prediction of cardiac risk of major noncardiac surgery. Circulation 1999;100(10):1043–9.

14. Fleisher LA, Fleischmann KE, Auerbach AD, et al. 2014 ACC/AHA guideline on perioperative cardiovascular evaluation and management of patients undergoing noncardiac surgery: executive summary: a report of the American College of Cardiology/American Heart Association Task Force on practice guidelines. Developed in collaboration with the American College of Surgeons, American Society of Anesthesiologists, American Society of Echocardiography, American Society of Nuclear Cardiology, Heart Rhythm Society, Society for Cardiovascular Angiography and Interventions, Society of Cardiovascular Anesthesiologists, and Society of Vascular Medicine Endorsed by the Society of Hospital Medicine. J Nucl Cardiol 2015;22(1):162–215.

15. Delamaire M, Maugendre D, Moreno M, et al. Impaired leucocyte functions in diabetic patients. Diabet Med 1997;14(1):29–34.

16. Black CT, Hennessey PJ, Andrassy RJ. Short-term hyperglycemia depresses immunity through nonenzymatic glycosylation of circulating immunoglobulin. J Trauma 1990;30(7):830–2 [discussion: 32–3].

17. Ziegler D, Dannehl K, Muhlen H, et al. Prevalence of cardiovascular autonomic dysfunction assessed by spectral analysis, vector analysis, and standard tests of heart rate variation and blood pressure responses at various stages of diabetic neuropathy. Diabet Med 1992;9(9):806–14.

18. Balcioglu AS, Muderrisoglu H. Diabetes and cardiac autonomic neuropathy: clinical manifestations, cardiovascular consequences, diagnosis and treatment. World J Diabetes 2015;6(1):80–91.

19. Wright RA, Clemente R, Wathen R. Diabetic gastroparesis: an abnormality of gastric emptying of solids. Am J Med Sci 1985;289(6):240–2.

20. Charlson ME, MacKenzie CR, Gold JP. Preoperative autonomic function abnormalities in patients with diabetes mellitus and patients with hypertension. J Am Coll Surg 1994;179(1):1–10.

21. Ewing DJ, Campbell IW, Clarke BF. The natural history of diabetic autonomic neuropathy. Q J Med 1980;49(193):95–108.

22. Maser RE, Mitchell BD, Vinik AI, et al. The association between cardiovascular autonomic neuropathy and mortality in individuals with diabetes: a meta-analysis. Diabetes Care 2003;26(6):1895–901.

23. Orchard TJ, LLoyd CE, Maser RE, et al. Why does diabetic autonomic neuropathy predict IDDM mortality? An analysis from the Pittsburgh Epidemiology of Diabetes Complications Study. Diabetes Res Clin Pract 1996;34(Suppl):S165–71.

24. Vinik AI, Maser RE, Mitchell BD, et al. Diabetic autonomic neuropathy. Diabetes Care 2003;26(5):1553–79.

25. Vinik AI, Ziegler D. Diabetic cardiovascular autonomic neuropathy. Circulation 2007;115(3):387–97.

26. Kitamura A, Hoshino T, Kon T, et al. Patients with diabetic neuropathy are at risk of a greater intraoperative reduction in core temperature. Anesthesiology 2000; 92(5):1311–8.

27. Sobotka PA, Liss HP, Vinik AI. Impaired hypoxic ventilatory drive in diabetic patients with autonomic neuropathy. J Clin Endocrinol Metab 1986;62(4): 658–63.

28. Ewing DJ, Campbell IW, Clarke BF. Assessment of cardiovascular effects in diabetic autonomic neuropathy and prognostic implications. Ann Intern Med 1980; 92(2 Pt 2):308–11.

29. Page MM, Watkins PJ. Cardiorespiratory arrest and diabetic autonomic neuropathy. Lancet 1978;1(8054):14–6.

30. Ko SH, Song KH, Park SA, et al. Cardiovascular autonomic dysfunction predicts acute ischaemic stroke in patients with type 2 diabetes mellitus: a 7-year follow-up study. Diabet Med 2008;25(10):1171–7.

31. Schumann R, Shikora SA, Sigl JC, et al. Association of metabolic syndrome and surgical factors with pulmonary adverse events, and longitudinal mortality in bariatric surgery. Br J Anaesth 2015;114(1):83–90.

32. Vreven R, De Kock M. Metformin lactic acidosis and anaesthesia: myth or reality? Acta Anaesthesiol Belg 2005;56(3):297–302.

33. Moghissi ES, Korytkowski MT, DiNardo M, et al. American Association of Clinical Endocrinologists and American Diabetes Association consensus statement on inpatient glycemic control. Endocr Pract 2009;15(4):353–69.

34. Radiologists RCo. Metformin: updated guidance for use in diabetics with renal impairment. 2009. Available at: https://www.rcn.org.uk/__data/assets/pdf_file/0011/258743/BFCR097_Metformin.pdf.

35. Nadal JL, Fernandez BG, Escobar IC, et al. The palm print as a sensitive predictor of difficult laryngoscopy in diabetics. Acta Anaesthesiol Scand 1998;42(2): 199–203.

36. Gustafsson UO, Thorell A, Soop M, et al. Haemoglobin A1c as a predictor of postoperative hyperglycaemia and complications after major colorectal surgery. Br J Surg 2009;96(11):1358–64.

37. Moitra VK, Greenberg J, Arunajadai S, et al. The relationship between glycosylated hemoglobin and perioperative glucose control in patients with diabetes. Can J Anaesth 2010;57(4):322–9.

38. Kitabchi AE, Umpierrez GE, Miles JM, et al. Hyperglycemic crises in adult patients with diabetes. Diabetes Care 2009;32(7):1335–43.

39. American Society of Anesthesiologists Committee. Practice guidelines for preoperative fasting and the use of pharmacologic agents to reduce the risk of pulmonary aspiration: application to healthy patients undergoing elective procedures: an updated report by the American Society of Anesthesiologists Committee on Standards and Practice Parameters. Anesthesiology 2011;114(3):495–511.

40. Association AD. Standards of medical care in diabetes. Diabetes Care 2015; 38(Suppl 1):S80–5.

41. van den Berghe G, Wouters P, Weekers F, et al. Intensive insulin therapy in critically ill patients. N Engl J Med 2001;345(19):1359–67.

42. Van den Berghe G, Wilmer A, Hermans G, et al. Intensive insulin therapy in the medical ICU. N Engl J Med 2006;354(5):449–61.

43. NICE-SUGAR Study Investigators, Finfer S, Chittock DR, et al. Intensive versus conventional glucose control in critically ill patients. N Engl J Med 2009; 360(13):1283–97.

44. Furnary AP, Wu Y. Clinical effects of hyperglycemia in the cardiac surgery population: the Portland Diabetic Project. Endocr Pract 2006;12(Suppl 3):22–6.

45. The Joint Commission. Secondary suspension of data collection for performance measure SCIP-Inf-4. Available at: http://www.jointcommission.org/assets/1/23/jconlinc_January_28_15.pdf. Accessed September 5, 2015.

Preoperative Assessment of Geriatric Patients

 CrossMark

Justin G. Knittel, MD, Troy S. Wildes, MD*

KEYWORDS

- Preoperative • Geriatric • Elderly • Surgery • Frailty • Functional status • Delirium
- Nutrition

KEY POINTS

- Geriatric patients, with their increased incidence of comorbidities and deficits seen with aging, require special preoperative consideration.
- Comprehensive preoperative assessment of geriatric patients includes systematic evaluation of comorbidities, neurocognitive function, sensory impairment, substance use, functional status, frailty, nutrition, and medications.
- Delirium represents a common perioperative complication with significant effects on patient outcomes; patient risk should be identified preoperatively.
- Comprehensive assessment is important for risk identification, but the identification of risk factors and deficits should be accompanied by problem-specific management plans to realize improvements in outcome.
- Surgical and other perioperative decisions in the geriatric patient should be goal-oriented in nature, incorporating a realistic assessment of potential benefits and risks in each individual.

INTRODUCTION

Individuals aged 65 years and older currently make up 13% of the US population and are expected to comprise more than 20% of the population by 2030.[1] This demographic utilizes healthcare resources in a disproportionate fashion, accounting for 43% of all hospital days, 32.1% of outpatient procedures, and 35.3% of inpatient procedures.[2,3] Geriatric patients are similarly over-represented in health care expenditures.[2] This pattern of health resource utilization is the manifestation of multiple age-related factors including increased prevalence of comorbid conditions, cumulative exposure to diseases, and the increasingly incapacitating effects of new health

Funding Sources: NIA 1U1I2AG050312-01 (Dr T.S. Wildes).

Conflicts of Interest: None.

Department of Anesthesiology, Washington University School of Medicine, Campus Box 8054, 660 South Euclid Avenue, St Louis, MO 63110, USA

* Corresponding author.

E-mail address: wildest@anest.wustl.edu

Anesthesiology Clin 34 (2016) 171–183

http://dx.doi.org/10.1016/j.anclin.2015.10.013
anesthesiology.theclinics.com

insults. In addition to well-known comorbidities, age-associated alterations in general function and independence further reduce an individual's resilience. When surgery is performed in aged patients, these vulnerabilities can result in compromised post-operative outcomes, including prolonged hospitalization, skilled nursing facility admission, progressive loss of independence, or death. Such a course is more likely if these risk factors are not recognized and mitigated in the pre- and perioperative period.

Recently published collaborative guidelines from the American College of Surgeons National Surgical Quality Improvement Program (ACS NSQIP) and American Geriatrics Society (AGS) propose a formal framework for routine multidomain preoperative assessment of geriatric patients.[1] For risk estimation, multidomain, procedure-specific tools like the online ACS NSQIP risk calculator increasingly allow preoperative characteristics to be translated into risk estimates for a variety of complications after specific surgeries, ranging from minimally invasive to major.[4,5] Along with the identification of specific risks, the preoperative evaluation should be used to ensure there is a shared understanding of likely outcomes, to reappraise the patient's care goals, and to ensure that therapeutic decisions are appropriately aligned. For patients who will proceed with surgery, likely complications should be anticipated and modifiable risk factors mitigated in advance.

NEUROCOGNITIVE AND BEHAVIORAL ASSESSMENT

An estimated 14% and 22% of US individuals over the age of 71 have dementia and nondementia cognitive impairment, respectively.[6] The recent ACS NSQIP-AGS Guidelines for Optimal Preoperative Assessment of the Geriatric Patient include recommendations for routine preoperative neurocognitive assessment to detect such deficits before surgery.[1] Early identification of neurocognitive deficits influences the entire preoperative evaluation, including the reliability of the medical history, perioperative educational needs, and decision making. Additionally, preoperative detection is critical for diagnosing new postoperative deficits and anticipating postoperative complications such as delirium and functional dependency. Although multiple viable cognitive assessment tools exist, the Mini-Cog Assessment is an example of a short (approximately 3 minutes), easily applicable, and well-studied tool that assesses attention and executive function.[7] In addition to a cognitive assessment, the ACS NSQIP-AGS guidelines strongly recommend preoperative depression and substance abuse screening.[1]

CARDIAC EVALUATION

Perioperative cardiac complications such as myocardial infarction are relatively common in adults undergoing major surgery and are associated with subsequent mortality,[8] but geriatric patients are even more vulnerable to perioperative cardiac events than other age groups.[9] Risk factors for perioperative cardiac events like diabetes mellitus are more prevalent in the geriatric population, and the duration of exposure to such risk factors is lengthier. Geriatric patients should undergo cardiac risk stratification, should have indicated cardiac tests performed, and should have evidence-based optimization strategies applied prior to surgery.[10] As in nongeriatric patients, preoperative cardiac optimization should center around applying risk-reduction therapies that would be independently indicated outside of the perioperative setting. Preoperative myocardial revascularization is rarely indicated before noncardiac surgery.[10] It may be an even less viable strategy in the geriatric patient, who may be a poor candidate for primary or repeat coronary bypass grafting and whose health goals may not align well with the expected postoperative course of surgical revascularization. More routinely useful preoperative strategies in aged patients include medical optimization and careful consideration of how increased cardiac risk may influence the decision to proceed with surgery. Multiple risk stratification indices exist for evaluating the risk of perioperative cardiac complications. The web-based NSQIP Risk Calculator[5] is one of the risk estimation tools recommended by the 2014 American College of Cardiology/American Heart Association Guideline on Perioperative Cardiovascular Evaluation and Management of Patients Undergoing Noncardiac Surgery,[10] and this tool includes patient age and functional dependence as factors.

PULMONARY EVALUATION

Respiratory complications are associated with increased hospital length of stay and increased cost,[11] as well as increased long-term mortality.[12] Age and functional dependence have been identified as among the most reliable risk factors for postoperative pulmonary complications.[13] Other risk factors are shown in **Box 1**. Preoperative serum albumin testing may help to identify patients at higher risk, but other diagnostic testing is generally not recommended for improving risk estimation,[13] and usually does not help to identify modifiable factors. Smoking is a modifiable risk factor; cessation should be encouraged whenever possible, but ideally more than 4 weeks before surgery.[14] There is evidence that preoperative physical rehabilitation can reduce pneumonia and length of stay, but evidence for a reduction in mortality is lacking.[15] Although functional dependence is a strong risk factor and more prevalent in aged patients, its potential to be modified and produce improvements in perioperative pulmonary events is unknown.

FUNCTIONAL ASSESSMENT

Limitations in function, such as being unable to perform both basic and complex tasks important for independence, are predictive of perioperative complications,[13] institutionalization,[16] and mortality.[17] Impaired mobility is also associated with postoperative delirium, pneumonia, and surgical site infection.[13,18,19] Such functional deficits are present in many aged individuals whether or not they have comorbid diseases.[20]

A patient's ability to maintain normal independent function can be measured with instruments that target specific tasks or skills; these may be assessed by interviews, observation, or objective testing (**Box 2**). The Katz Activities of Daily Living (ADLs) instrument scores basic activities viewed to be relevant to all individuals, such as independent ability to bathe, dress, and transfer.[21] Instrumental Activities of Daily Living (IADLs) tools capture higher levels of function including medication management, shopping, and transportation capabilities.[22] Additional functional assessments target other individual abilities or combinations thereof. For example, the Timed Up and Go test identifies fall risk by assessing a task that requires strength, mobility, and balance.[23]

Functional status assessment should be included in the preoperative assessment of aged patients.[1] Beyond contributing significantly to overall risk assessment, detection of issues such as mobility problems and sensory impairments can lead to specific interventions like home safety improvements to decrease the risk of falls. Discussions can also be initiated with patients and family members regarding likely needs for temporary or permanent assistance postoperatively, including possible nursing facility admission.

Box 1
Risk factors for postoperative pulmonary complications

Patient-related factors

- Age greater than 60 y
- Chronic obstructive pulmonary disease
- American Society of Anesthesiologists class II or greater
- Functional dependence[a]
- Congestive heart failure
- Obstructive sleep apnea
- Pulmonary hypertension
- Current cigarette use
- Impaired sensorium[b]
- Preoperative sepsis
- Weight loss >10% in 6 months
- Serum albumin less than 3.5 mg/dL
- Blood urea nitrogen ≥7.5 mmol/L (≥21 mg/dL)
- Serum creatinine greater than 133 μmol/L (>1.5 mg/dL)

Surgery-related factors

- Prolonged operation >3 h
- Surgical site[c]
- Emergency operation
- General anesthesia
- Perioperative transfusion
- Residual neuromuscular blockade after an operation

Not risk factors

- Obesity
- Well-controlled asthma
- Diabetes

[a] Total dependence was the inability to perform any activities of daily living. Partial dependence was the need for equipment or devices and assistance from another person for some activities of daily living.

[b] Acutely confused or delirious patient who is able to respond to verbal or mild tactile stimulation, or mental status changes or delirium in the context of current illness.

[c] Highest-risk procedures: upper abdominal, thoracic, neurosurgical, head and neck, vascular (eg, aortic aneurysm repair).

From Chow WB, Rosenthal RA, Merkow RP, et al. Optimal preoperative assessment of the geriatric surgical patient: a best practices guideline from the American College of Surgeons National Surgical Quality Improvement Program and the American Geriatrics Society. J Am Coll Surg 2012;215(4):456; with permission.

DELIRIUM

Delirium is a multifactorial disorder characterized by impaired attention and disorganized thinking that frequently occurs in the perioperative setting. It is one of the

---

Box 2
Functional assessments

Activities of Daily Living[21]

- Bathing

- Dressing

- Toileting

- Transferring

- Continence

- Feeding

Instrumental Activities of Daily Living[22]

- Telephone ability

- Shopping

- Food preparation

- Housekeeping

- Laundry

- Transportation

- Medication management

- Handling finances

Other

- Muscle strength

- Balance

- Gait

- Walking speed

- Transfer ability

Data from Katz S, Ford AB, Moskowitz RW, et al. Studies of illness in the aged: the index of ADL: a standardized measure of biological and psychosocial function. JAMA 1963;185(12):914–9; and Lawton MP, Brody EM. Assessment of older people: self-maintaining and instrumental activities of daily living. Gerontologist 1969;9(3):179–86.

---

most common postoperative complications seen among geriatric patients, with an incidence of up to 50%.[24] Delirium is strongly associated with other adverse outcomes, including increased length of hospital stay, increased health care costs, postoperative cognitive dysfunction, and mortality.[24] Unfortunately, delirium often goes undiagnosed, likely relating to inadequate detection strategies paired with the fact that most incident delirium is of the hypoactive type and accordingly lacks more prominent behavioral features. Even when anticipated or diagnosed, there is a paucity of evidence-supported strategies for prevention and treatment. For all of these reasons, delirium has recently become an intensive area of perioperative research, education, and quality improvement.

Although many inciting factors for postoperative delirium develop in the immediate perioperative period, other factors can be identified preoperatively. The American Geriatrics Society recently published best practice guidelines for the prevention and treatment of delirium,[25] including a recommendation that all geriatric surgical patients be screened for delirium risk factors preoperatively (**Box 3**). Although proven risk

---

Box 3
Risk factors for postoperative delirium

- Age greater than 65 y
- Cognitive impairment
- Severe illness or comorbidity burden
- Hearing or vision impairment
- Current hip fracture
- Presence of infection
- Inadequately controlled pain
- Depression
- Alcohol use
- Sleep deprivation or disturbance
- Renal insufficiency
- Anemia
- Hypoxia or hypercarbia
- Poor nutrition
- Dehydration
- Electrolyte abnormalities (hyper- or hyponatremia)
- Poor functional status
- Immobilization or limited mobility
- Polypharmacy and use of psychotropic medications (benzodiazepines, anticholinergics, antihistamines, antipsychotics)
- Risk of urinary retention or constipation
- Presence of urinary catheter
- Aortic procedures

From Inouye SK, Robinson T, Blaum C, et al. Postoperative delirium in older adults: best practice statement from the American Geriatrics Society. J Am Coll Surg 2015;220(2):138.e1; with permission.

---

mitigation strategies for delirium are few, a delirium risk assessment allows existing factors to be addressed, highlights the need to avoid other inciting factors, and can heighten postoperative detection plans. Patients with sensory deficits can be reminded to bring hearing aids to the hospital, high-risk outpatient medications may be put on hold, and focused delirium assessments can be performed postoperatively. Other specific interventions for management of postoperative delirium risk are listed in **Box 4**. The preoperative period is also an important time to inform the patient and family about postoperative delirium; this should include presenting features, the usual course, and how it can be managed. A patient's family is vital for promoting continual reorientation and cognitive stimulation, and their perioperative participation in delirium risk management should be strongly encouraged.

MEDICATION MANAGEMENT

Physiologic changes in geriatric patients that may impact drug response include impaired gastrointestinal absorption, decreased hepatic and renal blood flow, increased

---

Box 4
Management of delirium

- Reorientation
- Sensory assist devices (ie, hearing aids, eyeglasses)
- Sleep hygiene
- Early mobilization
- Adequate pain control
- Avoidance of high-risk medications and polypharmacy
- Minimization of catheters, invasive lines, restraints
- Cognitive stimulation
- Family support and interaction

---

adipose tissue, decreased total body water, and decreased muscle mass; these factors impact drug pharmacokinetics and pharmacodynamics, leading to adverse perioperative events.[26]

Geriatric patients may have lengthy home medication lists, often including nonprescription drugs and drugs prescribed by multiple providers. Several medications routinely used in the outpatient and perioperative period have sedating adverse effects that may be accentuated in geriatric patients, particularly when combined with other drugs with similar properties; these include benzodiazepines, medications used for insomnia, and analgesic medications. Other home medications, such as tricyclic antidepressants, antihistamines, and anti-incontinence medications, can increase the risk for falls and orthostatic hypotension in the perioperative period. Additionally, unique geriatric treatments can lead to specific interactions with anesthetic drugs; for example, the acetylcholinesterase inhibitor donepezil prescribed for dementia can interact with neuromuscular blocker drugs.[27] Medication appropriateness criteria such as Beer Criteria[28] and the Screening Tool of Older Persons' Prescriptions (STOPP) tool[29] highlight potentially inappropriate medications for geriatric individuals. Such tools should be used to identify medications that may need to be discontinued perioperatively to avoid adverse events. For some medications with potential adverse perioperative effects but important benefits, prudent management may be to continue the medication accompanied by increased vigilance for adverse effects and the avoidance of interacting medications.

NUTRITION

Surgery and the recovery process create a hypermetabolic state that taxes the reserves of any patient, but can be particularly dangerous in geriatric patients. The prevalence of malnutrition among geriatric patients is substantial, with 38.7% of geriatric hospital patients and more than 50% of geriatric rehabilitation patients classified as malnourished.[30] Malnourished patients are at increased risk for postoperative infection, poor wound healing, wound breakdown, lengthier hospital stay, and mortality.[31,32] Therefore it is important that all geriatric surgical candidates undergo preoperative nutritional screening. Many screening tools exist, such as the Subjective Global Assessment (SGA) and Nutritional Risk Screening (NRS) instrument, but fundamental factors are documentation of height and weight, simple laboratory markers such as albumin levels, and asking patients about recent weight loss.[33,34] Patients identified as malnourished on initial screening should be evaluated by a dietician for potential nutritional optimization prior to surgery. In addition, collaborative plans can be made for maintenance of perioperative nutritional needs and for identifying individuals who may be at risk for complications such as refeeding syndrome in the postoperative period.

FRAILTY

To some extent, preoperative evaluation has always extended beyond an evaluation of the patient's medical history to include a general appraisal of the patient's physical, social, and neuropsychological condition. An informal assessment of these factors could, based on one's experience in caring for aged patients, be used to identify patients who would not tolerate a given treatment. Still, age in itself has also been used as a cutoff for surgical treatment candidacy.

It is now widely appreciated that age is a poor independent marker of risk, and significant progress has been made in improving risk assessment within the geriatric population; one such methodology is the identification of frailty. Frailty is broadly defined as a vulnerable state present in aged individuals that predisposes to adverse health outcomes,[35] but the underlying construct of frailty and how it should be measured have been the subject of much discussion.[35,36] One framework is that frailty is a phenotype with biologic underpinnings manifested externally by slow walking speed, weakness, inactivity, exhaustion, and shrinking; at least three of these features must be present to diagnose frailty.[20] Frailty deficit indices are the alternate general approach, where frailty is marked by the accumulation of up to 75 reported or measurable deficits; the number of criteria evaluated, diagnostic threshold, and severity grading depend on the individual frailty index employed.[37] Although definition and measurement technique may vary between models, the diagnosis of frailty has been repeatedly demonstrated to identify individuals with a decreased probability of survival, with the effect size varying by both the model used and severity.[36,37] Frailty assessment is now being applied clinically, including as a part of the preoperative evaluation. The presence of frailty increases the risk of perioperative complications across various surgeries, including general; cardiac; thoracic, ear, nose, and throat; and urology.[38–43] Various frailty assessment methods have been reported, but an ideal instrument for clinical, and particularly preoperative, use has not been identified. In general, frailty assessment methods that employ more criteria produce more specificity regarding risk identification but come at the cost of being more challenging to employ.

Although various frailty assessment tools are able to identify increased perioperative risk, it remains unclear whether frailty can be modified preoperatively and whether such modification would translate into improved perioperative outcomes. One area of interest has been the potential role of prehabilitation prior to surgery.[44,45] Trials examining improving muscle mass with angiotensin enzyme-converting inhibitors, hormones such as testosterone, or supplements like vitamin D have not resulted in the expected benefits.[46–48]

COMPREHENSIVE GERIATRIC ASSESSMENT

The patient assessment components discussed in this article can be combined to formulate a multidomain preoperative assessment, as recommended in the recent ACS NSQIP-AGS recommendations.[1] Such multifaceted evaluations of geriatric patients are similar to the idea of comprehensive geriatric assessments, which were first used and studied outside of the perioperative setting. The deployment of comprehensive geriatric evaluations in community dwellers has been demonstrated to decrease mortality and prolong independent living.[49] However, importantly, there is significant variation in the implementation of comprehensive geriatric assessment-based care, with greater positive effects associated with programs that have more structured means of implementing recommendations derived from the patient assessment.[49] Comprehensive geriatric assessment has also been applied in the preoperative setting with mixed results, likely dependent on whether or not, and by what mechanism, patient issues were addressed once discovered during the assessment.[50] Therefore, critical aspects of deploying preoperative comprehensive geriatric assessment include planning for which domains will be included, how each domain will be assessed, and how the results will be translated into improved care; ideally, assessment results should impact risk estimation, decision-making, preoperative optimization, anesthetic planning, perioperative surveillance, the postoperative hospitalization, and the postdischarge plan.

THE DECISION FOR SURGERY

With the increased risk of complications and morbidity associated with surgical intervention in the geriatric patient, the decision to proceed with surgery cannot be taken lightly. The decision-making process frequently begins with the primary care or other referring physician, proceeds with the surgical consult, and often has not ended until the day of surgery. Surgeons often depend on preoperative consultants to assist in identifying and addressing patient risk factors that may impact surgical and long-term outcome. Anesthesiologists possess multidisciplinary knowledge regarding the implication of comorbidities and other deficits on the perioperative period and early recovery, and are thus well suited to contribute to the preoperative risk assessment and decision-making process. A recommended approach to decision making in geriatric patients is demonstrated in (http://jama.jamanetwork.com/article.aspx?articleid=1874486#jca140004f1).

Preoperative evaluations of geriatric patients should include decision-making capacity assessment. Decision-making capacity requires the ability to make a rational treatment choice after considering one's medical condition, the desired procedure, potential benefits, and potential risks.[51] Although age alone does not indicate loss of decision-making capacity, the higher prevalence of capacity limitations in individuals with neurocognitive decline and other comorbidities mandates a consideration of this issue in all aged patients.

It is important that preoperative decisions in the aged population incorporate a patient's priorities in combination with a realistic assessment of anticipated procedural benefits and perioperative risks. Although important in all age groups, geriatric patients undergoing high-risk surgeries in particular should be engaged preoperatively in goal-oriented discussions concerning health and life priorities, using a framework such as described by Reuben.[52] In some patients, the decision-making aspects of the preoperative evaluation may be a final endorsement of thoughtfully aligned patient goals and therapeutic plans. In many other patients preparing for high-risk surgery, it is evident that a patient has never had a chance to consider and elucidate his or her life priorities to family members, friends, and care providers. Patients place varying weight on prolongation of life, independence, mobility, control over bodily functions, freedom from pain, avoidance of hospitalization, avoidance of long-term care admission, and the ability to engage in valued pastimes. The prospect of such functional limitations affects patient's treatment decisions.[53] There is no simple or best approach to carrying out what can be a time-consuming and difficult discussion regarding health priorities. However, "The Conversation Project"[54] and "Five Wishes"[55] are examples of tools that can be used by patients to structure such discussions in a manner that provides helpful information to physicians and family members. These shared understandings are helpful preoperatively for assisting patients in aligning medical decisions with their priorities and also postoperatively when additional difficult decisions may have to be made on a patient's behalf. In addition to gaining understanding of patients' priorities, legal documents such as advance directives and decision-maker proxies should be obtained and discussed.[56] However, it is important to bear in mind that neither obtaining legal documents nor having shared discussions about health care priorities replaces the need for the other to occur.

Even when health priorities that would impact decision-making have been clarified, both surgeons and geriatric patients often fail to include these considerations in their own decisions about high-risk surgery.[57] Aged patients may choose to face unreasonable surgical risks for several reasons:

Because they feel obligated to choose potentially life-sustaining care
Because they believe surgery can be successfully aborted if complications might arise
Because they feel that should perioperative death occur it would be a painless outcome[57]

In patients facing high-stakes surgical decisions, it may be beneficial to structure the decision not as a choice for or against treatment, but instead as a choice between several treatment alternatives with varying health benefits and risks.

REFERENCES

1. Chow WB, Rosenthal RA, Merkow RP, et al. Optimal preoperative assessment of the geriatric surgical patient: a best practices guideline from the American College of Surgeons National Surgical Quality Improvement Program and the American Geriatrics Society. J Am Coll Surg 2012;215(4):453–66.
2. Hall MJ, DeFrances CJ, Williams SN. National hospital discharge survey: 2007 summary. Natl Health Stat Report 2010;(29):1–20, 24.
3. Cullen KA, Hall MJ, Golosinskiy A. Ambulatory surgery in the United States, 2006. Natl Health Stat Rep 2009;11:1–25.
4. Bilimoria KY, Liu Y, Paruch JL, et al. Development and evaluation of the universal ACS NSQIP surgical risk calculator: a decision aid and informed consent tool for patients and surgeons. J Am Coll Surg 2013;217(5):833–42.e1-3.
5. ACS NSQIP Surgical Risk Calculator. Available at: http://riskcalculator.facs.org/. Accessed August 14, 2015.
6. Plassman BL, Langa KM, Fisher GG, et al. Prevalence of cognitive impairment without dementia in the United States. Ann Intern Med 2008;148(6):427–34.
7. Borson S, Scanlan JM, Chen P, et al. The Mini-Cog as a screen for dementia: validation in a population-based sample. J Am Geriatr Soc 2003;51(10): 1451–4.
8. Devereaux PJ, Xavier D, Pogue J, et al. Characteristics and short-term prognosis of perioperative myocardial infarction in patients undergoing noncardiac surgery: a cohort study. Ann Intern Med 2011;154(8):523–8.
9. Davenport DL, Ferraris VA, Hosokawa P, et al. Multivariable predictors of postoperative cardiac adverse events after general and vascular surgery: results from the patient safety in surgery study. J Am Coll Surg 2007;204(6):1199–210.
10. Fleisher LA, Fleischmann KE, Auerbach AD, et al. 2014 ACC/AHA guideline on perioperative cardiovascular evaluation and management of patients undergoing

noncardiac surgery: a report of the American College of Cardiology/American Heart Association Task Force on Practice Guidelines. Circulation 2014;130(24):e278–333.

11. Dimick JB, Chen SL, Taheri PA, et al. Hospital costs associated with surgical complications: a report from the private-sector National Surgical Quality Improvement Program. J Am Coll Surg 2004;199(4):531–7.

12. Manku K, Bacchetti P, Leung JM. Prognostic significance of postoperative in-hospital complications in elderly patients. I. Long-term survival. Anesth Analg 2003;96(2):583–9.

13. Smetana GW, Lawrence VA, Cornell JE, American College of Physicians. Preoperative pulmonary risk stratification for noncardiothoracic surgery: systematic review for the American College of Physicians. Ann Intern Med 2006;144(8): 581–95.

14. Wong J, Lam DP, Abrishami A, et al. Short-term preoperative smoking cessation and postoperative complications: a systematic review and meta-analysis. Can J Anaesth 2012;59(3):268–79.

15. Hulzebos EHJ, Smit Y, Helders PPJM, et al. Preoperative physical therapy for elective cardiac surgery patients. Cochrane Database Syst Rev 2012;(11): CD010118.

16. Robinson TN, Wallace JI, Wu DS, et al. Accumulated frailty characteristics predict postoperative discharge institutionalization in the geriatric patient. J Am Coll Surg 2011;213(1):37–42.

17. Robinson TN, Eiseman B, Wallace JI, et al. Redefining geriatric preoperative assessment using frailty, disability and co-morbidity. Trans Meet Am Surg Assoc Am Surg Assoc 2009;127:93–9.

18. Brouquet A, Cudennec T, Benoist S, et al. Impaired mobility, ASA status and administration of tramadol are risk factors for postoperative delirium in patients aged 75 years or more after major abdominal surgery. Ann Surg 2010;251(4): 759–65.

19. Chen T-Y, Anderson DJ, Chopra T, et al. Poor functional status is an independent predictor of surgical site infections due to methicillin-resistant staphylococcus aureusin older Adults. J Am Geriatr Soc 2010;58(3):527–32.

20. Fried LP, Tangen CM, Walston J, et al. Frailty in older adults: evidence for a phenotype. J Gerontol A Biol Sci Med Sci 2001;56(3):M146–56.

21. Katz S, Ford AB, Moskowitz RW, et al. Studies of illness in the aged: the index of ADL: a standardized measure of biological and psychosocial function. JAMA 1963;185(12):914–9.

22. Lawton MP, Brody EM. Assessment of older people: self-maintaining and instrumental activities of daily living. Gerontologist 1969;9(3):179–86.

23. Shumway-Cook A, Brauer S, Woollacott M. Predicting the probability for falls in community-dwelling older adults using the Timed Up & Go Test. Phys Ther 2000;80(9):896–903.

24. Inouye SK, Westendorp RGJ, Saczynski JS. Delirium in elderly people. Lancet 2014;383(9920):911–22.

25. American Geriatrics Society Expert Panel on Postoperative Delirium in Older Adults. American Geriatrics Society abstracted clinical practice guideline for postoperative delirium in older adults. J Am Geriatr Soc 2014; 63(1):142–50.

26. Bressler R, Bahl JJ. Principles of drug therapy for the elderly patient. Mayo Clin Proc 2003;78(12):1564–77.

27. Crowe S, Collins L. Suxamethonium and donepezil: a cause of prolonged paralysis. Anesthesiology 2003;98(2):574–5.

28. American Geriatrics Society 2012 Beers Criteria Update Expert Panel. American Geriatrics Society updated Beers criteria for potentially inappropriate medication use in older adults. J Am Geriatr Soc 2012;60(4):616–31.
29. Gallagher P, Ryan C, Byrne S, et al. STOPP (screening tool of older person's prescriptions) and START (screening tool to alert doctors to right treatment). Consensus validation. Int J Clin Pharmacol Ther 2008;46(2):72–83.
30. Kaiser MJ, Bauer JM, Rämsch C, et al. Frequency of malnutrition in older adults: a multinational perspective using the mini nutritional assessment. J Am Geriatr Soc 2010;58(9):1734–8.
31. Hiesmayr M, Schindler K, Pernicka E, et al. Decreased food intake is a risk factor for mortality in hospitalised patients: the NutritionDay survey 2006. Clin Nutr 2009; 28(5):484–91.
32. Correia M, Waitzberg DL. The impact of malnutrition on morbidity, mortality, length of hospital stay and costs evaluated through a multivariate model analysis. Clin Nutr 2003;22(3):235–9.
33. Detsky AS, McLaughlin JR, Baker JP, et al. What is subjective global assessment of nutritional status? JPEN J Parenter Enteral Nutr 1987;11(1):8–13.
34. Kondrup J, Rasmussen HH, Hamberg O, et al. Nutritional risk screening (NRS 2002): a new method based on an analysis of controlled clinical trials. Clin Nutr 2003;22(3):321–36.
35. Walston J, Hadley EC, Ferrucci L, et al. Research agenda for frailty in older adults: toward a better understanding of physiology and etiology: summary from the American Geriatrics Society/National Institute on aging research conference on frailty in older adults. J Am Geriatr Soc 2006;54(6):991–1001.
36. Rockwood K, Andrew M, Mitnitski A. A comparison of two approaches to measuring frailty in elderly people. J Gerontol A Biol Sci Med Sci 2007;62(7): 738–43.
37. Shamliyan T, Talley KMC, Ramakrishnan R, et al. Association of frailty with survival: A systematic literature review. Ageing Res Rev 2013;12(2):719–36.
38. Bagnall NM, Faiz O, Darzi A, et al. What is the utility of preoperative frailty assessment for risk stratification in cardiac surgery? Interact Cardiovasc Thorac Surg 2013;17(2):398–402.
39. Patel KV, Brennan KL, Brennan ML, et al. Association of a modified frailty index with mortality after femoral neck fracture in patients aged 60 years and older. Clin Orthop Relat Res 2013;472(3):1010–7.
40. Cohen R-R, Lagoo-Deenadayalan SA, Heflin MT, et al. Exploring predictors of complication in older surgical patients: a deficit accumulation index and the braden scale. J Am Geriatr Soc 2012;60(9):1609–15.
41. Adams P, Ghanem T, Stachler R, et al. Frailty as a predictor of morbidity and mortality in inpatient head and neck surgery. JAMA Otolaryngol Head Neck Surg 2013;139(8):783–7.
42. Makary MA, Segev DL, Pronovost PJ, et al. Frailty as a predictor of surgical outcomes in older patients. J Am Coll Surg 2010;210(6):901–8.
43. Robinson TN, Wu DS, Pointer L, et al. Simple frailty score predicts postoperative complications across surgical specialties. Am J Surg 2013;206(4):544–50.
44. Gillis C, Li C, Lee L, et al. Prehabilitation versus rehabilitation: a randomized control trial in patients undergoing colorectal resection for cancer. Anesthesiology 2014;121(5):937–47.
45. Swank AM, Kachelman JB, Bibeau W, et al. Prehabilitation before total knee arthroplasty increases strength and function in older adults with severe osteoarthritis. J Strength Cond Res 2011;25(2):318–25.

46. Sumukadas D, Band M, Miller S, et al. Do ACE inhibitors improve the response to exercise training in functionally impaired older adults? A randomized controlled trial. J Gerontol A Biol Sci Med Sci 2014;69(6):736–43.

47. Laosa O, Alonso C, Castro M, et al. Pharmaceutical interventions for frailty and sarcopenia. Curr Pharm Des 2014;20(18):3068–82.

48. Rizzoli R, Boonen S, Brandi ML, et al. Vitamin D supplementation in elderly or postmenopausal women: a 2013 update of the 2008 recommendations from the European Society for Clinical and Economic Aspects of Osteoporosis and Osteoarthritis (ESCEO). Curr Med Res Opin 2013;29(4):305–13.

49. Stuck AE, Siu AL, Wieland GD, et al. Comprehensive geriatric assessment: a meta-analysis of controlled trials. Lancet 1993;342(8878):1032–6.

50. Partridge JSL, Harari D, Martin FC, et al. The impact of pre-operative comprehensive geriatric assessment on postoperative outcomes in older patients undergoing scheduled surgery: a systematic review. Anaesthesia 2014;69(Suppl 1):8–16.

51. Appelbaum PS. Clinical practice. Assessment of patients' competence to consent to treatment. N Engl J Med 2007;357(18):1834–40.

52. Reuben DB. Medical care for the final years of life:"when you're 83, it's not going to be 20 years." JAMA 2009;302(24):2686–94.

53. Fried TR, Bradley EH, Towle VR, et al. Understanding the treatment preferences of seriously ill patients. N Engl J Med 2002;346(14):1061–6.

54. The Conversation Project. Available at: http://theconversationproject.org/. Accessed August 14, 2015.

55. Five Wishes. Aging with Dignity: Five Wishes. Available at: https://www.agingwithdignity.org/five-wishes.php. Accessed August 14, 2015.

56. Grimaldo DA, Wiener-Kronish JP, Jurson T, et al. A randomized, controlled trial of advanced care planning discussions during preoperative evaluations. Anesthesiology 2001;95(1):43–50 [discussion: 5A].

57. Nabozny MJ, Kruser JM, Steffens NM, et al. Constructing High-Stakes Surgical Decisions. Ann Surg 2015;1–7. http://dx.doi.org/10.1097/SLA.0000000000001081.

Implantable Devices

Assessment and Perioperative Management

Ana Costa, MD*, Deborah C. Richman, MBChB, FFA(SA)

KEYWORDS

- Cardiovascular implantable electronic device (CIED)
- Automatic implantable cardioverter defibrillator • Pacemaker
- Electromagnetic interference (EMI) • Preoperative assessment
- Perioperative management • Ventricular assist devices (VAD)

KEY POINTS

Preoperative assessment of patients with implanted devices for unrelated surgeries includes

- The underlying disease and its associated comorbidities and presence of complications
- Treatment modalities and side effects
- Effect of surgery and anesthesia on the disease
- Effect of surgery and anesthesia on the implanted device
- Perioperative management plans to prevent
  - Patient injury
  - Device damage
  - Device malfunction.

INTRODUCTION

The twenty-first century has seen incredible progress in technology and this has affected the medical field as well. For years, instruments have been used for patient care; however, with advancement in knowledge, electronic device sophistication, and nanotechnology increasing numbers and types of implantable devices are being used. Much progress has been made since the first pacemaker that was partially implanted in a Bolivian priest in 1957, powered by a 9 V car battery with a total device

Disclosures: Authors have no financial disclosures.

D.C. Richman is vice president of Society for Perioperative Assessment and Quality Improvement (SPAQI).

Department of Anesthesiology, Stony Brook Medicine, 101 Nicolls Road, Stony Brook, NY 11794-8480, USA

* Corresponding author.

E-mail address: ana.costa@stonybrookmedicine.edu

weight of 80 lb. He probably did not have the cardiac reserve to carry that extra weight. Modern devices weigh a few grams and have remotely rechargeable batteries.

Patients with these devices are presenting for unrelated surgeries and their perioperative management requires understanding of these devices, the associated risks, the underlying comorbidity for which the device is implanted, and the medications the patient is taking. This article focuses on cardiac devices and neurostimulators. Other devices will be listed and briefly described.

Principles of assessment, risk, and management are similar with all devices.

CARDIOVASCULAR IMPLANTABLE ELECTRONIC DEVICES

There has been a paramount increase in the number of implantable cardiovascular devices. As the population lives longer and develops a multitude of cardiac conditions, medical science has developed a variety of devices that assist in the daily functioning and, possibly, life extension of individuals with cardiac problems. Cardiovascular implantable electronic device (CIED) is a broad term that includes permanent pacemaker (PPM), implantable cardioverter-defibrillator (ICD), cardiac resynchronization therapy device, and implantable loop recorder. In an analysis of CIED implantation in the United States between 1997 and 2004, implantation rates for PPMs and ICDs increased by 19% and 60%, respectively.[1]

The perioperative management of patients with CIEDs has changed dramatically as the types and functions of these devices have evolved in recent years. Ensuring patients' safety during surgical procedures is challenging when using CIEDs. Reviews and guidelines are required regarding the rapidly changing CIED technology, wide use of electromagnetic interference (EMI) sources, and obscure recommendations. The American College of Cardiology/American Heart Association/Heart Rhythm Society (HRS) provide guidelines and specific recommendations for CIED implantation.[2] The 2011 HRS/American Society of Anesthesiologists (ASA) Expert Consensus Statement created by the American Heart Association, the American College of Cardiology, and the Society of Thoracic Surgeons provides guidelines for the preoperative management of patients with CIEDs.[3] This article focuses on the actual preoperative assessment and management of patients with pre-existing CIEDs presenting for surgeries or any procedure requiring the care of an anesthesiologist.

The preoperative evaluation is extremely important in the assessment of a patient's past and present medical conditions, including the presence of and management plan for implantable devices. In patients presenting with CIEDs, the specific indication for implantation, type, function, and management of the device needs to be elicited directly from the patient's CIED team (electrophysiologist, cardiologist, primary care physician, and, possibly, the device manufacturer). The perioperative team, including the anesthesiologist and surgical group, need to communicate the exact nature of the procedure to the CIED team, including possible sources of EMI, fluid and electrolyte management, availability of telemetry perioperatively, and expected postoperative management. If the patient's own CIED team is unavailable, the institutional CIED team needs to be consulted to evaluate the patient, possibly interrogate the device, and provide specific recommendations. The CIED's manufacturer and an industry-employed allied professional (IEAP) may make expert suggestions about to the perioperative care. However, an IEAP may not determine the perioperative management of patients with CIEDs.[4]

Many physical and chemical factors affect the functioning of CIEDs. These include

- EMI, which is ubiquitous in the modern world and the operating room environment

- Myopotentials (shivering and fasciculations)
- Electrolyte disturbance
- Alterations in pH
- Blood transfusion
- Chemotherapy.

Possible Sources of Electromagnetic Interference and Its Consequences

Modern life is replete with potential sources of EMI, such as televisions, cell phones, computers, microwave ovens, metal detectors at airports, surgical equipment, and so forth.[5] EMI may interfere with CIEDs, causing possible rate interference, pulse generator damage, lead-issue damage, and inappropriate electrical reset mode. The exact impact of EMI depends on the type and function of the CIED, specific algorithms to minimize external interference, the patient's own rate and rhythm, and protective equipment available during the surgical procedure.

Electrosurgical energy in monopolar or bipolar configurations constitute the main source of EMI during standard surgical procedures in the United States. Electrosurgery applies radio frequency electrical current in a focused fashion to achieve coagulation, tissue cutting, or dissection. Monopolar electrocautery applies an electrical current to tissue via a small electrode device and is the most common source of EMI to CIEDs in the operating room. This interference may reprogram a PPM, cause inhibition because the CIED may perceive the monopolar signal as an intrinsic electrical stimulus from the patient, may cause unnecessary tachyarrhythmia therapy by the CIED, and may cause reset of the electrical pulse generator.[6–8] These interactions are very infrequent when appropriate precautions are taken before the start of the surgical procedure. However, various reports have identified cases in which monopolar electrocautery caused PPM failure despite standard precautions.[9] Bipolar electrocautery typically does not interfere with the function of CIEDs because the current is small and travels between the 2 poles of device.[10] However, bipolar is only helpful in coagulation, whereas monopolar can be used for tissue cutting, dissection, and coagulation. Device malfunctions, such as failure to pace and reprogramming, have become much less common with new advances in lead and generator designs, CIED algorithms, and EMI resistance in recent years. In the case of implantable loop recorders, EMI may cause the device to reset, losing all of its acquired data. Therefore, patients with implantable loop recorders scheduled for surgery should have their CIED team retrieve the recorded data before surgery.

It is imperative for the perioperative physician to understand how the intraoperative performance of CIEDs may be affected by EMI. The most common interactions are oversensing of the electrosurgery current, initiation of noise-reversion mode, and initiation of electrical reset mode; whereas damage or failure of the pulse generator, and damage to the interface between the lead and the myocardium increasing pacing thresholds are very rare unless the current is applied directly to the pulse generator or lead.[7] As long as the distance from the electrocautery path and the pulse generator and leads is greater than 6 inches, it is unlikely that interference will take place and that the pulse generator will be damaged. The location of the cautery dispersion pad on the patient should be along a path that ensures that the EMI current does not cross over the CIED generator.[11,12]

The most common interference from EMI in the operating room is oversensing, which refers to a CIED sensing that the current from electrosurgery is intrinsic cardiac activity. In the case of a PPM, oversensing may cause the inhibition of pacing. Oversensing by an ICD may result in inappropriate antitachycardic therapy (pacing or defibrillation), which in turn could trigger arrhythmic activity.[13] Because ICDs typically require several seconds of high-rate sensing to trigger antitachycardic therapy, short bursts limited to 4 to 5 seconds are typically recommended if monopolar cautery is necessary. The HRS/ASA consensus group states that the risk of oversensing and generator or lead damage is minimal for surgeries below the umbilicus; therefore, the CIED does not need to be reprogrammed and a magnet does not to be placed on the CIED.[3] However, it is necessary to have a magnet readily available throughout the perioperative period.

Magnets

Magnets evoke different responses depending on the type of device, manufacturer, and device programmer. A PPM can be programmed to have no response or to pace asynchronously when a magnet is placed over the pulse generator. The pacing rate when the magnet is placed depends on the manufacturer and the battery life of the generator. A low battery life will cause the PPM to pace at lower rates, which could be detrimental intraoperatively. The placement of a magnet on an ICD will prevent oversensing, disabling tachycardia therapy. In general, however, a magnet will not disable the pacing function of modern ICDs. In other words, a magnet will not place the ICD in asynchronous mode. Therefore, it is imperative that the CIED team be consulted, especially if a patient with an ICD depend on pacing and will undergo surgery with extensive use of EMI. In such cases, both tachycardia and bradycardia therapies can be reprogrammed by the CIED team. In patients with cardiac resynchronization therapy devices or biventricular ICDs, turning off the pacing feature may affect hemodynamic stability because ventricular pacing optimizes stroke volume.[14]

Cardiovascular Implantable Electronic Device Failure

CIED failure can result from damage to the generator, failure of the device to sense, or failure to pace. Modern pacemakers have minute ventilation sensors that allow for an increased pacing rate in response to exercise. If this feature is not disabled, it may be deemed as a PPM failure perioperatively because EMI can alter body impedance, leading the PPM to pace at a faster rate.[15,16] If EMI directly contacts the CIED, it can cause an electrical reset. This scenario is more common during radiation therapy.[17,18] The electrical reset will default the CIED to a specific setting depending on the device and its manufacturer. The device will need to be interrogated and, possibly, reprogrammed after the procedure.

MRI

It is generally accepted that MRI can interfere with pacing and cause total inhibition of output in CIEDs. Therefore, the presence of a CIED has been an absolute contraindication to obtaining MRI for many years. However, recent studies have suggested that MRI could be performed in patients with PPMs if certain criteria are met, such as MRI at 0.5 T, thorax placed outside of the magnet bore, PPM set to asynchronous mode, limited radio frequency exposure, and appropriate monitors in place.[19,20]

Other Factors That Affect Cardiovascular Implantable Electronic Device Function

Muscle movement that is interpreted as cardiac contraction should be avoided. For pacemakers, application of a magnet will change the PPM to asynchronous pacing and will avoid this complication. Automatic implantable cardioverter defibrillators will need to be deactivated to prevent unnecessary shock delivery (**Table 1**).

Chemical changes affecting capture threshold cannot be avoided; however, lack of mechanical capture will be seen on plethysmographic monitoring. Pacemaker

Table 1
Factors affecting implantable cardiovascular device function

Factor	Effect	Reason
Shivering	Inhibits pacing	Sensed as cardiac contraction
Fasciculations (succinylcholine)	Inhibits pacing	Sensed as cardiac contraction
Electrolyte changes	Affects capture	Alters myopotential threshold
Temperature	Affects capture Hypothermia	Alters myopotential threshold Increases arrhythmogenicity of myocardium
pH	Affects capture	Alters myopotential threshold
Blood transfusions	Alters pH, temperature, or electrolytes	Alters myopotential threshold
Chemotherapy[21]	Loss of capture	Elevation of capture threshold

amplitude may need to be increased. Patients on chemotherapy need to have their device interrogated and, if needed, reprogrammed before surgery.

Preoperative Assessment

Open communication between the surgical and CIED teams is paramount.

Information needed from the surgical team includes
- The specific surgical procedure and its anatomic location
- Possible use of monopolar electrosurgery and its anatomic location
- Other sources of EMI
- Patient positioning
- Anesthetic plan
- Anticipated large blood loss and/or fluid shifts
- Surgical venue (operating room with readily available medical support personnel and equipment, procedure suite)
- Postoperative care (home, inpatient admission, telemetry)
- Possible complications.

Information needed from the CIED team includes
- Plan for the management of the CIED perioperatively
- The type and function of the CIED
- Manufacturer and model
- The indication for its implantation
- Information about the device's last interrogation (within the past 12 months for PPMs, and the past 6 months for ICDs[3])
- Battery life
- CIED program details (pacing mode, programmed lower rate, ICD therapy, lowest rate for shock delivery)
- Patient dependency on pacer
- Underlying rhythm
- Pacing threshold
- Response of the device to the placement of a magnet
- Device reverting to its original program settings on removal of the magnet.

Intraoperative Management

Intraoperative management considerations include

- Whether monopolar electrosurgery or radio-frequency ablation will be used above the umbilicus, plan to inactivate the tachycardia feature of an ICD and turn the PPM to asynchronous mode by either reprogramming the device or placing a magnet over it (CIED team to provide recommendations on the most reliable method)
- For procedures that will not use monopolar electrosurgery or radio-frequency ablation above the umbilicus, it is not necessary to inactivate the ICD tachycardia feature or place a PPM into asynchronous mode
- Use of electrocardiogram (ECG) monitor throughout preoperative care and ECG monitor gain must be set to recognize pacing spikes
- Availability of external defibrillator is required for all patients with PPMs or ICDs in all areas of perioperative care
- Defibrillating pads must be placed on high-risk patients and on patients whose intraoperative positioning would prevent the placement of the pads quickly in case of an emergency
- Have a magnet readily available for all patients with a CIED
- All patients with PPMs or ICDs require plethysmographic or arterial pressure monitoring to confirm that electrical capture is converted to mechanical systole
- Exercise caution with the placement of upper body central lines to avoid false detections and lead damage.

An observational study published in Oct 2015, discussed the development of leadless nanopacemakers placed percutaneously into the right ventricle with the hope of reducing the rate of lead dislodgement and pocket infection. Comparison with conventional PPMs is pending but these devices are promising. Until further information is available, the preoperative recommendations and intraoperative precautions for patients with pacemakers presenting for surgery apply to these leadless pacemakers.[22]

VENTRICULAR ASSIST DEVICES

The most recent report by the Interagency Registry for Mechanical Assist Circulatory Support (INTERMACS) on ventricular assist devices (VADs) reported that more than 6500 adult patients received primary implants of left VADs (LVADs) between 2006 and 2012.[23] The incidence of heart failure has drastically increased as the elderly population in the United States continues to grow. For patients with end-stage heart failure, a VAD became an essential device used as a bridge to heart transplantation (BTT); bridge to candidacy (BTC); destination therapy (DT); or, in a very small minority, as bridges to recovery or rescue therapy. Although most VADs are inserted as BTT or BTC, VADs for DT have become quite common. According to INTERMACS, more than 40% of LVADs implanted in 2012 were DT. As the technology and management of VADs improve, the longevity of patients with VADs improves, leading to a larger population of patients with VADs presenting for noncardiac surgery.[24] Therefore, it is imperative that the surgical team become acquainted with the challenges present in the perioperative management of patients with VADs presenting for noncardiac surgery.

The perioperative assessment and management of a patient with a VAD should include a surgical team that is accustomed to managing patients with VADs for noncardiac surgery, including perfusionists and VAD technicians. Elements of the preoperative assessment must incorporate a thorough history and physical examination, medications, coagulation status, functional status, myocardial function of the right ventricle in patients with LVADs, electrical power needs, battery life, and appropriate electrical power supply in the perioperative area.

The perioperative management must consider anticoagulation, antibiotic prophylaxis, anesthetic technique, appropriate modifications for the specific procedure, and adequate monitoring. Monitoring is challenging in patients with nonpulsatile flow, making pulse oximetry and noninvasive blood pressure monitoring by oscillometry very difficult, if not impossible. Therefore, the placement of an arterial line is necessary for most procedures. Cerebral oximetry can provide information about frontal cortex oxygenation in patients with continuous flow (CF) devices.

All of the INTERMACS patients classified as DT since 2010 received CF devices. Patients with CF devices have better survival rates and fewer complications in DT patients than pulsatile devices.[25,26] Decreasing the continuous flow rate of CF devices intermittently, may allow for pulse oximetry and noninvasive blood pressure monitoring.

Indications for placement of central venous and pulmonary artery catheters remain the same as for non-VAD patients. Modern LVADs, such as the HeartMate II (Thoratec Corporation, Pleasanton, CA, USA), provide an estimate of cardiac output. Transesophageal echocardiography remains a crucial tool in the assessment of preload, VAD function, and right ventricular function.[27]

Specific Hemodynamic Considerations

In patients with LVADs, specific hemodynamic considerations include

- Preload dependency: LVADs depend on preload because they cannot adjust the cardiac output as a normal heart per Frank-Starling principles.
- Right ventricular dysfunction: Many patients with LVADs may have right ventricular dysfunction. LVADs decompress the left ventricle, leading to a leftward shift of the intraventricular septum, causing increased right ventricular compliance and decreased contractility.[28,29] Careful consideration should be given to maintain adequate preload, avoid overfilling, and avoid increases in pulmonary vascular resistance, which could place greater strain on the right ventricle. Patients with VADs have successfully undergone laparoscopic procedures but careful monitoring of end-tidal CO_2 throughout the perioperative period is recommended to avoid increases in pulmonary vascular resistance from hypercapnia.
- Afterload: This needs to be maintained within normal parameters established preoperatively because increased afterload may lead to decreased output in CF LVADs.
- Anticoagulation: Most patients with VADs need to be anticoagulated, often with warfarin. Patients with the Heartmate may be off anticoagulation for a certain amount of time.[30]
- EMI does not seem to affect the function of modern VADs. However, the preoperative assessment should include an analysis of all sources and location of EMI and communication with the manufacturer.[25]

NEUROSTIMULATORS

Have pulse generator, will stimulate. This may sound like a flippant comment but the proliferation of neurostimulators and ever-increasing on-label and off-label uses for them, has the twenty-first century anesthesiologist caring for patients with these devices on a regular basis. This section is not an exhaustive review of the devices and the diseases they are used for, rather it is an introduction to the principles of perioperative management and a list of examples of these devices (**Table 2**) and their implications for safe patient care.

Table 2
Types of neurostimulators

Device	Indications
Deep brain stimulator	Parkinson's disease Essential tremor Depression Obsessive compulsive disorder
Spinal cord stimulator	Chronic pain
Carotid baroreceptor activation therapy	Hypertension resistant to medication
Vagal nerve stimulator	Intractable seizures
Cochlear implants (cochlear branch of acoustic nerve stimulation)	Sensorineural hearing loss
Bladder stimulator	Neurogenic bladder symptoms
Hypoglossal nerve stimulator	Obstructive sleep apnea
Occipital nerve stimulator	Headache or migraine
Gastric pacemaker	Gastroparesis
Phrenic nerve stimulator	Diaphragmatic weakness Directly into muscle in amyotrophic lateral sclerosis

Risks specific to these devices (**Table 3**) are patient injury due to burns from inadvertent EMI resulting in abnormal current flow along the electrode; when these electrodes are in the central nervous system (CNS) this can be devastating. The neurostimulator can be damaged and require replacement, which causes pain and suffering and is very costly. The device may malfunction, causing recurrence of patient symptoms. Although this usually leads to patient discomfort, it can also be dangerous (eg, loss of seizure control). Other lesser effects are interference with bedside tests (eg, ECG artifact) and inability to do certain diagnostic procedures (MRI incompatibility in all older devices but newer ones may be MRI safe, and CT scan metal artifact). Device and therapy interactions are another concern and postprocedure interrogation

Table 3
Risks associated with implanted neurostimulators

Effect by Decreasing Severity		Outcomes
Injury to patient	Morbidity and mortality	Burns, infections
Damage to device	Cost	Pain and inconvenience
Malfunction of device	Patient discomfort	None, understimulation, or overstimulation
Interference with monitoring		Missed diagnosis
Certain procedures or tests contraindicated (ESWL/AICD/MRI/radiofrequency ablation)	Absolute Relative	Care plan modification

of any neurostimulator (or CIED) should be performed after radiofrequency ablation, defibrillation, electroconvulsive therapy, extracorporeal shock wave lithotripsy, or implantation of a second device with a pulse generator.

Deep Brain Stimulators

A deep brain stimulator (DBS) is used for bilateral stimulation of the internal globus pallidus or subthalamic nucleus by surgically implanted electrodes connected to a pulse generator by an extension lead. The pulse generator is usually in the upper chest. Stimulating these areas leads to reversal of the troubling symptoms of Parkinsonism: tremor and rigidity. Patients have a remote to turn off the device at night, which prolongs battery life. Those with rigidity, however, may leave the DBS activated at all times. The DBS replaces the irreversible pallidotomy procedure of the 1950s. The indication is primarily Parkinson's disease (PD); however, newer indications for DBS placement are chronic pain, obsessive compulsive disorder, dystonia, and depression.[31–33]

The PD patients enjoy great relief of symptoms and need less medication but still have the same perioperative risks of other PD patients, including bulbar dysfunction and aspiration risk, slower overall recovery, medication side effects and interactions (monoamine oxidase inhibitors and anesthesia), in addition to the risks that their neurostimulators confer. PD symptoms can often worsen postoperatively due to altered oral intake and poor absorption. Intravenous alternatives to PD medication are not available, so normal oral intake and gut function are crucial to recovery in these patients.

Literature review reveals a small but growing number of case reports of surgery and anesthesia in these patients. Some cases proceeded without the physicians being aware of the nature of the device until after the procedure. Most patients did not experience complications associated with their device; however, in a couple of instances, even though the device was identified, there were reported bad outcomes with neurologic injury.[34,35]

Using what little literature that there is available on the management of patients with DBS for subsequent surgeries, the authors developed a clinical pathway to guide management[33,36] (**Fig. 1**). This pathway can be modified for and applied to any other neurostimulator patient.

Spinal Cord Stimulators

The subcutaneous neurostimulator is usually placed in the lower abdomen or gluteal region with the electrode in the epidural space anywhere from the cervical to sacral area. Spinal cord stimulators are used for

- Chronic pain
  - Reflex sympathetic dystrophy
  - Ischemia
  - Degenerative spine disease
- Spasticity
- Arachnoiditis
- Neuropathy

Spinal cord stimulation blocks transmission of pain signals by the gate theory. The patient has a remote control and modern devices allow for remote charging and also modulation of stimulus depending on symptoms. Some patients have positional pain and, when the patient is not in the position that causes the pain, the stimulation can be turned down or off. The newest devices have automatic adaptive response to position change.[36] Patients with spinal cord stimulators are assessed for the underlying comorbidity and are often on multimodal analgesia with increased tolerance to opioid

Preoperative considerations

Contact treating neurologist	• Get latest clinical information • Recommendations for perioperative levodopa or carbidopa dosage • Postoperative follow-up
Ask patient	Indication for DBS A. PD • Tremor or rigidity • Result when DBS turned off B. Other: eg, essential tremor, OCD Generator location (or chest radiograph) Device card: copy for chart Identify battery type
Chest radiograph (as needed)	Identify generator location
Contact DBS team (anesthesia and neurology)	Maintain consistency in clinical care Name:_____Pager:_____ Name:_____Pager:_____
Copy this pathway to surgeon	• Coordinate patient, neurology assessment, and representative arrival time • Alert surgeon about intraoperative considerations
Contact device manufacturer	Have representative available to disable device (if needed) for the operating room Company:_____ Phone number: 1-800-_____
Scheduling	Allow time on day of surgery for • Neurology assessment • Device representative arrival (usually not 1st case) Notify operating room booking of presence of device Telephone number:_____ Notify presurgical admissions (to check final arrangements evening before) Telephone number:_____ Notify anesthesia division chief
Have patient bring remote	Can temporarily disable device during hospital stay (eg, ECG)

Intraoperative considerations

Use of bipolar electrocautery only	Minimize potential for device damage and CNS injury
	• Device must be disabled with patient's remote
	• Representative must set output voltage to 0
	  ○ This applies to Soletra (Medtronic, Inc. Minneapolis, MN, USA) and Kinetra batteries (Medtronic, Inc. Minneapolis, MN, USA)
	  ○ The newer Activa battery (Medtronic, Inc. Minneapolis, MN, USA) does not need this step

Prophylactic antibiotics	Minimize infection for CNS-implanted device
General anesthesia	Rigidity or hypoventilation may ensue when device is disabled
Appropriate antiemetic	Avoid droperidol and metoclopramide in PD patients

Post-Operative considerations:

Reactivation of device	Must have baseline frequency and amplitude settings restored
Close neurology follow-up	Dosages of medications may need to be adjusted • Erratic absorption postoperatively
Hypoventilation	Rigidity is usually rapidly reversed after device reactivation
Recovery	PD patients have longer recovery time after illness and surgery • Ambulatory surgery patients may need admission

Anesthesia 'team' members/ ph. #s:_____   Neurology 'team' members/ ph. #s:_____

Fig. 1. Clinical pathway for management of patients with deep brain stimulators presenting for surgery and anesthesia (developed and applied at Stony Brook Medicine, NY).

medications. The acute pain service should be closely involved postoperatively. Anxiety and depression are frequently associated with chronic pain. Chronic pain syndromes can be a result of chronic progressive neurologic diseases, such as multiple sclerosis. Muscle weakness, specifically respiratory and bulbar dysfunction, should be assessed for.

Neuraxial anesthesia and analgesia are relatively contraindicated due to risk of lead damage.

Vagal Nerve Stimulators

Intractable seizures nonresponsive to antiepileptic medications have been successfully treated or, at least, seizure frequency has been reduced by direct stimulation of the vagal nerve in the neck. The risk of injury, device damage, or dysfunction due to EMI is present as with all stimulators, and the recommendation is to turn the stimulator off intraoperatively.[37] Fortunately seizure control during this time is not a problem due to the effects of anesthetic agents. However, postoperatively, the device needs to be reactivated as soon as possible. There is still an increased risk of seizures after surgery because medications may not be taken regularly due to contraction NPO status and/or nausea and absorption can be erratic, even when medications are taken on schedule. Seizure threshold may also be lowered postoperatively, due to stress response to surgery.

Phrenic Nerve and Diaphragmatic Stimulators

Originally used to treat phrenic nerve lesions causing respiratory distress symptoms after coronary artery bypass graft–related thermal injury or other phrenic nerve trauma or cervical spine injury, this modality was not very successful and is now rarely used for this indication. More recently, diaphragmatic stimulators have been implanted into amyotrophic lateral sclerosis (ALS) patients. The stimulation here is directly to the muscle of the diaphragm, instead of the phrenic nerve in the thorax. To be eligible for diaphragmatic pacing, patients need to have evidence of a stimulatable diaphragm on neurophysiologic testing or fluoroscopy and chronic hypoventilation as evidenced by one of the following: (1) forced vital capacity less than 50% predicted, (2) maximum inspiratory pressure less than 60 cm H_2O, (3) P_{CO_2} greater than or equal to 45 mm Hg, or (4) arterial oxygen saturation less than 88% for 5 consecutive minutes while asleep. There is an adjustment period during which the patient uses the stimulator for increasing lengths of time each day. Initial results showed good outcomes of prolonged survival (16 months), delay to onset of noninvasive ventilation (9 months), and better sleep quality.[38,39] These are, however, high-risk patients who undergo general anesthesia for the diaphragmatic pacing insertion and their advance directive status needs to be discussed preoperatively because failure to wean after the procedure is a real risk. A recent review questions the need for further study because all study groups are small and have methodology flaws. In addition, ALS is rapidly progressive so it is hard to comment on long-term outcomes.[38] The study on diaphragm pacing in patients with respiratory insufficiency due to amyotrophic lateral sclerosis (DiPALS), the first randomized controlled trial in this population, was published in September, 2015. It concluded that, in this group of 74 ALS subjects, survival was shorter and more adverse events occurred in the group that had diaphragmatic pacers implanted. Diaphragmatic pacing is not recommended routinely in ALS patients, but may still be appropriate for a select group.[40]

Hypoglossal Nerve Stimulators

Hypoglossal nerve stimulators are a relatively new treatment modality used for increasing tone in the genioglossus muscle, causing the tongue to move anteriorly, and decreasing the obstruction in obstructive sleep apnea.[41] Although it works well, it is uncomfortable and not well tolerated.

These patients need to be assessed for severity of their obstructive sleep apnea. Associated comorbidities include obesity, difficult intubation, obesity hypoventilation syndrome, and so forth. Anesthesia management should include opiate-sparing techniques and appropriate postoperative monitoring.

OTHER IMPLANTABLE DEVICES

There are many other implantable devices, including intrathecal, intraperitoneal, intra-hepatic, intra-arterial, and intravenous medication pumps for

- Pain
- Spasticity
- Chemotherapy
- Insulin
- Anticoagulation.

In 1898, Augustus Bier performed the first spinal anesthesia on himself and his assistant using cocaine. In the early 1900s, investigators in Japan and the United States mixed morphine with the cocaine. It was not until 1973 that opiate receptors were first described in the CNS in an article in *Science* and 1976 when it was recognized that narcotics can act directly the spinal level.[42-44] Direct delivery of opiates into the cerebrospinal fluid provides effective analgesia at much lower doses than are needed by other routes and, consequently, with fewer side effects. The first intrathecal therapy for cancer pain[45] and the first continuous spinal analgesia for labor were used in 1979. The first implantable pain pump was described in 1981.[46] Technological advances in microelectromechanical systems and nanotechnology[47] have allowed implantable pumps to become a common and practical treatment modality for chronic pain. Subsequently, other drugs have been used for a variety of treatments at different sites, including targeted chemotherapy.[48,49]

Principles in preoperative assessment of these patients are

a. Evaluation of the underlying disease and its complications
b. Assessment of the medication infused and it is side effects and drug interactions
c. Pump malfunction due to perioperative EMI; risk of underdosing (withdrawal) or overdosing (increased side effects)
d. Draining drug and maintaining line patency by flushing with heparinized saline when the drug has to be stopped perioperatively.

SUMMARY

The recent advances in CIEDs and neurostimulator design and function have greatly improved survival and the quality of life of millions of people around the world. A surgical team familiar with the intricacies of the perioperative assessment and management with patients with these implanted devices is imperative. Open communication between the surgical team and CIED team or neurostimulator consultant is an essential element in the preoperative assessment of these patients. The intraoperative management of these patients relies on a comprehensive understanding of EMI sources and their consequences to the devices, techniques to optimize hemodynamics, safety mechanisms to prevent device malfunction, and availability of well-trained personnel.

The preoperative assessment of patients with implanted devices for unrelated surgeries includes the gathering of information about the underlying disease and its associated comorbidities and presence of complications, knowledge of treatment modalities and side effects of these medications or interventions, and understanding the effect of surgery and anesthesia on the disease as well as the effect of surgery and anesthesia on the implanted device. Thorough evaluation and planning of the perioperative management is needed to prevent poor outcomes, specifically patient injury, device damage, and device malfunction. This field is evolving continuously with technology updates and medical society guidelines. Device manufacturer recommendations are handy references for safe management of these patients.

REFERENCES

1. Zhan C, Baine WB, Sedrakyan A, et al. Cardiac device implantation in the United States from 1997 through 2004: a population-based analysis. J Gen Intern Med 2008;23(Suppl 1):13–9.
2. Epstein AE, DiMarco JP, Ellenbogen KA, et al. ACC/AHA/HRS 2008 Guidelines for Device-Based Therapy of Cardiac Rhythm Abnormalities: a report of the American College of Cardiology/American Heart Association Task Force on Practice Guidelines (Writing Committee to Revise the ACC/AHA/NASPE 2002 Guideline Update for Implantation of Cardiac Pacemakers and Antiarrhythmia Devices) developed in collaboration with the American Association for Thoracic Surgery and Society of Thoracic Surgeons. Circulation 2008;117(21): e350–408.
3. Crossley GH, Poole JE, Rozner MA, et al. The Heart Rhythm Society (HRS)/American Society of Anesthesiologists (ASA) Expert Consensus Statement on the perioperative management of patients with implantable defibrillators, pacemakers and arrhythmia monitors: facilities and patient management this document was developed as a joint project with the American Society of Anesthesiologists (ASA), and in collaboration with the American Heart Association (AHA), and the Society of Thoracic Surgeons (STS). Heart Rhythm 2011;8(7): 1114–54.
4. Lindsay BD, Estes NA 3rd, Maloney JD, et al, Heart Rhythm Society. Heart rhythm society policy statement update: recommendations on the role of industry employed allied professionals (IEAPs). Heart Rhythm 2008;5(11):e8–10.
5. Niehaus M, Tebbenjohanns J. Electromagnetic interference in patients with implanted pacemakers or cardioverter-defibrillators. Heart 2001;86(3):246–8.
6. Belott PH, Sands S, Warren J. Resetting of DDD pacemakers due to EMI. Pacing Clin Electrophysiol 1984;7(2):169–72.
7. Levine PA, Balady GJ, Lazar HL, et al. Electrocautery and pacemakers: management of the paced patient subject to electrocautery. Ann Thorac Surg 1986;41(3): 313–7.
8. Atlee J. Arrhythmias and pacemakers, practical management for anesthesia and Critical care medicine. 1st edition. Philadelphia: WB Saunders; 1996.
9. Mangar D, Atlas GM, Kane PB. Electrocautery-induced pacemaker malfunction during surgery. Can J Anaesth 1991;38(5):616–8.
10. Lee D, Sharp VJ, Konety BR. Use of bipolar power source for transurethral resection of bladder tumor in patient with implanted pacemaker. Urology 2005;66(1):194.
11. Chauvin M, Crenner F, Brechenmacher C. Interaction between permanent cardiac pacing and electrocautery: the significance of electrode position. Pacing Clin Electrophysiol 1992;15(11 Pt 2):2028–33.
12. Robinson TN, Varosy PD, Guillaume G, et al. Effect of radiofrequency energy emitted from monopolar "Bovie" instruments on cardiac implantable electronic devices. J Am Coll Surg 2014;219(3):399–406.
13. Casavant D, Haffajee C, Stevens S, et al. Aborted implantable cardioverter defibrillator shock during facial electrosurgery. Pacing Clin Electrophysiol 1998; 21(6):1325–6.
14. Ho JK, Mahajan A. Cardiac resynchronization therapy for treatment of heart failure. Anesth Analg 2010;111(6):1353–61.

15. Van Hemel NM, Hamerlijnck RP, Pronk KJ, et al. Upper limit ventricular stimulation in respiratory rate responsive pacing due to electrocautery. Pacing Clin Electrophysiol 1989;12(11):1720–3.

16. Wong DT, Middleton W. Electrocautery-induced tachycardia in a rate-responsive pacemaker. Anesthesiology 2001;94(4):710–1.

17. Katzenberg CA, Marcus FI, Heusinkveld RS, et al. Pacemaker failure due to radiation therapy. Pacing Clin Electrophysiol 1982;5(2):156–9.

18. Rozner M. Pacemaker misinformation in the perioperative period: programming around the problem. Anesth Analg 2004;99(6):1582–4.

19. Lauck G, von Smekal A, Wolke S, et al. Effects of nuclear magnetic resonance imaging on cardiac pacemakers. Pacing Clin Electrophysiol 1995;18(8):1549–55.

20. Sommer T, Vahlhaus C, Lauck G, et al. MR imaging and cardiac pacemakers: in-vitro evaluation and in-vivo studies in 51 patients at 0.5 T. Radiology 2000;215(3):869–79.

21. Web site SJ. Chemotherapy 2010. Available at: professional.sjm.com/emi/med-dental/. Accessed July 13, 2015.

22. Reddy VY, Exner DV, Cantillon DJ, et al. Percutaneous implantation of an entirely intracardiac leadless pacemaker. N Engl J Med 2015;373(12):1125–35.

23. Kirklin JK, Naftel DC, Kormos RL, et al. Fifth INTERMACS annual report: risk factor analysis from more than 6,000 mechanical circulatory support patients. J Heart Lung Transplant 2013;32(2):141–56.

24. Barbara DW, Wetzel DR, Pulido JN, et al. The perioperative management of patients with left ventricular assist devices undergoing noncardiac surgery. Mayo Clin Proc 2013;88(7):674–82.

25. Hessel EA 2nd. Management of patients with implanted ventricular assist devices for noncardiac surgery: a clinical review. Semin Cardiothorac Vasc Anesth 2014;18(1):57–70.

26. Slininger KA, Haddadin AS, Mangi AA. Perioperative management of patients with left ventricular assist devices undergoing noncardiac surgery. J Cardiothorac Vasc Anesth 2013;27(4):752–9.

27. Thunberg CA, Gaitan BD, Arabia FA, et al. Ventricular assist devices today and tomorrow. J Cardiothorac Vasc Anesth 2010;24(4):656–80.

28. Stone ME, Soong W, Krol M, et al. The anesthetic considerations in patients with ventricular assist devices presenting for noncardiac surgery: a review of eight cases. Anesth Analg 2002;95(1):42–9.

29. Santamore WP, Gray LA Jr. Left ventricular contributions to right ventricular systolic function during LVAD support. Ann Thorac Surg 1996;61(1):350–6.

30. Bhat G, Kumar S, Aggarwal A, et al. Experience with noncardiac surgery in destination therapy left ventricular assist devices patients. ASAIO J 2012;58(4):396–401.

31. Okun MS. Deep-brain stimulation for Parkinson's disease. N Engl J Med 2012;367(16):1529–38.

32. Davies RG. Deep brain stimulators and anaesthesia. Br J Anaesth 2005;95(3):424.

33. Poon CC, Irwin MG. Anaesthesia for deep brain stimulation and in patients with implanted neurostimulator devices. Br J Anaesth 2009;103(2):152–65.

34. Roark C, Whicher S, Abosch A. Reversible neurological symptoms caused by diathermy in a patient with deep brain stimulators: case report. Neurosurgery 2008;62(1):E256 [discussion: E256].

35. Nutt JG, Anderson VC, Peacock JH, et al. DBS and diathermy interaction induces severe CNS damage. Neurology 2001;56(10):1384–6.
36. Medtronic neurostimulator website. Available at: https://professional.medtronic.com/index.htm. Accessed August 8, 2015.
37. VNS website. Available at: http://us.cyberonics.com/en/vns-therapy-for-epilepsy/healthcare-professionals. Accessed August 8, 2015.
38. ALS-FDA page. Available at: http://www.accessdata.fda.gov/cdrh_docs/pdf10/H100006b.pdf. Accessed August 9, 2015.
39. Scherer K, Bedlack RS. Diaphragm pacing in amyotrophic lateral sclerosis: a literature review. Muscle Nerve 2012;46(1):1–8.
40. DiPALS Writing Committee, DiPALS Study Group Collaborators. Safety and efficacy of diaphragm pacing in patients with respiratory insufficiency due to amyotrophic lateral sclerosis (DiPALS): a multicentre, open-label, randomised controlled trial. Lancet Neurol 2015;14(9):883–92.
41. Strollo PJ Jr, Soose RJ, Maurer JT, et al. Upper-airway stimulation for obstructive sleep apnea. N Engl J Med 2014;370(2):139–49.
42. Bier A. Versuche über Cocainisirung des Rückenmarkes. Deutsche Zeitschrift für Chirurgie 1899;51(3):361–9.
43. Pert CB, Snyder SH. Opiate receptor: demonstration in nervous tissue. Science 1973;179(4077):1011–4.
44. Yaksh TL, Rudy TA. Analgesia mediated by a direct spinal action of narcotics. Science 1976;192(4246):1357–8.
45. Wang JK, Nauss LA, Thomas JE. Pain relief by intrathecally applied morphine in man. Anesthesiology 1979;50(2):149–51.
46. Onofrio BM, Yaksh TL, Arnold PG. Continuous low-dose intrathecal morphine administration in the treatment of chronic pain of malignant origin. Mayo Clin Proc 1981;56(8):516–20.
47. Meng E, Hoang T. MEMS-enabled implantable drug infusion pumps for laboratory animal research, preclinical, and clinical applications. Adv Drug Deliv Rev 2012;64(14):1628–38.
48. Stearns L, Boortz-Marx R, Du Pen S, et al. Intrathecal drug delivery for the management of cancer pain: a multidisciplinary consensus of best clinical practices. J Support Oncol 2005;3(6):399–408.
49. Deer TR, Smith HS, Burton AW, et al. Comprehensive consensus based guidelines on intrathecal drug delivery systems in the treatment of pain caused by cancer pain. Pain physician 2011;14(3):E283–312.

Preoperative Evaluation of the Patient with Substance Use Disorder and Perioperative Considerations

CrossMark

Debra Domino Pulley, MD

KEYWORDS

- Substance use disorder • Preoperative evaluation • Alcoholism
- Preoperative drug testing • Cocaine • Chronic opioid use • Addiction

KEY POINTS

- Preoperative evaluation should include routine questions about substance abuse (alcohol and nonmedical uses of prescription and illicit drugs).
- In patients with known or suspected substance abuse, an assessment of associated illnesses and end-organ damage from chronic use needs to be performed.
- Substances that are most commonly abused in the United States are alcohol, marijuana, and nonmedical use of prescription pain relievers.
- Order a preoperative urine drug screen only if the result will change clinical management.
- Postoperative pain management may be difficult in the substance use disorder patient (especially with patients on opioids).

SUBSTANCE USE DISORDER PATIENT

Incidence

Health care professionals encounter many patients with a history of current and/or former substance abuse. Each year the Substance Abuse and Mental Health Services Administration conducts a survey of substance use, abuse, and dependence among Americans 12 years and older titled the National Survey on Drug Use and Health. In 2014, a total of 21.5 million persons in the United States aged 12 or older (8.1%) were classified with substance dependence or abuse in the past year and 10.2% of the US population had used an illicit drug in the past month.[1]

Because of new substance availability and change in socioeconomic factors, substance use trends can change rapidly. The National Institute on Drug Abuse launched the National Drug Early Warning System in August 2014.[2] It reports on emerging

Disclosures: The author has nothing to disclose.
Department of Anesthesiology, Washington University School of Medicine in St. Louis, 660 South Euclid Avenue, Campus Box 8054, St Louis, MO 63110, USA
E-mail address: pulleyd@wustl.edu

Anesthesiology Clin 34 (2016) 201–211
http://dx.doi.org/10.1016/j.anclin.2015.10.015   anesthesiology.theclinics.com
1932-2275/16/$ – see front matter © 2016 Elsevier Inc. All rights reserved.

trends and patterns of drug use as problems arise. In addition, local or regional conditions can also cause variability in the substances used.

Impact and Associated Illnesses

Substance abuse is not just a problem in the United States, but occurs worldwide and places significant disease burden on society.[3] Chronic substance abuse can lead to other major health problems.[4] The particular health issue depends on the substance used. To complicate matters, often there are several substances being used. Intravenous drug abusers may develop infectious complications, such as endocarditis, abscesses, osteomyelitis, hepatitis, and human immunodeficiency virus infection.[5]

There is evidence of an association between specific drug use disorders and mood and anxiety disorders.[6] It is not clear what the exact mechanism is, but it has been proposed that drugs of abuse cause symptoms that mimic other mental illnesses, other mental illnesses can lead to drug abuse, or drug abuse/other mental illnesses share etiologies and risk factors (eg, brain deficits, genetic vulnerabilities, or exposure to stress/trauma).[7]

Perioperative Considerations

A thorough preoperative evaluation is essential. Unfortunately many of the substance abuse patients presenting for an operation may not be medically optimized. Many of these patients may not have access to primary care, and even if they do, they may not be compliant with their prescribed medications.[8,9] Interactions are challenging with mutual mistrust, compounded by a lack of understanding and compassion from health care professionals. In addition, many of these patients have not had treatment of their addiction. In 2013, 8.6% needed treatment for a problem related to drugs or alcohol but only 0.9% received treatment at a specialty facility.[10]

When developing an anesthetic plan, considerations need to incorporate the following potential consequences:

- Acute substance use may cause toxicity and these effects need to be recognized so that they are potentially mitigated. In general, acute use decreases the analgesic and anesthetic requirements.[11]
- Chronic substance use may cause tolerance to commonly used perioperative medications so adjustments to dosing may need to be made. In general, chronic use increases the analgesic and anesthetic requirements.
- Chronic substance use may cause pathophysiology and consequences of major organ damage need to be considered.
- Pain control may be especially difficult to manage.
- Be aware of withdrawal symptoms in hospitalized patients.[11]
- Substance abuse patients may not be appropriate candidates for office-based procedures.[12]

Postoperatively as preoperatively, there are similar concerns that may hinder recovery, such as medication noncompliance and drug-seeking behavior. Substance abuse patients (especially with illicit drugs) may be less likely to come to follow-up visits.[13] In-hospital integrative programs should be considered, because there has been some reported success in increasing treatment of substance abuse and increasing frequency of outpatient care.[14]

Screening for Substance Abuse

A routine preoperative history and physical examination should include assessment of substance abuse. Patients should be asked about use of alcohol and illicit drugs. A few clues as to possible substance abuse include refusing to grant permission to obtain old records, reluctance to undergo a urine drug screening test (UDS), multiple allergies to recommended medications, and requesting a specific drug.[15]

Many debate the pros and cons of testing patients preoperatively using the quick standard immunoassay UDS. The American Society of Anesthesiology Task Force on Preanesthesia Evaluation most recent practice advisory does not comment on UDS.[16] There is one study that surveyed chiefs of anesthesia departments in the Veterans Affairs health care system specifically addressing cocaine-abusing patients.[17] Very few had a formal policy (only 11%). Testing was done based on different criteria, such as history by patient or chart (34%), history by patient or chart plus clinical suspicion of toxicity (42%), and clinical suspicion alone (13%); 11% were never screened. If results were positive, two-thirds of the respondents cancel surgery, whereas one-third consider clinical signs of toxicity. Referring back to the American Society of Anesthesiology Task Force practice advisory, this advice is the best: "Preoperative tests may be ordered, required, or performed on a selective basis for purposes of guiding or optimizing perioperative management." Indication for ordering a UDS should be documented and plans of what to do if the results come back as positive should be thought of before ordering.

When a UDS is ordered it is important to understand the limitations of the test to properly interpret the results, such as false-positives, and the ability of the assay to detect all opioids (many do not detect methadone or fentanyl).[15] Also, a negative UDS does not mean a patient could not present acutely intoxicated to the operating room. Even while in a hospital waiting for surgery, motivated patients have taken substances when given the opportunity (eg, leaving the floor, going to the restroom) and complications can occur intraoperatively.

SPECIFIC ABUSED SUBSTANCES

In each section that follows, the incidence, effects, and perioperative concerns are discussed for several abused substances that are currently seen clinically.

Alcohol

Incidence
In 2014, the rate of alcohol use disorder in the United States was 17.0 million (6.4%).[1] Alcohol is one of the most commonly abused substances in the United States.

Effects of acute and chronic use
Alcohol is a central nervous system depressant and produces sedation and sleep, but at low concentrations it may produce "stimulation" because of suppression of inhibition.[18] In nonalcoholics, blood alcohol levels of 25 mg/dL can cause impaired cognition and coordination. At concentrations greater than 100 mg/dL, vestibular and cerebellar dysfunction occur. As blood levels increase sedation increases and coma, respiratory depression, and death can occur. In addition, severe hypoglycemia may occur with lack of food. Blood alcohol levels higher than 500 mg/dL are usually fatal.[11] Alcohol can also impair memory and cause "blackouts." There is variability in a person's tolerance or sensitivity to ingestion of alcohol. With chronic use, tolerance and physical dependency occurs. Cross-tolerance can develop to other sedatives. Medical conditions associated with chronic use include the following[11,18]:

- Central nervous system
  - Psychiatric disorders (depression, antisocial behavior)
  - Cognitive deficits (severe with thiamine deficiency [called Wernicke-Korsakoff syndrome])

- ○ Withdrawal syndrome when not drinking alcohol
- ○ Cerebellar degeneration
- ○ Cerebral atrophy
- Cardiovascular disease
  - ○ Hypertension
  - ○ Dysrhythmias
  - ○ Cardiomyopathy
- Pulmonary
  - ○ Hepatopulmonary shunt
  - ○ Pulmonary hypertension
- Gastrointestinal and hepatobiliary
  - ○ Esophagitis
  - ○ Esophageal varices
  - ○ Gastritis
  - ○ Pancreatitis
  - ○ Cirrhosis
  - ○ Portal hypertension
- Endocrine and metabolic disorders
  - ○ Decreased gluconeogenesis/hypoglycemia
  - ○ Ketoacidosis
  - ○ Hypoalbuminemia
  - ○ Hypomagnesemia
  - ○ Malnutrition
  - ○ Decreased testosterone
- Renal
  - ○ Hepatorenal syndrome
- Hematologic
  - ○ Anemia
  - ○ Leukopenia
  - ○ Thrombocytopenia
  - ○ Coagulopathies

Perioperative considerations

Preoperatively it is important to evaluate for end-organ damage from chronic alcohol use as listed previously. Anesthetic management needs to take these conditions into account. In the case of severe liver disease, it is especially important to weigh the benefits of surgery against the risks of increased morbidity and mortality before deciding to proceed with surgery. Interruption of regular alcohol ingestion patterns postoperatively may cause the chronic user to go into withdrawal. Chronic alcohol users frequently experience withdrawal symptoms. These are usually not severe and are self-treated by resumption of alcohol intake. **Box 1** shows a list of signs and symptoms of alcohol withdrawal. Severe and life-threatening withdrawal can occur in association with infection, trauma, malnutrition, or electrolyte imbalance.[18] Delirium tremens typically occurs 2 to 4 days after cessation of alcohol and symptoms include hallucinations, combativeness, hyperthermia, tachycardia, dysrhythmias, hypertension or hypotension, and grand mal seizures. Treatment includes benzodiazepines to sedate the patient and β-blockers to control the sympathetic hyperactivity.[11]

Former alcoholics may be treated with naltrexone (Revia, Vivitrol), which has been shown to decrease the rate of relapse in most clinical trials.[19] This can make perioperative opioid administration difficult and should be discontinued by the prescribing physician about 3 days before surgery.[5] Although not as common now, disulfiram is

---

Box 1
Alcohol withdrawal syndrome

Alcohol craving

Tremor, irritability

Nausea, diarrhea

Sleep disturbance

Tachycardia

Hypertension

Sweating

Perceptual distortion

Seizures (6–48 hours after last drink)

Visual (and occasionally auditory or tactile) hallucination (12–48 hours after last drink)

Delirium tremens (48–96 hours after last drink; rare in uncomplicated withdrawal)

Severe agitation

Confusion

Fever, profuse sweating

Dilated pupils

From O'Brien CP. Drug addiction. Chapter 24. Table 24-4 alcohol withdrawal syndrome. In: Brunton LL, Chabner BA, Knollmann BC, editors. Goodman & Gilman's the pharmacological basis of therapeutics. 12th edition. New York: McGraw-Hill; 2011; with permission.

---

also used to treat alcoholism. The anesthetic management needs to take into consideration sedation and hepatotoxicity from disulfiram. This drug can also inhibit metabolism of other drugs and alter response from sympathomimetic medications. Alcohol containing solutions for skin preparation should be avoided in disulfiram-treated patients.[11]

Cannabinoids

Incidence

In 2014, the rate of marijuana use disorder was 1.6% of the US population.[1] The number of current marijuana users in 2014 was higher at 22.2 million or 8.4% of the US population.

Effects of acute and chronic use

There are 61 pharmacologically active cannabinoids in the smoke of marijuana, but most of the characteristic pharmacologic effects are from Δ-9-tetrahydrocannabinol.[18] The acute effects vary greatly, but the most frequently sought after effects are a high and a feeling of mellowing out. There is a decrease in cognition, perception, and reaction time. In addition, memory and learning are impaired. It can also produce "giddiness" and increased hunger. There is an increase in the sympathetic nervous system activity and a decrease in the parasympathetic nervous system activity causing an increased resting heart rate.[11] Regular use of marijuana has been associated with an increased risk of anxiety, depression, and psychotic illness.[19] Smoking can cause deposits in the lungs, impaired pulmonary defense mechanisms, and decreased pulmonary function.[11] Tolerance can develop rapidly but with cessation decreases rapidly.[18] Withdrawal symptoms are usually mild and include irritability, insomnia, diaphoresis, nausea, vomiting, and diarrhea.[11]

Many report on the usefulness of smoking marijuana to treat various medical conditions. There was a recent systemic review and meta-analysis that reported on the quality of evidence.[20] The authors summarized that there was moderate-quality evidence supporting its use in treating chronic pain and reducing spasticity in patients with multiple sclerosis or paraplegia. There was low-quality evidence for use for chemotherapy-induced nausea and vomiting, weight gain in patients with human immunodeficiency virus, sleep disorders, and tics associated with Tourette syndrome. The most commonly reported short-term adverse events when using marijuana for medical conditions include disorientation, dizziness, euphoria, confusion, drowsiness, and dry mouth. These events are similar to those reported with recreational use.

Perioperative considerations

There is limited evidence of any major adverse perioperative outcomes from cannabinoid use. The main consequences from acute use are primarily sedation and decreased minimum alveolar concentration, although effects of inhaled use do not last longer than 2 to 3 hours.[11] From chronic use there are respiratory issues similar to patients who smoke tobacco.[21] There was a report in 1996 of acute uvular edema and postoperative airway obstruction possibly from marijuana inhalation.[22] More recently, there was a letter to the editor about a case of possible negative pressure pulmonary edema that became hemorrhagic from lung injury and coagulopathy from cannabis use.[23]

Opioids and Heroin

Incidence

In 2014, there were 1.9 million people in the United States with dependence or abuse of prescription pain medications and 586,000 for heroin.[1]

Effects of acute and chronic use

Besides the use for treatment of pain, opioids have been abused, in particular heroin and oxycodone.[18] This is in part because of the feeling of well-being or euphoria that can occur. The acute effect of each type of opioid can vary. With heroin, there is a "rush" characterized by warmth, "high," and intense pleasure. Morphine can cause histamine release. Meperidine can lead to more excitation or confusion. Hydromorphone is similar to heroin. Eventually there is sedation from the opioid. Side effects include respiratory depression, nausea and vomiting, and constipation.

Chronic use causes tolerance. This is seen especially early for the symptom of euphoria. It also occurs with respiratory, analgesic, sedative, and emetic effects. Tolerance does not occur with miosis and constipation. In general, there is a high degree of cross-tolerance to other opioids. Tolerance does wane rapidly when opioids are discontinued. Opioid withdrawal can occur with either abstinence or administration of opioid antagonists, such as naloxone. **Table 1** shows signs and symptoms of opioid withdrawal and these symptoms can last up to 6 months.[18] **Box 2** shows associated medical issues with chronic opioid abuse.[11]

Methadone and buprenorphine have been used to treat addiction to opioids. These agonists have been found to stabilize addiction, with less "highs and lows" and patients are better able to maintain a functional life. Methadone is a long-acting opioid and from cross-tolerance drug craving diminishes when taking methadone. Buprenorphine is a partial agonist and has a ceiling effect. Naltrexone is an antagonist and it is also used to treat opioid addiction.[18]

Table 1 Characteristics of opioid withdrawal	
Symptoms	Signs
Regular withdrawal	
Craving for opioids	Pupillary dilation
Restlessness, irritability	Sweating
Increased sensitivity to pain	Piloerection
Nausea, cramps	Tachycardia
Muscle aches	Vomiting, diarrhea
Dysphoric mood	Increased blood pressure
Insomnia	Yawning
Anxiety	Fever
Protracted withdrawal	
Anxiety	Cyclic changes in weight
Insomnia	Cyclic changes in pupils
Drug craving	Cyclic changes in respiratory center sensitivity

From O'Brien CP. Drug addiction. Chapter 24. Table 24-7 alcohol withdrawal syndrome. In: Brunton LL, Chabner BA, Knollmann BC, editors. Goodman & Gilman's the pharmacological basis of therapeutics. 12th edition. New York: McGraw-Hill; 2011; with permission.

Perioperative considerations

Preoperative assessment of associated medical issues should be made. Opioid agonist-antagonist drugs should be avoided. Long-term opioid use can lead to cross-tolerance to other central nervous system depressants.[11] Patients on chronic opioids may have postoperative pain that is difficult to treat. Not only do they require their maintenance dose of opioid so they do not experience withdrawal, but they also

Box 2 Medical problems associated with chronic opioid abuse
Superficial skin abscesses
Cellulitis
Septic thrombophlebitis
Systemic septic emboli
Endocarditis
Aspiration pneumonitis
Transverse myelitis
Human immunodeficiency virus
Tetanus
Malnutrition
Hepatitis
From Hines RL, Marschall KE. Psychiatric disease, substance abuse, and drug overdose. Table 25-12 from Chapter 25. In: Hines RL, Marschall KE, editors. Stoelting's anesthesia and co-existing disease. 6th edition. Philadelphia: Saunders; 2012; with permission.

require additional opiates for the acute pain. It is advocated to use regional techniques and nonopioid analgesics whenever possible. Patients on naltrexone or buprenorphine should have the medication discontinued by the prescribing physician if possible about 3 days before surgery.[5] If it is not discontinued preoperatively, patients require additional pain medication and if discontinued postoperatively they are at risk for opioid overdose. Patients on methadone may have QT prolongation.

Cocaine and Other Stimulants

Incidence
In 2014, there were 913,000 people in the United States with dependence or abuse of cocaine and 1.5 million current users of cocaine and 1.6 million users of other stimulants, such as amphetamines and methamphetamines.[1]

Effects of acute and chronic use
Acute effects of cocaine are increased heart rate and blood pressure, increased arousal, and a sense of self-confidence and well-being, and euphoria with higher doses. There is a risk for cardiac dysrhythmias (QT prolongation), myocardial ischemia, myocarditis, aortic dissection, cerebral vasoconstriction, hyperthermia, and seizures. β-Blockade can accentuate cocaine-induced coronary artery vasospasm.[11] With chronic use there can be sensitization, but this is primarily caused by conditioning. Tolerance can also develop. Cocaine withdrawal is generally mild.[18]

Amphetamines increase alertness, act as appetite suppressants, and decrease need for sleep. Long-term abuse can result in somnolence or anxiety.[11]

Perioperative considerations
The effects of acute cocaine use immediately preoperatively can be detrimental and elective surgery should not be performed. It is controversial whether to cancel when there is no sign of acute cocaine toxicity. In 2006, Hill and colleagues[24] published a prospective nonrandomized, blinded analysis study comparing 40 urine cocaine-positive patients with no indication of acute cocaine toxicity with matched drug-free control subjects. They found similar cardiovascular stability in both groups.

Hyperthermia and increased anesthetic requirements can occur with acute use of amphetamine. Long-term amphetamine use may be associated with markedly decreased anesthetic requirements and need for direct-acting vasopressors to treat hypotension from catecholamine depletion.[11]

Hallucinogens and Psychedelics

Incidence
Hallucinogens include lysergic acid diethylamide, phencyclidine, and methylenedioxymethamphetamine or "Ecstasy." In 2014, there were 1.2 million people in the United States who reported actively using hallucinogens.[1]

Effects of acute and chronic use
The acute effect of hallucinogen use is production of a disturbance of perception, thought, or mood. A "bad trip" can cause severe anxiety.[18] Tolerance is generally not commonly seen and frequent repeated doses are not usually taken.

Perioperative considerations
There have been reports of precipitating panic attacks perioperatively. Lysergic acid diethylamide can prolong the analgesic and respiratory depression effects of opioids.[11]

POSTOPERATIVE RISK OF NEW OR RELAPSED SUBSTANCE ABUSE
Opioid Addiction

There are many stories of patients reporting opioid addiction after surgery, but little evidence for this. Opioid dependence rarely develops from using opioids to treat acute postoperative pain; however, it is possible to become addicted to opioids in less than 14 days with daily administration in ever-increasing dosages.[11]

Similarly, former abusers especially former opioid abusers are concerned about the risk of relapse after undergoing surgery. These patients are vulnerable and it is important to get acute pain and addiction specialists involved early. Inadequate pain control can lead to further substance abuse.[5]

Alcohol and Food Addiction Transfer

Concerns have arisen about "addiction transfer" in patients after bariatric weight loss surgery, specifically that there is substitution from food to alcohol.[25] After Roux-en-Y gastric bypass, there is a change in the pharmacokinetics of alcohol that can lead to problematic use.[26] Canason and colleagues[27] published a prospective study in 2012 investigating substance use after bariatric weight loss surgery. They hypothesized that to compensate for a decrease in food intake, patients would increase substance use (drug, alcohol, or cigarette) following surgery. They did find an overall increase in composite substance use 24 months after weight loss surgery and a specific increase in alcohol use for the patients who underwent laparoscopic Roux-en-Y gastric bypass surgery. They recommended that patients be counseled before surgery, especially those with a personal or family history of alcohol abuse, and that patients be screened at follow-up visits. In 2013, Ashton and colleagues[28] published a preliminary evaluation of a pilot program for patients at risk with promising results. There has also been a report of obesity following liver transplantation in patients who are former alcohol abusers, hypothesizing transfer of addiction from alcohol to food.[25]

SUMMARY

The patient with a current or former history of substance use disorder can be challenging to adequately care for in the perioperative period. A thorough preoperative evaluation is essential. In addition to drug abuse screening, the evaluation should include an assessment of the effects of the substance abuse, associated diseases, end-organ damage, and an awareness of the potential perioperative risks so appropriate plans are developed to minimize the risks. Intraoperatively, anesthetic management needs to be appropriately modified. Postoperatively, signs of withdrawal should be monitored for, and pain management can be difficult. After discharge, this patient population is vulnerable and requires close follow-up and early referral to appropriate specialists as needed.

REFERENCES

1. Center for Behavioral Health Statistics and Quality. Behavioral health trends in the United States: results from 2014 National Survey on Drug Use and Health (HHS Publication No. SMA 15–44927 NSDUH Series H-50). 2015. Available at: http://www.samhas.gov/data/. Accessed October 13, 2015.
2. National Institute on Drug Abuse. National drug early warning system (NDEWS). 2015. Available at: http://www.drugabuse.gov/related-topics/trends-statistics/national-drug-early-warning-system-ndews. Accessed October 13, 2015.

3. Patel V, Chisolm D, Parikh R, et al. Addressing the burden of mental, neurological, and substance use disorders: key messages from Disease Control Priorities, 3rd Edition. Lancet 2015 [Epub ahead of print]. Available at: www.thelancet.com. Accessed October 13, 2015.

4. National Institute on Drug Abuse. Medical consequences of drug abuse. 2012. Available at: http://www.drugabuse.gov/related-topics/medical-consequences-drug-abuse. Accessed October 13, 2015.

5. Wijeysundera DM, Sweitzer BJ. Preoperative evaluation. Chapter 38. In: Miller RD, editor. Miller's anesthesia. Philadelphia: Saunders; 2015. p. 1085–155.e7.

6. Conway KP, Compton W, Stinson FS, et al. Lifetime Comorbidity of DSM-IV mood and anxiety disorders and specific drug use disorders: results from the National Epidemiologic Survey on Alcohol and Related Conditions. J Clin Psychiatry 2006; 67:247–57.

7. Comorbidity: addiction and other mental illnesses NIDA. Available at: http://www.drugabuse.gov/publications/research-reports/comorbidity-addiction-other-mental-illnesses/letter-director. Accessed October 2, 2105.

8. Sohler NL, Wong MD, Cunningham WE, et al. Type and pattern of illicit drug use and access to health care services for HIV-infected people. AIDS Patient Care STDs 2007;21:S68–76.

9. Owen RR, Fischer EP, Booth BM, et al. Medication noncompliance and substance abuse among patients with schizophrenia. Psychiatr Serv 1996;47:853–8.

10. Substance Abuse and Mental Health Services Administration. Results from the 2013 National Survey on Drug Use and Health: summary of national findings. NSDUH Series H-48, HHS Publication No. (SMA) 14–4863. Rockville (MD): Substance Abuse and Mental Health Services Administration; 2014.

11. Hines RL, Marschall KE. Psychiatric disease, substance abuse, and drug overdose. Chapter 25. In: Hines RL, Marschall KE, editors. Stoelting's anesthesia and co-existing disease. 6th edition. Philadelphia: Saunders; 2012. p. 533–57.

12. Rosenblatt MA, Hausman LM. Office-based anesthesia. Chapter 31. In: Barash PG, et al, editors. Clinical anesthesia. 7th edition. Philadelphia: Lippincott Williams & Wilkins; 2013.

13. Zelle BA, Buttacacavboli FA, Schroff JB, et al. Loss of follow-up in orthopedic trauma: who is getting lost to follow-up? J Orthop Trauma 2015;29(11): 510–5.

14. O'Toole TP, Starin EC, Wand G, et al. Outpatient treatment entry and health care utilization after a combine medical/substance abuse intervention for hospitalized medical patients. J Gen Intern Med 2002;17(5):334–40.

15. Standridge JB, Adams SM, Zotos AP. Urine drug screening: a valuable office procedure. Am Fam Physician 2010;81:635–40.

16. American Society of Anesthesiology Task Force on Preanesthesia Evaluation. Practice advisory for preanesthesia evaluation: an updated report by the American Society of Task Force on preanesthesia evaluation. Anesthesiology 2012; 116:1–17.

17. Elkassabany N, Speck RM, Oslin D, et al. Preoperative screening and case cancellation in cocaine-abusing veterans scheduled for elective surgery. Anesthesiol Res Pract 2013;2013:7, 149892.

18. O'Brien CP. Drug addiction. Chapter 24. In: Brunton LL, Chabner BA, Knollmann BC, editors. Goodman & Gilman's the pharmacological basis of therapeutics. 12th edition. New York: McGraw-Hill; 2011.

19. Pettinati HM, O'Brien CP, Rabinowitz AR, et al. The status of naltrexone in the treatment of alcohol dependence: specific effects of heavy drinking. J Clin Psychopharmacol 2006;26:610–5.
20. Whiting PF, Wolff RF, Deshpande S, et al. Cannaboids for medical use a systemic review and meta-analysis. JAMA 2015;313(24):2456–76.
21. Bryson EO, Frost EA. The perioperative implications of tobacco, marijuana, and other inhaled toxins. Int Anesthesiol Clin 2011;49:103–18.
22. Mallat A, Roberson J, Brock-Utne JG. Preoperative marijuana inhalation: an airway concern. Can J Anaesth 1996;43:691–3.
23. Murray AW, Smith JD, Ibinson JW. Diffuse alveolar hemorrhage, anesthesia, and cannabis. Ann Am Thorac Soc 2014;11:1338–9.
24. Hill GE, Ogunnaike BO, Johnson ER. General anaesthesia for the cocaine abusing patient. Is it safe? Br J Anaesth 2006;97:654–7.
25. Brunalt P, Salame E, Jaafari N, et al. Why do liver transplant patients so often become obese? The addiction transfer hypothesis? Med Hypotheses 2015;85:68–75.
26. Heinberg LJ, Ashton K, Coughlin J. Alcohol and bariatric surgery: review and suggested recommendations for assessment and management. Surg Obes Relat Dis 2012;8:357–63.
27. Conason A, Teixeira J, Juse CH, et al. Substance use following bariatric weight loss surgery. JAMA Surg 2013;148:145–50.
28. Ashton K, Heinberg L, Merrel J, et al. Pilot evaluation of a substance abuse prevention group intervention for at-risk bariatric surgery candidates. Surg Obes Relat Dis 2013;9:462–9.

The Pregnant Patient
Assessment and Perioperative Management

Heather McKenzie, MD, Debra Domino Pulley, MD*

KEYWORDS

- Pregnancy • Preoperative evaluation • Perioperative management
- Preoperative pregnancy testing • Fetal effects of perioperative medications

KEY POINTS

- Pregnant women should not be denied indicated surgeries or procedures; however, the benefits and risks (both what is known and not known) need to be communicated so that informed decisions are made.
- Per American Congress of Obstetricians and Gynecologists guidelines, elective surgery should be postponed until after delivery. If it cannot, nonurgent surgery should be done in the second trimester.
- When a pregnant woman has a surgery or procedure, it is important that the entire health care team work together for optimal patient and fetal outcomes, and that coordination of care be clearly delineated beforehand.
- It is reasonable to offer urine pregnancy testing before diagnostic tests and procedures in a woman of childbearing age.

Although not common, pregnant patients do have surgery and a thorough preoperative evaluation is vital for maintaining maternal and fetal wellbeing. To accomplish this, it is important to remember that pregnancy itself can cause physiologic changes and that there are 2 patients (patient and fetus) to consider. This article reviews the types of surgeries that can occur during pregnancy, the physiologic changes that occur during pregnancy, both the maternal and fetal effects of anesthesia and surgery, and current recommendations for perioperative management.

PHYSIOLOGIC CHANGES OF PREGNANCY

The state of pregnancy has multiple systemic effects. These can vary from what can be considered the body's normal physiologic response to pregnancy to the abnormal

Disclosures: The authors have nothing to disclose.
Department of Anesthesiology, Washington University School of Medicine in St. Louis, 660 South Euclid Avenue, Campus Box 8054, St Louis, MO 63110, USA
* Corresponding author.
E-mail address: pulleyd@wustl.edu

diseased state. When evaluating a pregnant patient, it is important to keep in mind the expected normal physiologic changes of the major systems. This will help the clinician recognize when the level of care should be escalated and other medical services consulted. The expected physiologic responses to pregnancy are reviewed briefly, emphasizing what a clinician may encounter in the preoperative setting:

- Cardiac changes (**Box 1**)[1]
  - Increased heart rate
  - Increased cardiac output
  - Audible S3 heart sound, midsystolic flow murmur
  - Left axis deviation on electrocardiogram
  - Aortocaval compression in the supine position resulting in hypotension and decreased uterine perfusion
- Respiratory changes (**Table 1**)[1]
  - Increased minute ventilation
  - Decreased functional residual capacity
  - Respiratory rate within normal limits
  - Respiratory alkalosis on arterial blood gas
  - Upper airway capillary and mucosal engorgement
- Hematologic changes[1]
  - Anemia: dilutional effect due to a large increase in plasma volume relative to red blood cell volume
  - Hypercoagulable state: laboratory test may reveal decreased prothrombin time, partial thromboplastin time, and normal platelet values
- Renal changes[1]
  - Increased glomerular filtration rate
  - Decreased blood urea nitrogen and creatinine levels
- Gastrointestinal changes[1]
  - Increased intragastric pressure
  - Decreased lower esophageal sphincter tone.

MATERNAL EFFECTS OF ANESTHESIA AND SURGERY OR PROCEDURES

Due to physiologic changes, additional anesthetic concerns are present for a pregnant patient compared with a nonpregnant patient. There is an increased risk of desaturation during periods of apnea (such as induction), increased risk of aspiration (second and third trimesters), increased risk of difficult intubation, decreased MAC, yet increased risk of awareness.[2–4] In addition, the gravid uterus (second and third

---

Box 1
Changes in physical examination with pregnancy

Accentuation of S1 heart sound and exaggerated splitting of the mitral and tricuspid components

Typical systolic ejection murmur

Possible S3 and S4 (no clinical significance)

Leftward displacement of point of maximal impulse

Adapted from Gaiser R. Physiologic changes of pregnancy. In: Chestnut DH, editor. Chestnut's obstetric anesthesia: principles and practice. 5th edition. Philadelphia: Saunders; 2014. p. 15–38; with permission.

Parameter	Nonpregnant	Trimester		
		First	Second	Third
$Paco_2$ in mm Hg (kPa)	40 (5.3)	30 (4.0)	30 (4.0)	30 (4.0)
Pao_2 in mm Hg (kPa)	100 (13.3)	107 (14.3)	105 (14.0)	103 (13.7)
pH	7.40	7.44	7.44	7.44
$[Hco_3^-]$ (mEq/L)	24	21	20	20

Table 1
Typical blood gas measurements

From Gaiser R. Physiologic changes of pregnancy. In: Chestnut DH, editor. Chestnut's obstetric anesthesia: principles and practice. 5th edition. Philadelphia: Saunders; 2014. p. 15–38; with permission.

trimesters) can cause maternal hypotension in the supine position from compression of the aorta and inferior vena cava.[5]

A 2012 review of complications after nonobstetric surgeries in pregnant women from the National Surgery Quality Improvement Program (NSQIP) data showed that 30-day mortality was very low (0.25%).[6] Mortality was associated with preoperative systemic infection and undergoing emergent procedures. Overall, postoperative complications were also low (5.8%). Major complications included cardiac arrest requiring cardiopulmonary resuscitation, myocardial infarction, coma, stroke, deep surgical site infection, wound dehiscence, deep vein thrombosis or pulmonary embolism, unplanned reintubation, prolonged mechanical ventilation greater than 48 hours, pneumonia, or sepsis. Predictors of complications included age, preoperative systemic infection, New York Heart Association Class III or IV, ventilator dependency, preoperative functional status, dependent or partially dependent for activities of daily living, and increased operative time.

A retrospective study published in 2009 showed that pregnant women had worse outcomes following thyroid and parathyroid surgery than nonpregnant women.[7] The outcomes measured showed higher rate of endocrine and general complications in the pregnant group (15.9% and 11.4% vs 8.1% and 3.6%), longer length of stay (2 days vs 1 day), and higher hospital costs ($6873 vs $5963). However, a more recent retrospective cohort study of general surgery patients from NSQIP data showed no significant difference in 30-day mortality or overall morbidity in pregnant and nonpregnant matched patients.[8] The pregnant patients had a low 30-day mortality rate (0.4%) and a low overall morbidity rate (6.6%).

Major depressive disorder can occur during pregnancy. Electroconvulsive therapy (ECT) has been shown to be relatively safe and effective for the pregnant patient. Endoscopic retrograde cholangiopancreatography (ERCP) during pregnancy has also been shown to be safe and effective.[9]

FETAL EFFECTS OF ANESTHESIA AND SURGERY OR PROCEDURES AND PREGNANCY OUTCOMES

One of the most concerning fetal effects is teratogenicity. The US Food and Drug Administration has required labeling of a drug to include a use-in-pregnancy category (A, B, C, D, or X) based on the medical evidence (**Box 2**).[10] In December 2014, the Pregnancy and Lactation Labeling Rule stated the pregnancy letter categories would be removed effective June 2015. This change was based on the argument that the categories were oversimplified.[11] Instead, under the pregnancy subsection, there will be a risk summary, clinical considerations, and data to help physicians and their

---

Box 2
US Food and Drug Administration drug classification system

Category A

Controlled studies have shown no risk. Adequate, well-controlled studies in pregnant women have failed to demonstrate a risk to the fetus in the first trimester (and there is no evidence of a risk in later trimesters) and the possibility of fetal harm seems remote.

Category B

No evidence of human fetal risk exists. Either animal reproduction studies have not demonstrated fetal risk, but no controlled studies in pregnant women have been reported or animal reproduction studies have shown an adverse effect (other than a decrease in fertility) that was not confirmed in controlled studies in women in the first trimester (and there is no evidence of risk in later trimesters).

Category C

Risk cannot be ruled out. Either studies in animals have revealed adverse effects on the fetus (teratogenic, embryocidal, or other) but no controlled studies in women have been reported, or studies in women and animals are not available. These drugs should be given only if the potential benefit justifies the potential risk to the fetus.

Category D

Positive evidence of human fetal risk exists. However, the benefits from use in pregnant women may be acceptable despite the risk (eg, if the drug is needed for a life-threatening condition or for a serious disease for which safer drugs cannot be used or are ineffective).

Category X

Contraindicated in pregnancy. Studies in animals or human beings have demonstrated fetal abnormalities, or evidence exists of fetal risk based on human experience, or both, and the risk in pregnant women clearly outweighs any possible benefit. These drugs are contraindicated in women who are or may become pregnant.

---

patients make clinical decisions based on the evidence. In addition, information about pregnancy registries will be required to be made available on the drug labels. Encouragement in the use of these registries should help collection of data and review of databases to make future recommendations. In general, no anesthetic drug or drugs commonly used in anesthesia are listed as human teratogens.[12] Maternal conditions, such as severe hypoglycemia, prolonged hypoxemia and hypercarbia, and hyperthermia, may be teratogenic in humans.[13] However, when discussing teratogenic risks, all that can be said is that overall teratogenic risk is low but data are limited and the best approach is to minimize drug exposure.

Other fetal concerns include demise and premature birth. A systemic review of the literature from 1966 to 2002 that involved nonobstetric surgery in pregnant women found the rate of delivery induced by the surgical intervention or the underlying condition was 3.5% and overall fetal death was 2.5%.[14] Of particular interest was a subanalysis that showed pregnant patients undergoing appendectomy were at a greater risk for surgery-induced delivery (4.6%) and fetal death (2.6%) compared with other procedures. However, the investigators recommended prompt diagnosis and treatment of appendicitis because when peritonitis was present the fetal death markedly increased to 10.9%. There have been multiple studies that have shown a higher incidence of preterm delivery with surgery especially involving uterine manipulation.[3] Jenkins and colleagues[15] confirmed that the lowest incidence was when surgery occurred in the second trimester.

Wellbeing of the fetus mostly depends on the wellbeing of the pregnant patient. Anything affecting the uteroplacental perfusion and transfer of infectious agents, toxins, and drugs that cross the placental membrane may affect the fetus.

Maternal depression can adversely affect the fetus with low birth weight and/or premature delivery.[16] There is little evidence that ECT is harmful to fetus. ECT can be a safe and effective treatment of major depressive disorder that fails to respond to antidepressants or is life-threatening.[17]

During an anesthetic on a pregnant patient, it is especially important to maintain adequate maternal oxygenation, ventilation, and uteroplacental perfusion to preserve fetal wellbeing. In addition, minimizing unnecessary drug exposure, and monitoring for and treating preterm labor and delivery are also important. It is reasonable to use regional techniques whenever appropriate.[2]

Risks of Commonly Prescribed Drugs in the Perioperative Period

Sedatives or hypnotics

There is some evidence that propofol and ketamine may exert neurodevelopmental effects in animals but the effect on a developing human fetus is not clear.[18] There was a report of diazepam causing cleft palate; however, this was disputed in a subsequent study.[19] If sedatives or hypnotics are given close to delivery, neonatal respiratory depression may occur and resuscitation may be required.

Inhaled anesthetics

Exposure to nitrous oxide, when scavenging systems are not in place, has been associated with increased risk of spontaneous abortion in dental workers.[20] There is also emerging evidence that inhaled anesthetics may have neurodevelopmental effects in animals but the effect on a developing human fetus is not clear.[18]

Muscle relaxants

Muscle relaxants do not cross the placenta.

Opioids

The National Birth Defects Prevention Study reviewed maternal treatment with opioid analgesics and risk for birth defects from 1997 to 2005. The study showed that there was an association between opioid use early in pregnancy and birth defects including congenital heart disease.[21] When the reason for opioid use was known, 41% reported the use of opioid was due to a surgical procedure. If opioids are given close to delivery, neonatal respiratory depression may occur and resuscitation may be required. Chronic maternal opioid use can also cause neonatal abstinence syndrome.[22]

Nonsteroidal anti-inflammatory drugs

A 2013 review of the use of nonsteroidal anti-inflammatory drugs (NSAIDs) during pregnancy summarizes the current literature.[23] In the first trimester, several studies have shown an increased risk of spontaneous abortion with NSAIDs. In the second trimester they are generally safe but there has been a reported association with congenital cryptorchism. In the third trimester, NSAIDs should be avoided due to fetal risks such as renal injury and constriction of the ductus arteriosus.

Local anesthetics

Most local anesthetics are safe except for cocaine, which is a teratogen.[12] When administered late in pregnancy, use of cocaine has been identified as a risk factor for placental abruption.[24]

Vasopressors

Historically, ephedrine has been the vasopressor of choice but multiple clinical studies have confirmed the safety and efficacy of phenylephrine in treating maternal hypotension.[2]

Ionizing radiation

The American Congress of Obstetricians and Gynecologists (ACOG) has issued a Committee Opinion on Guidelines for Diagnostic Imaging During Pregnancy.[25] Ionizing radiation has been found to be teratogenic in humans. Fortunately, exposure of 5 rad or less has not been associated with fetal anomalies or fetal demise. High-dose radiation has been reported to cause mental retardation, especially during 8 to 15 weeks gestation. There is also probably a very small increased risk of childhood leukemia from in-utero exposure to ionizing radiation, although this is unclear. The use of radioactive isotopes of iodine for the treatment of hyperthyroidism is contraindicated during pregnancy. As with any medication, the potential benefits of high-dose radiation from medically needed diagnostic testing needs to be weighed against the potential risks.

NONOBSTETRIC SURGERIES OR PROCEDURES REQUIRING ANESTHESIA THAT OCCUR DURING PREGNANCY

Published reviews have shown that most nonobstetric surgeries performed on pregnant women were either appendectomy or cholecystectomy (44% and 22%, respectively).[6,26] Less frequently are surgeries for cancer, neurosurgery, cardiac, or trauma. Nonsurgical procedures can include endoscopy (including ERCP) and ECT.

Before any procedure is performed, adequate counseling should occur and the patient should be aware of the risks of proceeding and the risks of waiting until after delivery. ACOG, in its 2011 Committee Opinion on Nonobstetric Surgery During Pregnancy, advises that there are little data to make specific recommendations; however, they do have generalizations to help make decisions. These include that a pregnant woman should not be denied indicated surgery but elective surgery should delayed until after delivery, and "nonurgent surgery should be performed in the second trimester."[27]

PREOPERATIVE RECOMMENDATIONS
Coordination of Care and Assurance of Fetal Wellbeing

During the preoperative evaluation of a pregnant patient, her primary obstetric care provider should be identified. The ACOG Committee recommends that the primary obstetric care provider should be notified before any surgery. When the surgery or procedure is planned at another institution where the provider does not have privileges, another obstetric provider should be involved.[27]

The gestational age of the fetus should be determined to help guide clinical management. In general, 24 weeks and greater is considered viable. With improvements in neonatal care, however, the threshold for fetal viability is decreasing and it is important that individualized plans be made for each clinical situation. Recommendation for monitoring of fetal wellbeing should be made with involvement of obstetric, anesthesia, and surgical services. The plans should be delineated beforehand and not the day of the procedure. Coordination of care can be problematic, especially when done as an outpatient, and may take time to complete. Many institutions have developed their own protocols for evaluation of a pregnant patient undergoing a procedure that help define the processes for involving the multiple specialists so there is consistent and appropriate care. Per the ACOG Committee Opinion, before a procedure, fetal heart rate by Doppler should be performed. If the fetus is viable, the ACOG Committee recommends simultaneous electronic fetal heart rate and contraction monitoring also be performed immediately before.[27]

NPO Guidelines and Aspiration Pneumonia

It is widely believed that pregnant patients are at an increased risk for aspiration because of several factors. These factors include

1. Increased intragastric pressure caused by the gravid uterus
2. Decreased lower esophageal sphincter tone, believed to be caused by a combination of increased intraabdominal pressure from the gravid uterus and smooth muscle relaxation by progesterone
3. Increased likelihood of difficult or failed intubation and the possibility of encountering a difficult airway is further increased in emergent situations.

Mendelson first reported aspiration among pregnant woman receiving anesthesia in 1946.[28] The incidence of aspiration in the obstetric population, however, is not well defined. There are a limited number of studies that have investigated this. Olsson and colleagues'[29] computer-aided study showed an incidence 0.15% in the obstetric patient undergoing cesarean delivery intubated. A more recent study by Ezri and colleagues[30] suggested that timing and the type of surgery should be taken into consideration on the incidence of aspiration and that the risk of aspiration during general anesthesia without tracheal intubation during and immediately after delivery may not be higher in obstetric patients, as has been reported in the past. Most studies have focused on investigating factors that may decrease the risk of aspiration. This includes studying the efficacy of antacids in raising gastric pH and lowering gastric volume.[31] Accepting that aspiration is possible and that aspiration pneumonitis can be life threatening, the authors suggest clinicians continue efforts to ensure patient safety.

In accordance with American Society of Anesthesiologist and ACOG guidelines,[32,33] it is not recommended that patients consume solid foods during labor. For scheduled procedures, patients should be fasting from solid foods for 6 to 8 hours depending on the fat content of the meal. The latter being preferred when patients consume meals with a high fat content. Patients may consume clear liquids up to 2 hours before a scheduled procedure.

Frequently, during pregnancy patients experience new onset or increased severity of symptoms of acid reflux. The presence and/or severity of these symptoms should be determined preoperatively through a thorough history. In preparation for surgery, clinicians may choose to provide aspiration prophylaxis to decrease the severity and likelihood of aspiration pneumonitis. Examples of such medications are

1. Histamine H2 receptor antagonists such as famotidine and ranitidine that work by increasing gastric pH through blocking histamine H2 receptors in gastric parietal cells
2. Prokinetic agents, such as metoclopramide, which promotes increased upper gastrointestinal motility and increases lower esophageal sphincter tone
3. Nonparticulate antacid, sodium citrate, which increases gastric pH to more than 2.5 (should aspiration pneumonitis occur, the severity is decreased when compared with particulate antacids).

INTRAOPERATIVE RECOMMENDATIONS

As stated previously, immediately before the procedure, the Doppler fetal heart rate should be documented. If the fetus is viable, ACOG recommends simultaneous electronic fetal heart rate and contraction monitoring be performed immediately before and after.[27] They also state that intraoperative fetal monitoring may be appropriate when all the following conditions apply:

- Viable fetus
- Physically possible to monitor
- Health care provider with obstetric surgery privileges available and willing to intervene during the procedure for fetal indications
- Patient consents to emergency cesarean delivery
- Procedure can be interrupted for emergency delivery.

ACOG emphasizes that if any fetal monitoring is to be performed, the appropriate personnel need to be readily available to interpret the fetal heart rate tracing, intervene with emergency cesarean delivery if indicated, and have appropriate neonatal services.

The choice of anesthetic needs to be determined on a case-by-case basis. Anesthetic management should avoid fetal asphyxia, which can be caused by maternal hypoxemia, maternal hypotension, or any other causes of decreased uteroplacental perfusion.[2] Stimulating the myometrium should be avoided.[3] Difficult airway equipment should be readily available and the patient should be in a position to reduce aortocaval compression such as left uterine tilt or lateral.[13]

POSTOPERATIVE RECOMMENDATIONS

Per the ACOG Committee Opinion, after a procedure, Doppler should be performed to assess fetal heart rate. If the fetus is viable, simultaneous electronic fetal heart rate and contraction monitoring should ensue. Again, plans need to already be in place for the appropriate personnel to interpret the fetal monitoring and intervene with appropriate obstetric management and neonatal services, if indicated.[27]

PREOPERATIVE PREGNANCY TESTING

There are many changes that occur during pregnancy and changes in clinical care when a patient is known to be pregnant. When is pregnancy testing appropriate and indicated? There still remains some question about the correct answer. In the most recent update of the practice advisory for the American Society of Anesthesiology Task Force on Preanesthesia Evaluation, it stated that there are insufficient data to adequately inform patients of the risk of anesthesia or surgery in early pregnancy and pregnancy testing may be offered if the result will change management.[34] Review of the literature found that the incidence of positive urine human chorionic gonadotropin results was reported as 0.3% to 1.3% and, more importantly, in 100% of the cases with positive results, there were changes in clinical management.[35-38] Many institutions have developed their own policy making testing mandatory for any woman of childbearing age. Others make it required if the date of the last menstrual period is greater than 1 month but less than a year. It is best to know the institutional policy and base decisions to test on that policy.[39]

SUMMARY

Pregnant patients need special consideration when undergoing any surgery or procedure. An understanding of normal physiologic changes of pregnancy, knowledge of the current evidence (or lack of evidence) of the effects of anesthesia and the surgery or procedure on both the pregnant patient and her fetus, and organizational guidelines that help in coordination of perioperative care are vital to helping patients not only make informed decisions but also improve their overall outcome.

REFERENCES

1. Gaiser R. Physiologic changes of pregnancy. In: Chestnut DH, editor. Chestnut's obstetric anesthesia: principles and practice. 5th edition. Philadelphia: Saunders; 2004. p. 15–38.
2. Reitman E, Flood P. Anaesthetic considerations for non-obstetric surgery during pregnancy. Br J Anaesth 2011;107(S1):i72–8.
3. Van de Velde M. Nonobstetric surgery during pregnancy. In: Chestnut DH, editor. Chestnut's obstetric anesthesia: principles and practice. 5th edition. Philadelphia: Saunders; 2014. p. 358–437.
4. Anderson EL, Reti IM. ECT in pregnancy: a review of the literature from 1941 to 2007. Psychosom Med 2009;71:235–42.
5. Lanni SM, Tillinghast J, Silver HM. Hemodynamic changes and baroreflex gain in the supine hypotensive syndrome. Am J Obstet Gynecol 2002;187:1636–41.
6. Erekson EA, Brousseau EC, Dick-Biascoechea MA, et al. Maternal postoperative complications after nonobstetric antennal surgery. J Matern Fetal Neonatal Med 2012;25(12):2639–44.
7. Kuy S, Roman SA, Desai R, et al. Outcomes following thyroid and parathyroid surgery in pregnancy. Arch Surg 2009;144(5):399–406.
8. Moore HB, Juarez-Colunga E, Bronsert M, et al. Effect of pregnancy on adverse outcomes after general surgery. JAMA Surg 2015;150(7):637–43.
9. Fine S, Beirne J, Delgi-Esposti S, et al. Continued evidence for safety of endoscopic retrograde cholangiopancreatography. World J Gastrointest Endosc 2014;6:352–8.
10. Gin T, Yankowitz J. Pharmacology and nonanesthetic drugs during pregnancy and lactation. In: Chestnut DH, editor. Chestnut's obstetric anesthesia: principles and practice. 5th edition. Philadelphia: Saunders; 2014. p. 303–25.
11. FDA News Release. FDA issues final rule on changes to pregnancy and lactation labeling information for prescription drug and biological products. Silver Spring (MD): U. S. Food and Drug Adminstration; 2014.
12. Shepard TH, Lemire RJ. Catalog of teratogenic agents. Baltimore (MD): Johns Hopkins University Press; 2010.
13. Walston NKDW, Melachuri VK. Anaesthesia for non-obstetric surgery during pregnancy. Contin Educ Anaesth Crit Care Pain 2006;6:83–5.
14. Cohen-Kerem R, RAilton C, Oren D, et al. Pregnancy outcome following non-obstetric surgical intervention. Am J Surg 2005;190:467–73.
15. Jenkins TM, Macley SF, Benzoni EM, et al. Non-obstetric surgery during gestation: risk factors for lower birthweight. Aust N Z J Obstet Gynaecol 2003;43:27–31.
16. Diego MA, Field I, Hernandez-Reif M, et al. Prenatal depression restricts fetal growth. Early Hum Dev 2009;85:65–70.
17. Yonkers KA, Wisner KL, Stewart DE, et al. The management of depression during pregnancy: a report from the American Psychiatric Association and the American College of Obstetricians and Gynecologists. Gen Hosp Psychiatry 2009;31:403–13.
18. Palanisamy A. Maternal anesthesia and fetal neurodevelopment. Int J Obstet Anesth 2012;21:152–62.

19. Rosenberg L, Mitchell AA, Parsellis JL, et al. Lack of relation of oral clefts to diazepam use during pregnancy. N Engl J Med 1983;309:1282–5.
20. Rowland AS, Baird DD, Shore DL, et al. Nitrous oxide and spontaneous abortion in female dental assistants. Am J Epidemiol 1995;141:531–8.
21. Broussard CS, Rasmussen SA, Reefhuis J, et al. Maternal treatment with opioid analgesics and risk for birth defects. Am J Obstet Gynecol 2011;204:314.e1–11.
22. Patrick SW, Schumacher RE, Benneyworth BD, et al. Neonatal abstinence syndrome and associated health care expenditures: United States, 2000-2009. JAMA 2012;307(18):1934–40.
23. Bloor M, Paech M. Nonsteroidal anti-inflammatory drugs during pregnancy and the initiation of lactation. Anesth Analg 2013;116:1065–73.
24. Hulse GK, Milne E, English DR, et al. Assessing the relationship between maternal cocaine use and abruptio placentae. Addiction 1997;92:1547.
25. Guidelines for diagnostic imaging during pregnancy. ACOG Committee Opinion No. 299. American College of Obstetricians and Gynecologists. Obstet Gynecol 2004;104:647–51.
26. Gilo NB, Amini D, Landy HJ. Appendicitis and cholecystitis in pregnancy. Clin Obstet Gynecol 2009;52:586–96.
27. ACOG. Nonobstetric surgery during pregnancy. Committee opinion No. 474. American College of Obstetricians and Gynecologists. Obstet Gynecol 2011;11:420–1.
28. Mendelson CL. The aspiration of stomach contents into the lungs during obstetric anesthesia. Am J Obstet Gynecol 1946;52:191–205.
29. Olsson GEL, Hallen B, Hambraeus-Jonzon K. Aspiration during anaesthesia; a computer aided study of 185,358 anaesthetics. Acta Anaesthesiol Scand 1986; 30:84–92.
30. Ezri T, Szmuk P, Stein A, et al. Peripartum general anaesthesia without tracheal intubation: incidence of aspiration pneumonia. Anaesthesia 2000;55:421–6.
31. Pisegna JR, Martindale RG. Acid suppression in the perioperative period. J Clin Gastroenterol 2005;39:10–6.
32. American Society of Anesthesiologists Task Force on Obstetric Anesthesia. Practice guidelines for obstetric anesthesia: an updated report by the American Society of Anesthesiologists Task Force on Obstetric Anesthesia. Anesthesiology 2007;106:843–63.
33. Committee on Obstetric Practice, American College of Obstetricians and Gynecologists. ACOG Committee Opinion No. 441: oral intake during labor. Obstet Gynecol 2009;114:714.
34. American Society of Anesthesiology Task Force on Preanesthesia Evaluation. Practice advisory for preanesthesia evaluation: an updated report by the American Society of Task Force on Preanesthesia Evaluation. Anesthesiology 2012;116:1–17.
35. Azzam FJ, Padda GS, DeBoard JW, et al. Preoperative pregnancy testing in adolescents. Anesth Analg 1996;82:4–7.
36. Manley S, de Kelaita G, Joseph NJ, et al. Preoperative pregnancy testing in ambulatory surgery: incidence and impact of positive results. Anesthesiology 1995;83:690–3.
37. Pierre N, Moy LK, Redd S, et al. Evaluation of a pregnancy-testing protocol in adolescents undergoing surgery. J Pediatr Adolesc Gynecol 1998;11:139–41.
38. Wheeler M, Coté CJ. Preoperative pregnancy testing in a tertiary care children's hospital: a medico-legal conundrum. J Clin Anesth 1999;11:56–63.
39. Maher JL, Mahabir RC. Preoperative pregnancy testing. Can J Plast Surg 2012; 20:e32–4.

Non-operating Room Anesthesia

The Principles of Patient Assessment and Preparation

Beverly Chang, MD[a], Richard D. Urman, MD, MBA[b],*

KEYWORDS

- Non-operating room • Anesthesia • Preoperative • Evaluation • Assessment
- Procedural sedation

KEY POINTS

- Non-operating room (OR) anesthetics are becoming increasingly commonplace, which often entails taking care of patients who are more medically challenging than patients in the OR.
- Preoperative assessment may require a greater degree of resource coordination.
- Non-OR procedures present significantly different challenges for anesthesiologists during preprocedure, intraprocedure, and postprocedure periods.
- There are significant ways in which anesthesiologists can add value and optimize efficiency in the non-OR realm.

INTRODUCTION

Over the last decade, there has been a shift from procedures being performed strictly in the operating room (OR) to less familiar locations within the far reaches of the hospital as well as outside of the hospital setting. Especially given an increase in the aging population with a significant disease burden, more procedures are being performed in non-OR locations to take advantage of noninvasive techniques that potentially impart less risk. Increasingly complex procedures are being performed in these settings in a population that may not be amenable to traditional surgical correction. In addition, a growing number of urgent and emergent procedures with medically unstable patients are increasingly common occurrences in these areas.

There are no disclosures or conflicts of interest.
[a] Department of Anesthesiology, Perioperative and Pain Medicine, Stanford Hospital and Clinics, 300 Pasteur Drive H3580, Stanford, CA 94305, USA; [b] Department of Anesthesiology, Perioperative and Pain Medicine, Brigham and Women's Hospital, 75 Francis Street, Boston, MA 02115, USA
* Corresponding author.
E-mail address: RURMAN@partners.org

Anesthesiology Clin 34 (2016) 223–240
http://dx.doi.org/10.1016/j.anclin.2015.10.017
1932-2275/16/$ – see front matter © 2016 Elsevier Inc. All rights reserved.

anesthesiology.theclinics.com

CHALLENGES OF NON-OPERATING ROOM PROCEDURES

Performing procedures outside of the OR creates a new set of challenges for anesthesiologists. Patients scheduled for non-OR procedures are often selected by the severity of their disease, which prevents them from undergoing a major procedure in the OR. These patients are sometimes more medically compromised and less optimized compared with the general OR population. For some practitioners, the firmly established familiarity with the OR and its resources is suddenly stripped away. Many of the non-OR sites are located deep within the trenches of hospitals that often require guides to locate for first-time visitors. Resources such as space, monitors, anesthesia equipment, and medications may oftentimes be scarce or hidden. These locations are often built without an anticipation for anesthesia needs and equipment, and additional skilled personnel may be located far away. All of these difficulties create a unique challenge that each anesthesiologist faces when delivering anesthetics in these locations.[1,2]

As the interventional medical technology continues to advance, increasingly complex procedures are being performed in all areas of non-OR specialties. In each hospital setting, the number of non-OR cases performed is growing at a startling pace. A medically complex patient population is often seen, and emergent procedures are commonplace. Anesthesiologists are tasked with providing anesthetic care to patients who are "too sick" or too frail for the OR in procedure rooms that are sometimes not staffed or equipped to handle these patients. There is significant pressure to perform fast evaluations with oftentimes only limited information, because many patients first present on the day of the procedure or are scheduled as urgent or emergent cases. Anesthesiologists may be expected to recover patients in busy recovery suites without dedicated extended postoperative monitoring capabilities and with staff who may not routinely recover patients from general anesthetics. In other instances where anesthetic care by anesthesiologists was not originally anticipated, anesthesiologists often become the first responders to emergent situations where little to no information about the patient is available. Many patients are referred directly to the proceduralist by their regular providers, without the benefit of a thorough preoperative evaluation until the day of the procedure; this is also true of urgent and emergent add-on cases, where little time is available to properly prepare the patient for anesthesia and optimize their comorbid conditions.

The reality is that many interventional procedures do not require anesthesia care, but rather sedation by nonanesthesia providers. However, compliance with existing standards of care for procedural sedation needs to be assured, regardless of the location or the administering staff. Anesthesiologists will need to be the advocates for setting standards and assuring compliance during procedures involving sedation by nonanesthesiologists, in accordance with American Society of Anesthesiologists (ASA) procedural sedation guidelines.[3,4] There is also a growing involvement of state and federal regulatory agencies. By monitoring outcomes and procedural events, these agencies will continue to scrutinize non-OR areas where sedation or anesthesia is being administered. Anesthesia and nonanesthesia physicians working in the non-OR environment must ensure that the goals of medical optimization and regulatory compliance that OR staff face are met in other areas. By the same token, anesthetic care is mandated to be held to the same standard regardless of the location where it is administered, as decreed by the Joint Commission on Accreditation of Healthcare Organizations and the Center for Medicare and Medicaid Services.[5]

With the growing number of non-OR procedures, a significant number of patients now require assessment before their procedural date. Many hospitals have a preoperative clinic or some kind of preoperative process in place to assess patients scheduled for the OR, but many may not have the resources to handle this additional influx of patients. Anesthesiologists usually play an important role in initiating and maintaining a preoperative clinic. However, funding and staffing of such clinics may be challenging due to concerns of where the financial backing of such clinics should fall: should it be the hospital, anesthesiology, surgery, or procedural departments? Non-OR consults often create a strain on anesthesia departments, as "curbside" consults are generally not billable. Official anesthesia consults are billable but do not generate substantial value while requiring a significant amount of staff time. Many non-OR evaluations are performed on the day of the procedure, but this may be more costly by increasing the risk of procedural cancellations or delays.[6] In addition, establishing an organized process with a buy-in from all involved specialties and hospital administration establishes more efficacy, patient safety, and satisfaction for all stakeholders involved.

A formal triage process with protocols needs to be established. The staff placed in the preoperative assessment role, such as physicians and nurses, needs to be educated on proper triaging and selection of patients appropriate for each procedure and sedation.[7,8] Each facility needs to develop criteria that would automatically trigger an anesthesia consult for patients at risk of failing procedural sedation. Stringent education efforts are necessary to provide nonanesthesiologists with key preoperative assessment points and proper sedative selection. An additional challenge is the urgency of some procedures that oftentimes precludes a proper preoperative assessment. A process needs to be in place to triage these patients and provide the proper anesthetic and procedural care under emergent situations. Most importantly, a process needs to be established to communicate and notify treatment teams of concerning findings and comorbid conditions that may affect the procedure and anesthetic offered.

QUALITY ASSURANCE

Continued quality assessments of the preoperative process need to be performed to maintain appropriate patient selection and evaluation for non-OR cases.[9] The number of anesthesia preoperative consults per day should be quantified as should the number and reason for case delays and cancellations. The number of intraprocedural consultations requested and urgency of the procedure should be noted. These measures will allow for a periodic review of institutional guidelines and processes related to the appropriateness of each selected procedural modality and the involvement of anesthesia providers. A multidisciplinary committee should be formed to review each incident report related to sedation and anesthesia complications. Many of these initiatives can be championed by anesthesiologists who are familiar with the unique challenges of patient comorbidities and sedation techniques.

ADDING VALUE AS ANESTHESIOLOGISTS

Anesthesiologists are the natural safeguards for patients requiring any type of procedural sedation. With unique training in preoperative triaging and other aspects of perioperative management, anesthesiologists ensure a smooth transition for both patients and proceduralists in the perioperative process whether in or out of the OR. Studies have demonstrated cost savings and increased efficiency when preoperative evaluation and testing is performed by anesthesiologists.[10,11] Hospitals place significant effort into increasing the efficiency of the OR, setting up preoperative clinics, pain management teams, and after-anesthesia care unit resources to maximize revenues. These same efforts now need to be directed to the non-OR realm. Supporting a preoperative assessment system reduces the costs of non-OR cancellations and delays, leading to increased efficiency and an ability to perform more procedures per day. Numerous studies have demonstrated the financial justifications of establishing an organized preoperative assessment process.[12,13] Cost reductions can be seen in decreasing nonreimbursed preoperative laboratory and diagnostic tests as well as unnecessary preoperative consultations by specialty clinics. Reimbursements can be maximized by standardization and accuracy of documentation, compliance with pay-for-performance measures, and reimbursements for preoperative assessments. Preoperative medical management reduces potential complications, hospital costs, and length of stay. Lastly, a smoother, safer, and more streamlined process contributes to greater patient satisfaction.[6]

ANESTHESIA VERSUS PROCEDURAL SEDATION

Traditionally, most non-OR procedures have been performed without the presence of anesthesiologists but under sedation administered by nonanesthesiologists. However, as increasingly complex procedures are introduced and patients with more severe comorbidities are being scheduled, anesthesiologists have an increasing presence in non-OR procedural rooms. With the advent of new technologies, whether a patient or a proceduralist requires an anesthesiologist is a key question to ask during each preoperative assessment. Numerous studies have demonstrated the complications of sedation and anesthesia in the non-OR setting.[1,14,15] A recent review of approximately 63,000 non-OR cases in a tertiary care center described adverse events associated with all types of sedation and anesthesia, advocating for a robust quality assurance system to track and report such events.[16]

For example, the ASA Closed Claims analysis by Metzner and colleagues[17] revealed that the most common non-OR anesthesia (NORA) claims were related to severe respiratory events leading to death and permanent brain damage, which occurred twice as frequently as in the OR. NORA was associated with a greater degree of injury compared with OR claims, whereas patient mortality was almost double that observed in the OR (54% in NORA vs 29% for OR claims). Respiratory depression as a result of anesthetic overdose accounted for 30% of all monitored anesthetic care claims. In most cases, the care was deemed to be substandard and preventable with improved monitoring, such as adherence to basic ASA monitoring standards. Furthermore, in 15% of the cases, monitoring with a pulse oximeter was absent. Fifty-four percent of care in NORA locations was deemed to be substandard, and injury was determined to be preventable in up to 32% of the cases. Most of the OR claims occurred in the gastroenterology, cardiology, or emergency departments and involved significantly elderly and medically complex patients.[17,18] A large database analysis of the National Anesthesia Clinical Outcomes Registry of the Anesthesia Quality Institute revealed cardiology and gastroenterology patients to be more medically complex and older as compared with the OR population. Although overall rates of complications were still greater in the OR, subgroup analysis revealed an increase in both major and minor complications as well as higher mortalities among cardiology and radiology patients in NORA locations.[19] Karamnov and colleagues[20] demonstrated that more than 5% of cases associated with adverse events were related to incomplete history taking in the preoperative process. Greater than 10% of cases were due to lack of proper intravenous (IV) moderate sedation certification in the administrating staff. Overall data from both closed claims and database analysis from the AQI indicate that many NORA complications may be preventable with increased vigilance and adherence to the same standards of anesthetic care that is required in the OR.

The inclusion of an anesthesiologist is typically made by the request of the proceduralist. Many institutions have guidelines in place for certain comorbidities or certain procedures that identify the need for anesthesia assistance.[21] Long procedures that have the potential for needing surgical backup and cases that may precipitate instability should at least warrant an anesthesia assessment.[22] In some high-risk sedation cases, it is important to ensure that anesthetic backup is readily available, even if there is no continuous anesthesia presence initially required for the procedure. However, patients should be carefully evaluated and selected to receive anesthesia consultation in order to maximize efficiency in workflow and in use of both anesthesia and hospital resources. If cases or consultations are not appropriately scheduled, the ability to provide anesthesiology services to out-of-OR locations may not be financially feasible.[23] Ultimately, this decision for anesthesia or procedural sedation with a nonanesthesiologist needs to be made on an individual basis. Certain procedures mandate the presence of an anesthesiologist to deliver general anesthetics and paralytics. Other procedures, such as endoscopies and colonoscopies, may commonly be performed with nonanesthesia sedation. However, specific patient characteristics may require the presence of anesthesia staff even in the most routine procedures. **Box 1** outlines patient-specific factors that may require an anesthesia consultation to evaluate for a need for anesthesia services during the procedure. However, one recent report acknowledged that even though there are numerous studies on sedation practices in the non-OR setting, there is a dearth of high-quality studies, especially the ones comparing patient outcomes between different types of practitioners and specialties.[24]

Box 1
Patients who may require an anesthesia consult

ASA class III, IV

Anticipated difficult airway (dysmorphic facial features, oral abnormalities, neck abnormalities, jaw abnormalities)

Severe pulmonary disease

Obstructive sleep apnea

Obesity (body mass index >35)

Coronary artery disease, prior myocardial infarction, angina, valvular disease

Congestive heart failure

Pacemaker/defibrillator

Extremes of age

Pregnancy

Substance abuse

Failed procedural sedation

Unable to assume position needed for procedure

Patients with chronic opioid use

Patients who request an anesthesiologist

Personal or family history of significant problems with anesthesia (ie, malignant hyperthermia)

Adapted from Bader AM, Pothier MM. Out-of-operating room procedures: preprocedure assessment. Anesthesiol Clin 2009;27(1):121–6.

Anesthesiologists are known for their contingency planning for the worst possible outcome or scenario and for devising ways to prevent or minimize complications. Careful examination of each patient's history and comorbidities during the preoperative assessment can provide the means to anticipate adverse events, ideally tailored to each patient and procedure. This type of planning is just as important in the non-OR setting. Preoperative planning in the non-OR setting should be focused on a few important points.[23] These include the following:

1. Familiarity with the location and resources of the anesthetizing location
2. Understanding the planned procedure and the requirements to perform it, such as type of positioning, duration, necessary level of immobility and sedation, and so forth
3. A thorough medical screening of the patient and medical optimization for all disease states
4. Determination of the need for an anesthesiologist to perform the procedure

There are several guidelines related to providing care in the non-OR locations. For example, according to the ASA Statement of Non-operating Room Anesthetizing Locations, minimum requirements for providing care include the following[25]:

1. A reliable source of oxygen adequate for the length of the procedure as well as a backup supply. A central oxygen source is preferred and a back-up source should include at least a full E cylinder
2. A reliable suction source
3. An adequate system for scavenging waste anesthetic gases
4. A self-inflating resuscitator bag capable of administering at least 90% O_2 as a means to deliver positive pressure ventilation
5. Adequate anesthetic drugs, supplies, and equipment for the intended anesthetic care
6. Adequate monitoring equipment that adheres to the ASA Standards for Basic Anesthetic Monitoring, which should be applied to all cases involving general anesthesia, regional anesthesia, and monitored anesthesia care[26]
   a. Qualified anesthesia personnel should be present throughout to conduct any anesthetics
   b. During all anesthetics, oxygenation, ventilation, circulation, and temperature should be continually (regularly and frequently) monitored using the following:
      i. Oxygenation: oxygen analyzer, pulse oximeter
      ii. Ventilation: chest excursion, breath sounds, expired carbon dioxide monitoring, capnography, disconnection monitors
      iii. Circulation: electrocardiogram, arterial blood pressure and heart rate monitoring, palpation of a pulse, auscultation of heart sounds, intra-arterial pressure monitoring, peripheral pulse monitoring or pulse oximetry
      iv. Temperature probe
7. In any location where inhaled anesthetics are used, there should be an anesthesia machine equivalent in function to that used in the OR and maintained to current OR standards
8. Sufficient electrical outlets that adhere to facility standards
9. Adequate illumination of the patient and equipment
10. Sufficient space to accommodate necessary equipment and personnel to allow fast access to the patient and equipment when needed
11. Immediate access to an emergency cart with a defibrillator, emergency drugs, and other equipment to provide cardiopulmonary resuscitation
12. Adequate anesthesia support staff should be readily available at each location

13. Appropriate provision of after-anesthesia management and recovery with properly trained staff and monitoring equipment

ASSESSMENT OF OUT-OF-THE-OPERATING ROOM ENVIRONMENT

Providing anesthesia in the non-OR setting requires flexibility and a thorough understanding of the resources that are both present and absent. **Box 2** lists examples of NORA sites. The out-of-OR environment may differ significantly from the regular flow of the OR, and it is important for anesthesiologists to familiarize themselves with the objectives, structure, and workflow of these locations. These spaces are often not built with anesthesiologists in mind. The procedure room may have limited space and a plethora of procedural equipment. Many rooms contain a procedure room with a control room used to monitor patients when radiation-based procedures are being administered. Other locations contain bulky MRI and computed tomographic machines that shield the patient from the anesthesiologist's view. Fluoroscopy suites have moveable parts that may interfere with monitoring and equipment requiring long extensions for IVs, medication lines, O_2 tubing, and breathing circuits. MRI suites have unique requirements for nonferrous equipment, limiting what can be brought into the procedure room. Interference with continuous monitoring from these radiology modalities can cause additional challenges in providing care to these patients.

Equipment that is often taken for granted in the OR, such as scavenging systems, oxygen/air delivery systems, or suction may not be readily available or located in unreachable areas of the room. Many anesthesiologists may have to bring portable equipment to these locations. Each piece of equipment should be identified and checked before use. Monitoring should also be visually accessible to the anesthesia

---

Box 2
Non-operating room anesthetizing sites

Radiology
- Interventional
- MRI
- Computed tomography
- Ultrasound
- Radiation oncology

Gastroenterology

Cardiac interventions
- Electrophysiology
- Catheterization
- Interventional cardiology
- Transesophageal echocardiography

Lithotripsy

Electroconvulsive therapy sites

Emergency room

Intensive care units

Obstetric labor and delivery

Hospital wards

Ambulatory procedure rooms

Outpatient offices

team. The anesthesia provider should take note of the location of the difficult airway, malignant hyperthermia, and Code Blue cardiopulmonary carts. A careful perusal of each unfamiliar location should be performed before the start of the procedure. It is important to determine where backup personnel are located and the means to reach them. A process must be established to quickly retrieve additional medications and equipment, if necessary. For example, having an automated medication dispensing cabinet located inside the procedure room can facilitate quick access to the necessary medications for the anesthesiologist and other staff. The careful planning and monitoring that has made anesthesiologists pioneers of patient safety in the OR should be adhered to, just as, if not more stringently than, one does in OR-based locations.

Other considerations during procedure site reconnaissance include the following[27,28]:

1. Where will the patient be induced: procedural bed, stretcher, other area?
2. Are the anesthesia equipment and O_2 source close enough to the patient?
3. Is it possible to monitor the patient from a further distance when hazards such as radiation require this?
4. Will additional portable monitors be necessary?
5. Does everyone in the procedure room know how to call a code and use the code cart?
6. Are all personnel aware of what constitutes an anesthetic emergency?

Performing anesthetics at NORA locations requires intense communication and teamwork. Many of the procedural staff may not be familiar with the unique requirements of anesthesia provision, which may impede workflow and cause unintended harm. Team leadership should be emphasized and a collaborative environment needs to be fostered, especially when taking care of a medically complex patient population. These patients are often referred to interventional procedures as a last resort, when more invasive procedures are not indicated or carry a higher risk. Therefore, both proceduralists and anesthesiologists can be faced with unexpected patient challenges during the procedure, requiring quick responses and teamwork. Both patient and procedural concerns should be identified to the procedural team before the initiation of the case.

Radiation safety must be a focus in the out-of-OR setting. Personnel operating in these sites are routinely exposed to radiation doses higher than what most medical personnel experience. The vast majority of occupational exposure is through fluoroscopy. Long-term complications may involve thyroid disease, skin conditions, cataracts, bone marrow suppression, and malignancy if radiosensitive cells (fast-growing, undifferentiated cells) are not protected; this involves protecting the reproductive organs, lenses of the eye, and thyroid gland. Fluoroscopy can introduce 20 times the radiation than a single exposure. Anesthesiologists who work close to the patient and the radiation beam must take care of shielding themselves. Because even with proper leaded apparel up to 18% of all active bone marrow is still exposed to the effects of radiation, it is important to protect as much body surface area as possible.[29] A protective panel of at least 0.25-mm lead equivalent should be positioned between the patient and all other staff. By law, no one less than the age of 18 should be allowed into the room during exposure. Lead aprons and thyroid shields that offer at least 0.5 m of lead should be worn at all times and should be checked annually for damage. Radiation beam attenuates are based on the inverse square law ($1/d^2$); therefore, placing a safe distance between the radiation beam is the safest way to decrease radiation exposure.[30] Radiation dosimeters should be worn outside of protective clothing. Distance from the patient and radiation beam is the best form of protection.

PREOPERATIVE PATIENT ASSESSMENT

The health assessment should begin with a careful history of patient's comorbidities. The ASA has developed a Practice Advisory for Preanesthesia Evaluation, an evidence-based guideline that outlines all aspects of preoperative assessment and testing.[31] Each disease condition should be explored, noting severity, exacerbating factors, and stability. Physician functional status should be assessed. Medications, including over the counter and herbal supplements, should be reviewed. Social history including substance, alcohol, and smoking use as well as a personal and/or family history of anesthetic complications should be noted. A targeted physical examination should include, at the minimum, obtaining vital signs, auscultating the heart and lung fields, abdominal examination, extremity examination, and a focused neurologic examination. Last, a thorough airway examination with a dental assessment should be completed, as outlined in **Box 3**.

Cardiovascular System

Cardiopulmonary events are the most feared complications during procedures, and therefore, a thorough assessment should be performed. Although most non-OR procedures can be performed under less invasive means and do not require a general anesthetic, any anesthetic may turn into a general anesthetic and any procedure may require emergent resuscitation and transport to the OR for a surgical intervention.

Box 3
Basic elements of patient assessment

Age

Height

Weight

Allergies: reactions to allergens

Current medications, including over the counter medications and herbal supplements

Smoking status: how frequent, how long, and when was the last use

Illicit substance use: how frequent, how long, and when was the last use

Alcohol use: how frequent, how long, and when was the last use

Family history

Previous hospitalizations

Previous surgeries

Pregnancy status

Current medical conditions

Functional status

Focused physical examination

Airway examination
- Mouth opening
- Mallampati score
- Thyromental distance
- Dental condition
- Neck mobility
- Prior anesthesia records

According to the most recent American College of Cardiology and the American Heart Association Guidelines for cardiovascular evaluation for noncardiac surgery, the patient should be cleared for the OR based on their disease status and current condition of disease, risk factors, and the type and urgency of the procedure.[32] Active cardiac conditions include acute myocardial ischemia (within 7 days of onset), unstable or severe angina, decompensated heart failure, severe valvular disease, or significant arrhythmia.

CARDIOVASCULAR ASSESSMENT

Approximately one American experiences a coronary event every 34 seconds, and coronary disease has caused approximately 1 of every 7 deaths in the United States in 2011.[33] The spectrum of symptoms range from asymptomatic to unstable, frequent angina, and functional impairment. Each patient's cardiovascular record should be requisitioned with prior echocardiography, electrocardiography, and stress tests. Baseline blood pressure and heart rate should be recorded, and these parameters should be maintained within 10% of baseline under anesthesia. Patients with concerning symptoms or risk factors without recent evaluation should receive an electrocardiogram, and further testing may be considered. The benefits of coronary revascularization before a procedure are controversial, and the risks need to be balanced with the risks of a procedure with significant disease burden.

Revascularized patients typically have either bare-metal or drug-eluting stents that require a period of antiplatelet therapy that may cause increased bleeding risks during procedures. Current guideline for therapy recommends at least a 1-month duration for bare-metal stents and a 6-month duration for drug-eluting stents, although the optimal period of therapy is still not completely clear.[34] Many patients are maintained on these medications for much longer than the officially suggested duration, and the risk of holding these medications before instrumentation needs to be considered against each patient's risk factors. For patients who are anticipating surgery, there may be discussions with the cardiology team regarding the patient's candidacy for bare-metal stents due to the shorter mandatory therapy time. Elective procedures should be postponed until this period of therapy has been reached to prevent complications. Aspirin should be continued during the perioperative period with the exception of certain procedures on closed spaces such as neurosurgical/neurologic interventional procedures. These concerns should be discussed with the procedural team. Both invasive and noninvasive procedures can increase a patient's risk of stent thrombosis, which is associated with high mortality.

Patients with congestive heart failure should be assessed for the presence of decompensation based on both symptoms and physical examination. Prior echocardiograms should be evaluated to determine anatomic dysfunction. Although systolic cardiac dysfunction is often the most worrisome type of heart failure, more than half of all heart failure incidences are caused by diastolic failure. These patients should be on salt restriction, β-blockers, and angiotensin-converting enzyme medications and should have a well-managed blood pressure.

Severe valvular dysfunction often manifests with symptoms of heart failure. These patients will require a thorough assessment of functional status and symptoms. With severe valvular conditions, changes in either heart rate or blood pressure may cause sudden and severe cardiac dysfunction. Maintenance of normal sinus rhythm for atrial kick, volume status, heart rate, and blood control needs to be tailored for the specific valvular abnormality. Finally, some patients may require endocarditis prophylaxis during the procedure; the latest guidelines are outline in **Box 4**.

> **Box 4**
> **Conditions requiring endocarditis prophylaxis**
>
> Prosthetic cardiac valve or prosthetic material used for cardiac valve repair
>
> Prior history of infective endocarditis
>
> Congenital heart disease (CHD)
> - Unrepaired cyanotic CHD
> - Completely repaired CHD with prosthetic material or device during the first 6 months after the procedure
> - Repaired CHD with residual defects at the site or adjacent to the site of a prosthetic patch or prosthetic device
>
> Cardiac transplant patients who develop cardiac vavulopathy
>
> *Adapted from* Wilson W, Taubert KA, Gewitz M, et al. Prevention of infective endocarditis: guidelines from the American Heart Association: a guideline from the American Heart Association Rheumatic Fever, Endocarditis, and Kawasaki Disease Committee, Council on Cardiovascular Disease in the Young, and the Council on Clinical Cardiology, Council on Cardiovascular Surgery and Anesthesia, and the Quality of Care and Outcomes Research Interdisciplinary Working Group. Circulation 2007;116(15):1745.

Patients with pacemakers and implantable cardioverter-defibrillators are seen with increasing frequency in procedural rooms. Each anesthesiologist should be familiar with the setting of each pacer, the patient's condition that required its placement, and the level of their pacemaker dependence. Each patient should be queried about the frequency of defibrillation, and if there are any concerns, the pacemaker should be interrogated. Each device reacts differently to magnet placement, including some that do not revert to its original settings after magnet placement, making it even more important to understand this function. Not all procedures require the placement of a magnet, and this decision must be made on an individual basis, depending on the patient's device dependence and location of the procedure. For patients who are pacemaker-dependent, having the device changed to an asynchronous mode instead of a sensed mode by a cardiologist on the day of surgery is recommended. Magnets should only be used as a last resort during emergencies. In the devices with both pacemaker and defibrillation capabilities, magnet placement may cause variable changes in function. In many devices, only the antitachyarrhythmia function is disabled without changes to the underlying pacemaker function. Therefore, reliance on magnet placement is not recommended, and actual interrogation and disabling of functions by cardiologists should be performed. Any device that has been deactivated by a magnet should be interrogated and re-enabled before the patient leaves the recovery room.[35]

PULMONARY ASSESSMENT

Despite the focus given to perioperative cardiac complications, pulmonary complications can contribute significantly to perioperative morbidity and mortality. Hypoxia and desaturation are the most common occurrences seen in the perioperative period. Risk factors include advanced age, chronic obstructive pulmonary disease (COPD), smoking (current and prior history), heart failure, higher ASA class, impaired sensorium, functional dependency, and obstructive sleep apnea.[36] Surgical risk factors include upper abdominal surgeries and any abdominal surgeries, duration of procedure, general anesthesia, and emergent procedures. Elective procedures should be postponed for patients with active respiratory disease for 6 weeks to decrease the risk of pulmonary events. Patients with asthma or COPD should be assessed for medical optimization and functional status. Although pulmonary function tests, radiographs, and arterial blood gas provide information on a patient's baseline status, these tests are not necessary to perform during the preoperative assessment and have demonstrated little benefit. Patients with severe disease and functional limitations may be candidates for regional or neuraxial anesthesia in an effort to avoid airway manipulation as well as perioperative bronchodilator therapy. Patients with sleep apnea should be instructed to bring with them their home continuous positive airway pressure devices on the day of the procedure.

GASTROINTESTINAL ASSESSMENT

Patients should be evaluated for conditions causing decreased gastric motility or full stomach precautions. Severity of gastroesophageal reflex should be determined and acid suppressants should be taken on the day of the procedure. Patients with concerns for delayed gastric emptying, such as intestinal obstruction, gastroparesis, trauma, emergent procedures, full stomachs, or opioid use, should be assessed for rapid sequence inductions and the need for gastric decompression after induction. For example, although many of the diagnostic gastrointestinal endoscopies (upper endoscopy, colonoscopy) are performed while maintaining a natural airway, some of these patients may pose a higher aspiration risk.

RENAL ASSESSMENT

Many non-OR procedures involve the use of fluoroscopy and IV dye, which can increase the risk of renal injury. Contrast-induced nephropathy (CIN) has been associated with up to 11% of all hospital-acquired acute renal failure. CIN is defined as a greater than 0.5 mg/dL increase in creatinine in patients with baseline creatinine less than 1.9 mg/dL occurring within 48 to 72 hours after contrast administration in the absence of other causes for renal injury.[37] Patients without history of renal disease have very low risk of CIN and do not require routine monitoring or prophylaxis.[38,39] The single most important risk factor for CIN is chronic kidney disease (serum creatinine >1.5 mg/dL), which imparts more than 20 times the risk compared with patients with normal renal function. Additional risk factors include diabetes, male gender, diabetes, volume of contrast agent, and renal impairment.[40] Procedures that are most commonly associated with CIN include coronary angiograms, angioplasties, and computed tomographic scans.[37] Strategies for prevention of CIN are outlined in **Table 1**.

Dialysis-dependent patients should have dialysis on the day before the procedure but generally avoid dialysis on the day of procedure because of concerns for electrolyte abnormalities and volume depletion.

OBSTETRIC ASSESSMENT

Pregnant patients should be assessed for the current status of their pregnancy, complications, and need for intervention. Because of the potentially devastating complications associated with pregnancy, elective procedures should be postponed until after delivery or until the second trimester. Procedures and medications administered during the first trimester coincide with fetal organogenesis and they are best avoided, while more invasive procedures during the third trimester may precipitate premature labor.[42] Abdominal procedures increase this risk.

All women of child-bearing age should be assessed for the possibility of pregnancy. This assessment of the possibility of pregnancy is especially important for procedures

Table 1	
Guidelines for prevention of contrast-induced nephropathy	
Glomerular filtration rate (GFR) >60 mL/min, normal or near normal renal function	Low risk for CIN, no follow-up or prophylaxis required
GFR <45–59 mL/min	Low risk for CIN without risk factors, no specific prophylaxis or follow-up required. If intra-arterial contrast is administered, preventative measures are recommended
GFR <45 mL/min	Moderate risk for CIN, preventative measure recommended
CIN prevention strategies[41]	IV hydration • For inpatients, 0.9% saline solution at 1 mL/kg/h for 12 h before the procedure and 12 h after the procedure • For outpatients, isotonic saline or sodium bicarbonate solution at 3 mL/kg/h, a minimum of 1 h before the procedure and 6 h after the procedure is a reasonable abbreviated alternative N-acetylcysteine: inconclusive results but often administered due to low cost and lack of major adverse effects Discontinue nephrotoxic medications 8 h before administration of contrast Avoid dehydration Avoid high osmolar contrast Dialysis patients do not require fluid hydration before contrast administration

Adapted from Nicola R, Shaqdan KW, Aran K, et al. Contrast-induced nephropathy: identifying the risks, choosing the right agent, and reviewing effective prevention and management methods. Curr Probl Diagn Radiol 2015;44(6):503.

that involve high levels of radiation exposure. A pregnancy test should routinely be a part of each assessment if there is any uncertainty about the woman's menstrual history.

PROCEDURAL ASSESSMENT

Many procedures performed in the non-OR setting involve creative techniques and maneuvering to access anatomic locations that may not be amendable for surgery. A careful discussion of the planned procedure, the involved components, the need for immobility, duration, and positioning should occur among the care team members. The need for IV contrast, medications, and invasive blood pressure monitoring should be ascertained before the procedure so that preventative measures can be taken.

DIAGNOSTIC TESTING

Diagnostic testing before each procedure must be individualized based on patient risk factors and the procedure itself. For patients without baseline laboratory tests in whom there are possible bleeding risks or renal injury risks, baseline laboratory tests assessing coagulation status, hemoglobin, and renal function should be drawn and blood typing should be obtained. Dialysis patients should have electrolyte levels drawn after their last dialysis run. Diabetics should have documented preoperative glucose levels on the day of the procedure, and glucose levels should be monitored during the procedure, depending on its duration. Patients with concerns for cardiac

Table 2
Perioperative medication administration

Medication	Perioperative Administration Instruction
Aspirin	Continue unless contraindicated by the procedure (ie, neurologic, ophthalmic interventions) or by the proceduralist
β-Blockers	—
Angiotension converting enzyme inhibitors and angiotension receptor blockers	Hold 12–24 h before procedure due to concerns of causing vasoplegia
Other antihypertensives	Continue the day of surgery
Diuretics	Hold on the day of surgery
Pulmonary inhalers	Continue the day of surgery, bring to the preoperative assessment center and administer before the procedure
Gastrointestinal reflex medications	Continue on the day of surgery
Neurologic therapies (dementia, Parkinson, seizure prophylaxis)	Continue the day of surgery
Antianxiety medications	Continue on the day of procedure
Monoamine oxidase inhibitors	Continue on the day of procedure unless risk for serotonin syndrome is high and patient at low risk for rebound from discontinuation. Complete clearance requires 3 wk
Autoimmune and immunosuppressant medications	Continue the day of procedure
Steroids	Continue the day of procedure Patients using ≤5 mg a day of prednisone equivalent for ≤3 wk have low risk of adrenal suppression ≥5–20 mg per day of prednisone equivalent for ≥3 wk may cause adrenal suppression ≥20 mg/d for ≥3 wk will cause adrenal suppression that may continue for a year after cessation
Insulin	Administer 1/3 to 1/2 dose the evening or morning of procedure depending on frequency of dosing. Hold short-acting insulin If insulin pump, continue lowest basal night time rate Measure blood glucose the morning of procedure. These patients should be scheduled as the first morning cases
Opioid and pain medications	Take normal morning dose before procedure Hold nonsteroidal anti-inflammatory medications 48 h before procedure
Oral antiglycemic medications	Hold on the day of surgery Hold metformin on the day of surgery, risk of lactic acidosis most prominent in renal or hepatic failure
Herbal medication and supplements	Hold for 7–14 d before procedure

disease should have an electrocardiogram, whereas further testing should be decided based on patient's symptoms. Routine preoperative tests have rarely been shown to impact patient management and improve patient care.[31] In fact, instances of harm have been documented due to pursuit of otherwise unknown abnormalities based on these tests. Tests should only be ordered if they will impact the care provided.[11]

PREPROCEDURAL MEDICATION MANAGEMENT

The patient's current medication list should be carefully examined to make sure it is up to date, the dosages correspond to the actual amount of each medication taken, and instructions by the patient's providers, including the proceduralist, have been followed. Some medications should be continued on the day of surgery, while others should be held before the procedure, as outlined in **Table 2**. The risk of stopping certain medications should be weighed against the risk of continuing them during the periprocedural period; this is especially true for the management of anticoagulants and antiplatelet medications.[43]

FUTURE DIRECTIONS

As non-OR procedures increase in frequency and complexity, a scientific approach to triaging patients for proper selection of sedation by nonanesthesiologists or anesthesia care needs to be developed. Algorithms that identify patient and procedural risk factors that would benefit from further assessment or the presence of anesthesia staff will aid physicians in providing the best care for each patient. Ideally, risk stratification strategies can be developed that take patient, procedural, anesthesia, and location factors into consideration. National standards and protocols for non-OR anesthetics for each subspecialty and procedure will need to be further developed and evaluated against patient outcomes. The standardization of patient assessment should be a result of interdisciplinary efforts by proceduralists, anesthesiologists, nurses, and hospital administrators. Lastly, there is a need to develop financial models to demonstrate the value of NORA evaluation process and how creating an infrastructure for this process can positively impact periprocedural efficiency and patient outcomes.

SUMMARY

As the pioneers of patient safety, anesthesiologists should strive to maintain the same standard of care throughout all anesthetizing locations. As the demand for NORA continues to increase, it is becoming more important than ever for the anesthesiologist to deliver the same standard of care that is expected in the OR. In the NORA environment, where both proceduralists and support staff may have limited knowledge of the patient's history and anesthetic needs, an increased emphasis on proper patient triaging and preoperative assessment by the anesthesia care team becomes imperative. As procedures and techniques rapidly evolve, preoperative assessments need to adapt concurrently. Oftentimes, this means that novel and unique management plans need to be tailored to each patient for each specific procedure. Communication and teamwork in these locations are equally important because many unknowns may arise due to increasingly complex techniques and comorbidities. In this exciting new era of medical advancement, anesthesiologists need to be at the forefront of promoting patient safety. In collaboration with medical specialists of all specialties, anesthesiologists are ushering in a new era of improved patient care where they can add significant value.

REFERENCES

1. Eichhorn V, Henzler D, Murphy MF. Standardizing care and monitoring for anesthesia or procedural sedation delivered outside the operating room. Curr Opin Anaesthesiol 2010;23(4):494–9.
2. Evron S, Ezri T. Organizational prerequisites for anesthesia outside the operating room. Curr Opin Anaesthesiology 2009;22(4):514–8.
3. American Society of Anesthesiologists. Statement on Granting Privileges for Administration of Moderate Sedation to Practitioners Who Are Not Anesthesia Professionals. 2011. Available at: http://www.asahq.org/quality-and-practice-management/standards-and-guidelines#. Accessed August 5, 2015.
4. American Society of Anesthesiologists. Statement on Granting Privileges to Nonanesthesiologist Physicians for Personally Administering or Supervising Deep Sedation. 2012. Available at: http://www.asahq.org/quality-and-practice-management/standards-and-guidelines#. Accessed August 5, 2015.
5. Cutter TW. Chapter 19: preoperative assessment for specific procedures or locations. In: Sweitzer B, editor. Preoperative assessment and management. 2nd edition. Philadelphia: Lippincott, Williams and Wilkins; 2008. p. 433–48.
6. Bader AM, Correll DJ. Chapter 18: organizational structure of preoperative evaluation center. In: Sweitzer B, editor. Preoperative assessment and management. 2nd edition. Philadelphia: Lippincott, Williams and Wilkins; 2008. p. 420–32.
7. Antonelli MT, Seaver D, Urman RD. Procedural sedation and implications for quality and risk management. J Healthc Risk Manag 2013;33(2):3–10.
8. Caperelli-White L, Urman RD. Developing a moderate sedation policy: essential elements and evidence-based considerations. AORN J 2014;99(3):416–30.
9. Lemay A, Shyn PB, Foley R, et al. A procedural sedation quality improvement audit form tool for interventional radiology. J Med Pract Manage 2015;30(6 Spec No):44–7.
10. Starsnic MA, Guarnieri DM, Norris MC. Efficacy and financial benefit of an anesthesiologist-directed university preadmission evaluation center. J Clin Anesth 1997;9(4):299–305.
11. Allison JG, Bromley HR. Unnecessary preoperative investigations: evaluation and cost analysis. Am Surg 1996;62(8):686–9.
12. Cima RR, Brown MJ, Hebl JR, et al. Use of lean and six sigma methodology to improve operating room efficiency in a high-volume tertiary-care academic medical center. J Am Coll Surg 2011;213(1):83–92 [discussion: 93–4].
13. Harnett MJ, Correll DJ, Hurwitz S, et al. Improving efficiency and patient satisfaction in a tertiary teaching hospital preoperative clinic. Anesthesiology 2010; 112(1):66–72.
14. Biber JL, Allareddy V, Gallagher SM, et al. Prevalence and predictors of adverse events during procedural sedation anesthesia-outside the operating room for esophagogastroduodenoscopy and colonoscopy in children: age is an independent predictor of outcomes. Pediatr Crit Care Med 2015;16(8):e251–9.
15. Cravero JP, Beach ML, Blike GT, et al. The incidence and nature of adverse events during pediatric sedation/anesthesia with propofol for procedures outside the operating room: a report from the Pediatric Sedation Research Consortium. Anesth Analg 2009;108(3):795–804.
16. Pino RM. The nature of anesthesia and procedural sedation outside of the operating room. Curr Opin Anaesthesiology 2007;20(4):347–51.
17. Metzner J, Posner KL, Domino KB. The risk and safety of anesthesia at remote locations: the US closed claims analysis. Curr Opin Anaesthesiology 2009; 22(4):502–8.

18. Metzner J, Posner KL, Lam MS, et al. Closed claims' analysis. Best Pract Res Clin Anaesthesiol 2011;25(2):263–76.
19. Chang B, Kaye AD, Diaz JH, et al. Complications of non-operating room procedures: outcomes from the national anesthesia clinical outcomes registry. J Patient Saf 2015. [Epub ahead of print].
20. Karamnov S, Sarkisian N, Grammer R, et al. Analysis of adverse events associated with adult moderate procedural sedation outside the operating room. J Patient Saf 2014. [Epub ahead of print].
21. Gross WL, Faillace RT, Shook DC, et al. Chapter 19: new challenges for anesthesiologists outside of the operating room: the cardiac catheterization and electrophysiology laboratories. In: Urman RD, Gross WL, Philip BK, editors. Anesthesia outside of the operating room. 1st edition. New York: Oxford University Press; 2011. p. 179–97.
22. Shook DC, Gross W. Offsite anesthesiology in the cardiac catheterization lab. Curr Opin Anaesthesiology 2007;20(4):352–8.
23. Bader AM, Pothier MM. Out-of-operating room procedures: preprocedure assessment. Anesthesiol Clin 2009;27(1):121–6.
24. Metzner J, Domino KB. Risks of anesthesia or sedation outside the operating room: the role of the anesthesia care provider. Curr Opin Anaesthesiology 2010;23(4):523–31.
25. American Society of Anesthesiologists. Statement on nonoperating room anesthetizing locations. 2013. Available at: http://www.asahq.org/quality-and-practice-management/standards-and-guidelines#. Accessed August 5, 2015.
26. American Society of Anesthesiologists. Standards for basic anesthetic monitoring. 2011. Available at: http://www.asahq.org/quality-and-practice-management/standards-and-guidelines#. Accessed August 5, 2015.
27. Gross WL, Urman RD. Chapter 1: challenges of anesthesia outside the operating room. In: Urman RD, Gross WL, Philip BK, editors. Anesthesia outside of the operating room. 1st edition. New York: Oxford University Press; 2011. p. 1–7.
28. Russell GB. Alternate-site anesthesia. 1st edition. Oxford (England): Butterworth-Heinemann; 1997.
29. Katz JD. Radiation exposure to anesthesia personnel: the impact of an electrophysiology laboratory. Anesth Analgesia 2005;101(6):1725–6.
30. Bashore TM, Bates ER, Berger PB, et al. American College of Cardiology/Society for Cardiac Angiography and Interventions Clinical Expert Consensus Document on cardiac catheterization laboratory standards. A report of the American College of Cardiology Task Force on Clinical Expert Consensus Documents. J Am Coll Cardiol 2001;37(8):2170–214.
31. Apfelbaum JL, Connis RT, Nickinovich DG, et al. Practice advisory for preanesthesia evaluation: an updated report by the American Society of Anesthesiologists Task Force on Preanesthesia Evaluation. Anesthesiology 2012;116(3):522–38.
32. Fleisher LA, Fleischmann KE, Auerbach AD, et al. 2014 ACC/AHA guideline on perioperative cardiovascular evaluation and management of patients undergoing noncardiac surgery: executive summary: a report of the American College of Cardiology/American Heart Association Task Force on practice guidelines. Developed in collaboration with the American College of Surgeons, American Society of Anesthesiologists, American Society of Echocardiography, American Society of Nuclear Cardiology, Heart Rhythm Society, Society for Cardiovascular Angiography and Interventions, Society of Cardiovascular Anesthesiologists, and Society of Vascular Medicine Endorsed by the Society of Hospital Medicine. J Nucl Cardiol 2015;22(1):162–215.

33. Mozaffarian D, Benjamin EJ, Go AS, et al, American Heart Association Statistics Committee and Stroke Statistics Subcommittee. Heart disease and stroke statistics—2015 update: a report from the American Heart Association. Circulation 2015;131(4):e29–322, 434–41.

34. Grines CL, Bonow RO, Casey DE Jr, et al. Prevention of premature discontinuation of dual antiplatelet therapy in patients with coronary artery stents: a science advisory from the American Heart Association, American College of Cardiology, Society for Cardiovascular Angiography and Interventions, American College of Surgeons, and American Dental Association, with representation from the American College of Physicians. Circulation 2007;115(6):813–8.

35. Sweitzer BJ. Chapter 2: preoperative patient evaluation for anesthesia care outside of the operating room. In: Urman RD, Gross WL, Philip BK, editors. Anesthesia outside of the operating room. 1st edition. New York: Oxford University Press; 2011. p. 8–19.

36. Smetana GW, Lawrence VA, Cornell JE. Preoperative pulmonary risk stratification for noncardiothoracic surgery: systematic review for the American College of Physicians. Ann Intern Med 2006;144(8):581–95.

37. Nash K, Hafeez A, Hou S. Hospital-acquired renal insufficiency. Am J Kidney Dis 2002;39(5):930–6.

38. Thomsen HS, Bush WH Jr. Adverse effects of contrast media: incidence, prevention and management. Drug Saf 1998;19(4):313–24.

39. Nicola R, Shaqdan KW, Aran K, et al. Contrast-induced nephropathy: identifying the risks, choosing the right agent, and reviewing effective prevention and management methods. Curr Probl Diagn Radiol 2015;44(6):501–4.

40. Rudnick MR, Goldfarb S, Wexler L, et al. Nephrotoxicity of ionic and nonionic contrast media in 1196 patients: a randomized trial. The Iohexol Cooperative Study. Kidney Int 1995;47(1):254–61.

41. Owen RJ, Hiremath S, Myers A, et al. Canadian Association of Radiologists consensus guidelines for the prevention of contrast-induced nephropathy: update 2012. Can Assoc Radiol J 2014;65(2):96–105.

42. Canadian Agency for Drugs and Technologies in Health. Anaesthetic agents in pregnant women undergoing non-obstetric surgical or endoscopic procedures: a review of the safety and guidelines. Ottawa (Canada): 2015. Available at: http://www.ncbi.nlm.nih.gov/pubmedhealth/PMH0078411/. Accessed November 8, 2015.

43. Narouze S, Benzon HT, Provenzano DA, et al. Interventional spine and pain procedures in patients on antiplatelet and anticoagulant medications: guidelines from the American Society of Regional Anesthesia and Pain Medicine, the European Society of Regional Anaesthesia and Pain Therapy, the American Academy of Pain Medicine, the International Neuromodulation Society, the North American Neuromodulation Society, and the World Institute of Pain. Reg Anesth Pain Med 2015;40(3):182–212.

Index

Note: Page numbers of article titles are in **boldface** type.

Anesthesiology Clin 34 (2016) 241–254
http://dx.doi.org/10.1016/S1932-2275(16)00028-8   **anesthesiology.theclinics.com**
1932-2275/16/$ – see front matter © 2016 Elsevier Inc. All rights reserved.

Moving?

Make sure your subscription moves with you!

To notify us of your new address, find your **Clinics Account Number** (located on your mailing label above your name), and contact customer service at:

Email: journalscustomerservice-usa@elsevier.com

800-654-2452 (subscribers in the U.S. & Canada)
314-447-8871 (subscribers outside of the U.S. & Canada)

Fax number: 314-447-8029

Elsevier Health Sciences Division
Subscription Customer Service
3251 Riverport Lane
Maryland Heights, MO 63043

*To ensure uninterrupted delivery of your subscription, please notify us at least 4 weeks in advance of move.

Printed and bound by CPI Group (UK) Ltd, Croydon, CR0 4YY

08/05/2025

01864682-0002